Pharmacy Technician Certification Exam Review

3rd Edition

by

Lorraine C. Zentz, CPhT, PhD.

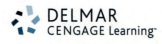

DELMAR
CENGAGE Learning

Australia • Brazil • Japan • Korea • Mexico • Singapore • Spain • United Kingdom • United States

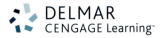

Pharmacy Technician Certification Exam Review, 3rd Edition
Lorraine C. Zentz, CPhT, PhD.

Vice President, Editorial: Dave Garza

Director of Learning Solutions: Matthew Kane

Senior Acquisitions Editor: Tari Broderick

Managing Editor: Marah Bellegarde

Associate Product Manager: Meghan E. Orvis

Editorial Assistant: Ian J. Lewis

Vice President, Marketing: Jennifer Baker

Marketing Director: Wendy Mapstone

Senior Marketing Manager: Michele McTighe

Associate Marketing Manager:
    Jonathan Sheehan

Marketing Coordinator: Scott Chrysler

Production Director: Carolyn Miller

Production Manager: Andrew Crouth

Senior Content Project Manager:
    Kenneth McGrath

Senior Art Director: Jack Pendleton

Technology Project Manager: Brain Davis

For product information and technology assistance, contact us at
Cengage Learning Customer & Sales Support, 1-800-354-9706
For permission to use material from this text or product,
submit all requests online at **www.cengage.com/permissions**.
Further permissions questions can be e-mailed to
permissionrequest@cengage.com

Library of Congress Control Number: 2011920072

ISBN-13: 978-1-4283-2062-8

ISBN-10: 1-4283-2062-8

Delmar
5 Maxwell Drive
Clifton park, NY 12065-2919
USA

Cengage Learning is a leading provider of customized learning solutions with office locations around the globe, including Singapore, the United Kingdom, Australia, Mexico, Brazil, and Japan. Locate your local office at:
international.cengage.com/region

Cengage Learning products are represented in Canada by Nelson Education, Ltd.

To learn more about Delmar, visit **www.cengage.com/delmar**

Purchase any of our products at your local college store or at our preferred online store **www.CengageBrain.com**

NOTICE TO THE READER

Publisher does not warrant or guarantee any of the products described herein or perform any independent analysis in connection with any of the product information contained herein. Publisher does not assume, and expressly disclaims, any obligation to obtain and include information other than that provided to it by the manufacturer. The reader is expressly warned to consider and adopt all safety precautions that might be indicated by the activities described herein and to avoid all potential hazards. By following the instructions contained herein, the reader willingly assumes all risks in connection with such instructions. The publisher makes no representations or warranties of any kind, including but not limited to, the warranties of fitness for particular purpose or merchantability, nor are any such representations implied with respect to the material set forth herein, and the publisher takes no responsibility with respect to such material. The publisher shall not be liable for any special, consequential, or exemplary damages resulting, in whole or part, from the readers' use of, or reliance upon, this material.

Printed in the United States of America
1 2 3 4 5 6 7 14 13 12 11

Contents

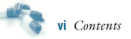

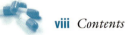

Preface

Welcome to one of the fastest growing fields in medical care—the pharmacy technician. The rapid growth in the field of pharmaceutical therapeutics has created opportunities for a variety of well-trained technical personnel: physician's assistants, medical assistants, nursing assistants, and pharmacy technicians.

The position of pharmacy technician has expanded from a simple assistant position to one of great responsibility in patient care. The pharmacy technician is now responsible for a variety of duties in the pharmacy—legal record-keeping, dispensing of prescriptions, proper inventory, storage, and maintenance of drugs, to name a few. In addition, the technician plays a role in patient care by assisting the pharmacist in evaluating the various aspects of patient care. The growing demand for these trained technical personnel is due, in large part, to the rapidly expanding area of drug research and drug discovery. The pharmacist simply does not have enough time to keep up with recent advances in drug therapy and new dosage delivery systems, counseling patients and physicians, and other duties such as drug dispensing and ordering, and the record-keeping that is required by law.

The CPhT Examination

The growing need for well-qualified technicians to perform sophisticated duties has created the requirement for a standardized examination to ensure that the technicians working within a pharmacy uphold an acceptable level of knowledge and integrity. Thus, a national examination for the certification of pharmacy technicians has been created to replace state certification examinations. There are two certified examinations available for technicians today. The Pharmacy Certification Training Board (PCTB), and the Institute for the Certification of Pharmacy Technicians (ICPT) offer these exams.

Since the PCTB exam was first implemented in 1994, the test material has become increasingly more difficult, which reflects the changing duties of the technician. The ICPT exam was developed in 2005. With the growing number of drugs available and the increasing number of patients that require medical care, the technician is now required to know an extensive amount of pharmacology in order to monitor for possible drug interaction or other harmful effects of the prescribed drug regimen on the patient.

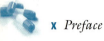

Both exams are offered with continual registration windows and on-line testing. They must be proctored, so they are offered throughout the country at licensed testing centers.

Why This Book?

The high standards and increasing difficulty of this examination have created a need for a text that, in addition to being useful for the student of pharmacy technology, will address the main features of the examination and provide information, a comprehensive review, and a basis for understanding the concepts addressed in the examination. The third edition of *Pharmacy Technician Certification Exam Review* was written to fill this need. This text was designed for a twofold purpose: to function as a review for technicians familiar with the material and to serve as a learning tool both for students of pharmacy technology and for technicians who have been trained to perform a limited number of duties (such as within a retail pharmacy). These technicians must now become familiar with more sophisticated concepts, such as pharmacology and advanced pharmaceutical calculations, in order to become certified. The text is written in conversational style to facilitate understanding of difficult concepts among many levels of readers. Foremost in the text is an examination of the routine procedures in the pharmacy: accepting prescriptions, creating patient profiles, processing and filling prescriptions, and maintaining inventory. This portion of the text covers procedures in both the retail and institutional pharmacy settings, and provides comparisons between them. Special care has been taken to discuss not only the procedures themselves but the reasoning behind the procedures—why are they done in a particular way? This approach is not only necessary to understand work within a pharmacy but is critical to doing well on the certification examination.

A large block of chapters dealing with pharmaceutical calculations has also been provided, which covers a variety of types of calculations that will appear on the examination. These have been presented in a simple, easy-to- understand manner and are designed to take the fear out of math. Topics include not only simple dosage conversions but also intravenous calculations, pediatric dosages, compounding, and commercial calculations. An entire chapter is included consisting only of math problems, with answers and worked-out solutions.

Organization of the text

This exam review guide is organized in the best possible presentation to maximize student learning and comprehension of the scope of the pharmacy technician profession. It consists of three sections, four parts that contains 38 chapters.

The textbook opens with Section I: Assisting the Pharmacist in Serving Patients, which is broken down into the following parts:

Part A: Filling the Medication Order introduces the learner to working within a professional setting and the responsibilities that are required to accurately set-up patient profiles and proper procedures in processing medication orders, including handling and storing medications.

Part B: Pharmaceutical Calculations prepares the learner by providing complete coverage of necessary mathematical concepts and formulas that are crucial for success on the national exam. This part is concluded by a practice math exam that tests the learner's knowledge of all mathematical concepts and principles that were introduced in this section of the textbook.

Part C: Pharmacology provides an introduction to the importance of pharmacology and the role of the technician. This part of the textbook follows a chapter format that groups together pharmacology medications according to the types of disease that needs to be treated or by body system. The learner's knowledge is tested with a practice pharmacology review test to ensure complete understanding and industry knowledge.

Part D: Pharmacy Law covers influential and mandatory state and federal regulations, governing bodies and provides the learner with a foundation of understanding about the laws and ethics surrounding the practice of pharmacy.

Section II: Maintaining Medication and Inventory Control System expands upon the role of the pharmacy technician in controlling inventory and the upkeep of medications within the pharmacy stock.

Section III: Administration and Management of Pharmacy Practice delves deeper into the technologies that are an integral part of a functioning pharmacy and the importance of accurate communication between patients, pharmacists, and pharmacy technicians.

The usefulness of this textbook is enhanced with several appendices, including an updated Too 200 Frequently Prescribed Drugs and Their Uses, Abbreviations list, and a sample exam that will help learners assess their comprehension of core concepts. There is also a corresponding appendix that provides answers for all of the chapter activities.

Features

Each chapter includes a variety of learning aids designed to help the learner further a basic understanding of key concepts. Each chapter begins with a **Quick Study** that condenses the chapter content into a learner friendly outline of what will be covered in the chapter. This will help learners focus their study and use time efficiently. Another important feature that enhances this textbook is **Notes**, which are found throughout each chapter in the left hand margin. They succinctly draw out the most important concepts presented within the content of the chapter. A **Physiology Review** is included in chapters where a refresher in physiology is influential to understanding chapter subject matter.

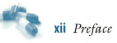

Concluding each chapter are **Chapter Review Questions** that assist the learner in retaining and directly applying the material presented in the chapters for preparation of the national exam. Detailed **solutions** and answers, which will help the learner understand the thought processes that are crucial to understanding and correctly answering the questions on the examination, are given in Appendix E.

New to the third edition

New material added in this revision includes:

- updated chapters on pharmacy practice and law offers the learner the most current industry standards and practices according to state and federal guidelines, including current HIPPA regulations.
- updated chapters on pharmacy math enhances a challenging core learning area. New and updated problems are presented in each chapter as well as corresponding solutions.
- back of book CD with randomized practice exams provides learners with an unlimited amount of practice exams and mimics the national examination for as close as the actual experience as possible.
- updated and expanded section on pharmacology with new market medications and substantial updates to medications included in the second edition when applicable. This section covers not only the principles of pharmacology, drug dosage, and dosage forms, but also the mechanism of action of drugs, adverse effects, and potential drug interactions.

Extensively updated chapters:
Section I: Assisting the Pharmacist in Serving Patients

- Part A: Filling the Medication Order; Chapters 1–6: These chapters have been updated to reflect new guidelines for labeling and dispensing drugs based on state and federal laws. The chapter review sections of chapters 1–5 have been expanded to 10 questions.
- Part B: Pharmaceutical Calculations; Chapters 7–20: Typographical errors have been corrected, updated examples have been added, and the chapter review sections of chapters 7–18 now have a minimum of 10 questions. Chapter 20 is a 60-question math test for further practice. All the review questions in Part B, including the math test, have the solutions worked out in addition to providing the correct answers (Appendix E).
- Part C: Pharmacology; Chapters 21–31: These chapters have been greatly re-worked to include new drug products and dosage forms in each of the drug classes represented. The chapter review sections of chapters 21–30 now have a minimum of 10 questions. Chapter 31 is a pharmacology exam that includes 50 questions.

- Part D: Pharmacy Law; Chapters 32–34: These chapters have been updated to reflect the changing state and federal regulations, including HIPAA. Each chapter review section has been expanded to a minimum of 10 questions.

Section II: Maintaining Medication and Inventory Control Systems

- Chapter review questions have been updated for chapters 35–36.

Section III: Administration and Management of Pharmacy Practice

- Chapter 37 has been updated to reflect the newer computer technologies now available in pharmacy.
- Chapter 38 has an updated chapter review with more questions.

Appendices:

- Appendix A: The Top 200 list has been revised to reflect the current dispensing trends.
- Appendix B: The commonly used abbreviations has been updated to reflect the currently accepted abbreviations used in the medical field today.
- Appendix C: This pretest has been updated. Obsolete questions have been removed and newer questions have been added. The answer key has been adjusted to reflect the new exam.
- Appendix D: This sample exam has been reformatted to reflect the PTCB exam. The questions have been reduced to 90 questions to match the current PTCB format.
- Appendix E: The solution choices for each of the chapter review sections were changed from a numeric format (1, 2, 3, 4) to an alpha format (A, B, C, D) for better clarity. The solutions have been updated to reflect the new questions and the math questions have the problems worked-out for further student learning.

Also Available

Book only
- Pharmacy Technician Certification Exam Review (1111321159)

CD only
- Practice Exam Software to accompany Pharmacy Technician Certification Exam Review (1111535744)

About the Author

The author of *Pharmacy Technician Certification Exam Review* third edition, Dr. Lorraine C. Zentz, is a certified pharmacy technician with a bachelor's

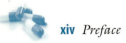

degree in biology and minor in chemistry. She also holds her master's degree in curriculum and instruction as well as her doctorate degree in adult education. She has authored, and currently instructs, her own pharmacy technician-training program offered through Cengage Learning's Ed2Go division, and has also authored a math textbook. She has presented continuing education at the NPTA annual convention and many programs locally in her home state of Colorado.

Acknowledgements

The author wishes to thank the reviewers and editors for their invaluable input. The author would also like to thank her husband for providing the time and much needed support, which made the production of this text possible.

About the CPhT Examination

Structure of the Examination

The PTCB examination consists of 90 questions. It is a timed test, which lasts for two hours. This means that you must pace yourself in answering the questions. There are three general areas in which competency will be assessed:

1. *Assisting the pharmacist in serving patients.* This section includes a discussion of the day-to-day procedures in pharmacy practice, such as:
   - interpretation of the prescription order;
   - preparation and use of the patient profile; and
   - the dispensing, labeling, storage, and delivery of medications

   Also included are discussions on the various aspects of preparing a dosage form for administration, such as:
   - pharmaceutical calculations, including:
   - dosage conversions
   - intravenous medications
   - preparation of IV admixtures
   - administration of drug dose per time
   - commercial calculations

   Computation of markup and selling price is also covered in this section, along with a thorough discussion of pharmacology. This will prepare the technician for assisting the pharmacist in the evaluation of proper prescribing procedures, identifying possible drug interactions and therapeutic duplications, and evaluation of the treatment regimen to assure that the patient has received a prescription for the correct drug in the correct dosage for his or her needs.

   The questions pertaining to assisting the pharmacist will make up 66% of the exam. Both hospital and retail settings will be discussed, and the student will be expected to know the differences in procedures between the different practice settings.

The questions following the chapter material will require you to think about why things are done a certain way (with responsibility comes challenge).

> ### EXAMPLE
>
> Why is certain information required to be placed onto the prescription order and patient profile? Why do we have the patient profile at all? Why do we use aseptic technique when preparing intravenous medications? This book will train you to think about the reasoning behind procedures as you answer the questions.

2. *Maintaining medication and inventory control system.* This portion addresses the proper way to store medication and drug products in the pharmacy; procedures for ordering and inventory of drugs, drug products, and devices; drug prepackaging and distribution; and unit dose distribution, labeling, and mandatory record-keeping. These questions will make up 22% of the exam.

3. *Administration of and management of pharmacy practice.* This section addresses safety concerns, cleanliness, infection control, pharmacy law, communications, and automation (e.g., computers). These questions make up 12% of the exam.

The ICPT examination consists of 110 questions. It is a timed test, which last two hours. This means you must pace yourself in answering the questions. The competency will be assessed in three general areas:

1. *Regulations and technician duties.* This section will include an overview of technician duties and general information, including:

   - Roles of pharmacists and technicians
   - Functions a technician may perform
   - Prescription work flow
   - Security
   - Inventory control
   - Stocking medications
   - Expired products
   - Controlled substances, including:
   - Drug schedules
   - Refills, filing and transfers
   - Procedure for schedule V sales
   - Control Substance Act
   - DEA numbers
   - Other laws and regulations, including:
   - Federal laws

- Generics substitutions
- Roles of government agencie
- Prescribing authority
- Manufacturer drug package labeling
- OTC labeling

The questions pertaining to the regulations and technician duties will make up 25% of the exam.

2. *Drugs and drug therapy.* This section will include the following:
   - Drug classification
   - Major drug classes
   - Dosage forms
   - OTC products
   - NDC numbers
   - Frequently prescribed medications, including:
   - Brand and generic names
   - Pharmacology and classifications
   - Indications
   - Adverse drug reactions and contraindications

The questions pertaining to drugs and drug therapy will make up 23% of the exam.

3. *Dispensing process.* This section will include the following:
   - Prescription information
   - Valid prescription information
   - Telephone/fax prescriptions
   - Refill requirements
   - Patient information
   - Common abbreviations
   - Preparing/dispensing prescriptions, including:
   - Avoiding errors
   - Checking prescriptions
   - Automated dispensing systems
   - Procedures for data entry
   - Labeling properly
   - Use of patient records
   - Packaging and storage
   - Managed care prescriptions
   - Calculations, including:

- Conversions
- Calculating prescription ingredients
- Calculating quantity to be dispensed
- Calculating daily doses
- Compounding calculations
- IV calculations
- Business calculations
- Sterile products, unit dose and repackaging, including:
- Drug distribution systems
- Repackaging medications
- Compliance aids
- Aseptic technique and laminar flow hoods
- Chemotherapy
- Routes of administration for parenteral products
- Types of sterile products
- Procedures for maintaining sterile environments
- Accurate compounding and labeling of sterile products

The questions in this section will make up approximately 52% of the exam.

Taking the Examination

You should read the booklet that came with your application carefully. It contains a lot of useful information, such as what you should bring to the exam. You should also be aware that the actual examination will not simply test on memorized information. Questions and problems will require the student to think and synthesize information. It is also helpful if you know how to take the test (see below).

> **NOTE**
>
> When using this text to prepare for the exam, bear in mind that the certification examination is now a national examination, and, since laws vary from state to state, information that may be considered correct for the examination may not be exactly the same as what you have learned in practice.

Answering Questions on the Examination

Since the test is in multiple-choice format, you must know how to take multiple-choice tests. You will not know all of the information; however, you can use what you do know to choose the correct answer.

Take the time to look at the question. Perhaps a question asks which of the following drugs is a diuretic. The potential answers are: streptomycin, penicillin, tobramycin, and mannitol. You panic because you have no clue. Instead, you should look carefully at the answers, bearing in mind that only one is correct. Everyone (hopefully) knows that penicillin is an antibiotic. Scratch that one. Two of the answers end in the same thing: strepto*mycin* and tobra*mycin:* It is likely (but not necessarily a given fact) that they do similar things. The only one that is left is mannitol, which happens to be the right answer.

> **NOTE**
>
> If you take the time to look at the question and all of the answers given, and think your way through the problem using the knowledge that you do have, it is time well spent.

Read the question. Another thing that you must be sure to do is read the question *carefully.* Ask yourself "What is the question asking?" Then, if you can, *answer the question in your head before looking at the answers provided.* If you do not, the answers will confuse you. A standard way of making up multiple-choice tests is to ask a question and then think of all the ways a student could interpret the question, or the mistakes that could easily be made, and then make the incorrect answers from that. It is not that the exam is unfair; the questions are simply testing your knowledge, which includes the ability to distinguish fine points. So always answer the question first in your head, and then look for your answer in the choices given.

Don't panic. Do not let the questions or answers intimidate you. Let's say you are answering a math problem. You come up with an answer and find it in the list, but the other answers are the same as yours, except for a zero or decimal place. If you did the calculation correctly, your answer is correct. Do not second-guess yourself. More wrong answers are made on exams because students get nervous and change their initial (correct) answer to another (in- correct) answer. You have prepared for this exam—act like it! Have confidence in what you can do.

> More wrong answers are made on exams because students get nervous and change their initial (correct) answer to another (incorrect) answer.

Scoring. This exam, like many standardized exams, does not have one passing score. The passing score is different for each exam, because the people who make up the questions assign a difficulty rating to each question, and the average difficulty rating for all of the questions on a particular exam determines the passing score. Thus, the passing score for an exam given in one session will not be the same as another, as the examinations will vary in difficulty. Bear this in mind, and **if the questions seem to be extremely difficult, don't despair.** This may mean that the passing score is lower as well. Don't panic—attack the exam logically.

Preparing for the Examination

First, take the "pretest" to determine which sections of the book to review first. There is a Quick Study guide at the beginning of each chapter for quick review. Study this first, then read through the chapters for approaches to thinking and important details. Then, as you continue to go through the book, practice doing the problems in each section, even if they seem too easy or too hard. The answers are explained for you, so use these to channel your thinking about how to approach the questions in a certain way. Ask yourself questions about the material, and see if you can come up with the answers either on your own or from the text material. *Ask yourself why!* Finally, take the practice test.

Taking the Practice Test

When you take the practice test, you should sit in a room with conditions that may not be the best for you. The examination center may not be as warm or as cool as you like, and there will be many other people there who will be making at least a small amount of noise (excessive erasing, drumming fingers or tapping feet, clearing throats, heavy breathing, etc.). Practice concentrating under the worst conditions—anyone can concentrate in a climate-controlled, comfortable, quiet room! If you can do well under the worst conditions, you will do even better if the conditions are most favorable for you. If possible, have some others next to you when taking the practice test. These exams are often in close quarters. Finally, grade the exam, using the answer key. Determine which questions you missed and why. Study those parts again.

Now you will have prepared for many things that can come your way (one can never be prepared for everything—that's where the thinking part comes in). You are ready to take the exam.

Before the Examination—Helpful Hints

Get a good night's sleep before the exam. Know where the exam is to be held, exactly how to get there, and where to park. Make a dry run, in order to find out how much time it will take you to get there, park, and get to the examination room—then add an extra few minutes. This way, when the test day arrives, you will arrive on time with a minimum of frustration.

Get adequate nutrition before the exam. Remember, the brain runs on glucose. If you do not feed it, it will not work. So, on the morning of the exam, be sure to eat a good breakfast, even if you are not hungry. This is more important than you might think! Avoid drinking a lot of coffee; substitute juices instead. You may wish to bring a sweater, in case the examination room is cold.

You have prepared, so you should not be nervous. If you are, try looking over the section outlines in the book or notes that you have taken for yourself. If it all looks too familiar, you should be ready.

Good luck!

Assisting the Pharmacist in Serving Patients

THIS SECTION of the book reviews the content in the first functional area as tested in the ICPT or PTCB exam. This comprises 52% (ICPT), and 66% (PTCB) of the examination questions. Due to the length of this section, it will be broken down into four parts:

Part A.   Filling the Medication Order

Part B.   Pharmaceutical Calculations

Part C.   Pharmacology

Part D.   Pharmacy Law

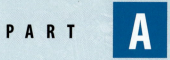

Filling the Medication Order

CHAPTER 1

Receiving the Medication Order

Quick Study

I. The retail medication order

    A. Information required to be present on the prescription at the time of acceptance—written in ink or typed on the prescription form

- The patient's full name
- The date of issue of the prescription: Prescriptions are typically valid for one year, depending on state regulations, with the exception of prescriptions for controlled substances (Schedules II–V), which are valid for three days to six months depending on the drug, state of issue, and the classification (II–V)
- The name and title of the prescriber
- The Drug Enforcement Agency (DEA) number assigned to the prescriber (this information is required for controlled substances only, and may be added by pharmacy personnel)
- The name of the drug prescribed (generic or brand name)
- The strength and dosage form of the drug prescribed (see exceptions)
- The quantity of drug to be dispensed
- The instructions for dosage (SIG)
- The signature of the prescriber, in ink
- Authorization to dispense a generic substitution: required for substitution of proprietary label only. When "dispense as written" (DAW) or "brand name medically necessary" designation is present, there is to be no substitution of any kind, including the substitution of another proprietary label.
- Refill information: must be clearly written in the appropriate blank on the form (or the number of refills circled). A refill authorization may be made to extend

the original prescription, but a new prescription must be written. This is the responsibility of the pharmacist in most states.

- Instructions for preparation of the drug, if applicable: If preparation of the drug is required, detailed instructions must be given; otherwise it is considered extemporaneous compounding and must be done by the pharmacist.

B. Information to be added to the prescription form at the time of acceptance
- The address and telephone number of the patient: used to identify the patient and assist in medication recalls
- Age or date of birth of the patient: used to identify the patient and to verify that the dose prescribed is appropriate
- Allergies and concurrent medications: used to prevent potential allergic reactions, drug interactions, adverse effects, and therapeutic duplications (information is found in patient profile)
- The insurance coverage of the patient may also be noted

C. Authentication and clarification of the prescription order
- Verification of medication and the amount prescribed
- Signature verification
- Verification of DEA number

D. Accepting prescriptions for controlled substances
- Prescriptions for drugs classified under Schedule II
- Some states require that all information be present on triplicate form: No writing on the form is allowed.
- Prescriptions for controlled substances expire quickly—based on state regulations, those for Schedule II drugs may expire within a few days in some states or up to six months in other states, and those for drugs falling under Schedules III–IV may be valid for six months following the date the prescription was written.

E. Receiving prescriptions by electronic means (telephone, fax machine, modem, or e-mail)
- May be accepted by licensed practitioner (i.e., pharmacist, intern, nurse) only
- Must be immediately transcribed onto a "hard copy"

F. Accepting refill requests: A refill request by a patient can be accepted by the technician. Changes in amount or form of the drug dispensed can only be made by the pharmacist.

II. The institutional medication order and MAR

A. The hospital medication order may include:
- More detail than the retail prescription
- Patient location, billing number, diagnosis, height, weight, diet, and medical tests
- Directions for use of medications and/or instructions for compounding
- The times of initiation and discontinuation of drug therapy are specified

B. Structure and use of the MAR
- The MAR is prepared in the pharmacy from the medication order.
- Medications are administered by work schedule, according to the 24-hour clock.
- The MAR serves as a legal record of drug administration for administrative and billing purposes.

C. Filling the medication order
- Calculation of the amount of drug required per dose (unit dose)
- Preparation of the correct amount of drug in the correct vehicle for delivery
- Preparation and placement of the appropriate label
- Placement of the prepared daily doses into an appropriately labeled cassette for placement into the medication cart
- Preparation of the MAR from the medication order

D. Preparation of unit dose medications

III. Comparison of medication orders in retail and institutional settings

- Differences in amount of detail presented: instructions, dosing schedules, etc.
- More detailed identifying information is presented on the hospital order: This helps ensure the administration of drugs to the proper patient.
- More information is present on the hospital order (e.g., laboratory tests, diet).
- DEA numbers of individual prescribers are not required.
- Special documentation for controlled substance prescription is not required on the hospital order.

The Retail Medication Order

The retail **medication order** (prescription) may be communicated to the pharmacy by several means—it may be presented by the patient or communicated by telephone, fax, or e-mail. Schedule II Drugs have specific criteria for presenting a prescription.

The Written Prescription Order

At the retail pharmacy window, the medication order (prescription order) is received written on a form that is normally preprinted with certain information. If the required information is not preprinted, it may be written in or typed on the form. The prescription order *must be completed in ink or typed* to avoid possible alteration, and it must contain specific information when it is received in the pharmacy. If the prescription is incomplete or illegible, it cannot be filled, and the patient should be referred back to the prescriber or to the pharmacist.

Required Information on the Prescription Order

Information on the upper portion of the prescription form must include the following (see Figure 1-1):

> The date the prescription was written helps to determine if the prescription may be filled.

> Prescriptions are valid only for one year after being written. Exceptions are prescriptions for controlled substances, which may be valid for as little as three days.

- *The patient's full name*: This is required for positive identification.
- *The date of issue of the prescription*: The date of writing helps to determine if the prescription may be filled. It should be noted that the laws regarding prescription filling do vary from state to state. However, since the certification exam is based on *federal* laws, the normal rule of thumb to remember is this: Prescriptions are valid only for one year after being written with the exception of prescriptions for controlled substances (Schedule II–Schedule V), which are valid for six months or less. If the prescription is presented after the allotted time (i.e., one year), the prescription cannot be filled.
- *The name and title of the prescriber*: The prescriber may be a doctor of medicine (MD), osteopathic medicine (DO), optometry (OD), dentistry (DDS), veterinary medicine (DVM), or podiatry. Other individuals licensed to prescribe drugs include the physician's assistant and nurse practitioner.
- *The Drug Enforcement Agency (DEA) number assigned to the prescriber (required for controlled substances only)*: The DEA number is a seven-digit number issued to the prescriber or institution by the

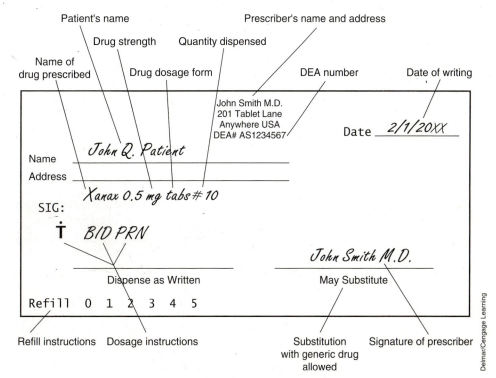

Figure 1-1: The Retail Prescription

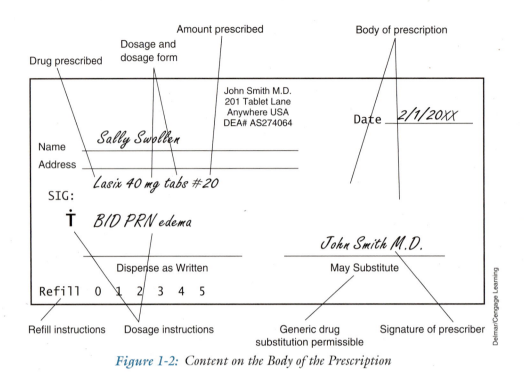

Figure 1-2: *Content on the Body of the Prescription*

DEA. It should begin with two letters. The first letter, an A, B, F, or M, designates the status of the prescriber. The second letter of the DEA number is the first letter of the prescriber's last name.

On the body (middle part) of the prescription, you should find all of the following (see Chapter 2 for discussion) (Figure 1-2):

- *The name of the drug prescribed* (generic or brand name).
- *Strength and dosage form* of the drug prescribed (e.g., 40 mg tablets).
- *Quantity of drug to be dispensed* (e.g., 20 tablets, or 80 mL if the drug is to be administered in liquid form).
- *Instructions for dosage (SIG)*: These should be clear and understandable. Dosage instructions on the prescription form are normally written in "medical shorthand," which the technician should be familiar with. For example, numerical designations of the number of tablets, teaspoons, etc. are written in lowercase Roman numerals (e.g., i, ii, iv, etc.). The way you will actually see this written on a prescription is shown below.

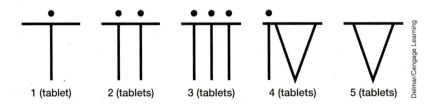

Further discussion of the abbreviations seen on the prescription blank is found in Chapter 2. See also Appendix B.

- *Instructions for labeling*: The prescriber may not want certain information on the prescription form to be shown on the label. In this case, instructions for what information is to be printed on the label are included.

- *Signature of the prescriber, in ink*: No prestamped facsimiles are acceptable.

- *Authorization to dispense a generic substitution*: The way in which a generic substitution is authorized or disallowed varies from state to state. Some states have an open box printed on the prescription form in which the prescriber writes the letters **DAW (for "dispense as written")** or **Brand Medically Necessary** if the prescription is to be filled exactly as it is written. In other states, the prescription blank has two lines for signature, and the line on which the prescriber signs designates how the prescription is to be filled. (See Figure 1-2.) Generic substitutions are further discussed in Chapter 2.

> If the prescriber designates the dispense as written (DAW) option, the prescription must be filled exactly as written!

- *Refill information*: The number of refills should be clearly designated on the prescription form.

- *Instructions for the preparation of a drug*: This is rarely seen on a prescription form; however, if a drug needs to be made a certain way, such as a cream, lotion, or suppository instead of a tablet, the prescriber may write out instructions for preparation of the drug. If specific, written instructions exist for preparation of the drug, it may be prepared by the technician.

Verification of the DEA Number

At present, top-level prescribers (e.g., MD, DO, DDS, and OD) are assigned either a capital letter "A", "B" or "F" as the first letter of the DEA number. No particular significance is attached to the letter. Letters are simply assigned according to the date that the application for the DEA number was made. As more DEA numbers are assigned, the letter designation will continue to move through the alphabet. Mid-level practitioners (e.g., physician's assistants, nurse practitioners) are assigned the letter "M."

The second letter of the DEA number is the first letter of the prescriber's last name. Thus, it is easy to check the validity of the prescription: If the prescriber's name is Smith, for example, and the DEA number starts with **AU**, it is invalid (it should be **AS**, not **AU**), unless the practitioner has gotten married and changed their last name since receiving a DEA number. A valid DEA number can also be verified mathematically by adding the odd-numbered digits (the first, third, and fifth) to the sum of the even numbered digits (the second, fourth, and sixth), multiplied by two. The last digit of this number should be the same as the seventh number in the prescriber's DEA number.

> ### EXAMPLE
>
> You receive a prescription at the pharmacy window, and the prescriber's DEA number is listed as AU3284065. First, add the odd-numbered digits (the first, third, and fifth positions):
>
> $$3 + 8 + 0 = 11$$
>
> Then, add the even-numbered digits (the second, fourth, and sixth positions): and multiply by two
>
> $$2 + 4 + 6 = 12 \times 2 = 24$$
>
> Adding the two sums together we have:
>
> $$11 + 24 = 35$$

The last digit in the calculated sum is 5, which matches the last digit of the DEA number. It thus appears to be a valid number.

The authenticity of the DEA number can thus be verified in two ways: by comparing the letters in the DEA number against the name and status of the practitioner and by numerical calculation.

Adding Information to the Prescription Form

Information to be placed onto a prescription form at the time of acceptance includes:

- The patient's address and contact information
- Age or date of birth of the patient
- Allergies and concurrent medications
- Medical conditions
- Method of payment/insurance coverage

This information is then transferred to the patient profile.

There is some information that is necessary for the pharmacy to have in order to protect the patient (and also to protect the pharmacy from liability). This information should be obtained from the patient by the technician and written on the prescription form.

Exception: Prescriptions for Schedule II drugs, such as morphine (MSContin), meperidine (Demerol), or oxycodone (Roxicet), must have all information complete on the form before acceptance at the pharmacy window.

Information that may be placed on a prescription form at the time of acceptance includes the following:

- *The patient's address and telephone number:* This will help identify the patient and provide a contact in case of drug recall.
- *Age or date of birth:* This will assist in identification and assure an appropriate drug regimen.
- *Allergies and concurrent medications:* This will prevent adverse reactions to medication.

- *The insurance coverage of the patient.* How does the patient intend to pay? Payment might be in the form of cash (self-pay), co-pay (the pharmacy bills the insurance company directly), or receipt for reimbursement, for example.

Authentication and Clarification of the Prescription Order

> If the prescription form is illegible or questionable, the technician should ask the pharmacist for clarification.

In the event that the prescription form is unreadable or questionable, the technician should ask the pharmacist for clarification. Often the handwriting of the prescriber is illegible, or the signature or other information is questionable. In this case, the pharmacist will be aware of normal prescribed amounts for the drug in question and will be able to easily clarify the instructions and verify the prescription by telephone with the prescriber. This is especially important in the case of written prescriptions for Schedule II drugs, as they may be altered in order to obtain more drugs for abuse or sale.

Accepting Refill Requests

> Refills are normally spaced out over an appropriate amount of time. However, at the discretion of the pharmacist, medication may be dispensed in larger or smaller increments, if the patient requests it (except for refills on prescriptions for controlled substances).

Refill requests for prescriptions other than Schedule II drugs may be made by the patient either over the telephone, by fax, or in person. These requests may be accepted by the technician. After filling the refill prescription, the appropriate amount of drug is then deducted from the number of remaining prescription refills listed in the patient profile (see Chapter 3).

Refills are normally spaced out over an appropriate amount of time; however, they may be given all at one time (at the discretion of the pharmacist) if the patient requests it. Sometimes, when the drug is taken for a long period of time (e.g., antiseizure drugs and anxiolytics), it is less expensive for the patient to buy larger quantities at one time. Conversely, the patient might not be able to afford the entire quantity of drug prescribed and may be allowed to purchase only part of the prescription at a time. Changes in the amount of drug dispensed are made *at the discretion of the pharmacist,* as the pharmacist is legally responsible for everything that happens in the pharmacy.

Controlled substances, such as Schedule II drugs, are treated in a very different way. These prescriptions may be filled by the technician, but any refills (available on Schedules III–V drugs only) must be dispensed within a specific time frame to prevent misuse of the drug. In other words, if a prescription is for three months, refills may only be dispensed every 30 days. Five refills in six months are allowed on prescriptions for drugs classified as Schedules III–IV. No refills may be dispensed on a prescription for a Schedule II drug.

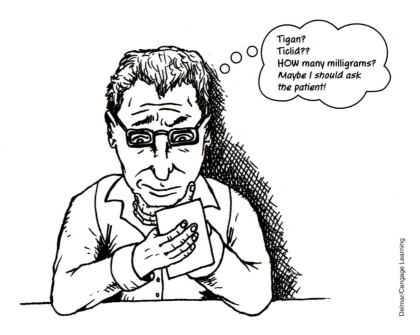

Tigan?
Ticlid??
HOW many milligrams?
Maybe I should ask
the patient!

Delmar/Cengage Learning

Refill Authorizations

> Prescription refills may be accepted and filled by the technician. However, refill authorizations may be taken only by a licensed pharmacist or pharmacy intern.

Sometimes a patient runs out of a needed medication and has not obtained a new prescription. In this case, the pharmacy may contact the physician/prescriber to extend the original prescription. This is called a **refill authorization** and may be obtained only by a licensed pharmacy practitioner (e.g., the pharmacist or pharmacy intern). Some states now allow technicians to do this also.

Prescriptions for Schedule II (Controlled Substance) Drugs

> Prescriptions for drugs classified as Schedule II must be complete when presented. No corrections or additions are permitted.

A state may require a special prescription form for Schedule II drugs. In some states, this is a triplicate form, with the copies of the form serving as records for dispensing: one copy is sent to the Drug Enforcement Agency, one is sent to the prescriber, and one is filed in the pharmacy.

As discussed previously, prescriptions for controlled substances must be filled exactly as prescribed. Again, no errors, corrections, or write-overs should be present on the form. If any corrections or extra writing appears on the form when it is presented, the prescription should not be filled and it should be brought to the attention of the pharmacist.

Receiving Prescriptions by Electronic Means

> Prescriptions received electronically must be transcribed onto a prescription form ("hard copy") for purposes of documentation. This may only be done by a licensed practitioner (i.e., the pharmacist).

Some states grant licensure to pharmacy interns. In this case, telephone prescriptions may also be legally taken by a licensed pharmacy intern. The technician may not take prescription orders from electronic devices.

Prescriptions received electronically must be transcribed onto a hard-copy form before filling. This must be done by the pharmacist or pharmacy intern in most states.

The Institutional Pharmacy

The Medication Order and Medication Administration Record

The inpatient **medication order** is found only in a hospital or institutional pharmacy and serves as the drug order. It is very detailed, much more so than a retail prescription. From the medication order, the **Medication Administration Record (MAR)** is generated (Figure 1-3).

The Medication Order

> Information regarding the patient and the patient's medical condition allows the pharmacist to verify that the drugs prescribed and dosage schedule are appropriate.

> The drug dosage form must be clearly specified and must be appropriate to the patient's medical condition. If only one dosage form exists, specification of dosage form is not required.

The list of medications ordered for the patient includes a *schedule* for the administration of the drugs, and, if necessary, *instructions for preparation of the drugs.* By looking at the dosage schedule and the age, height, weight, medical history, diet, and diagnosis of the patient, the pharmacist can determine whether the patient is receiving the appropriate drug and dose for the diagnosis and also that the drug is compatible with the patient's diet and will not adversely affect existing medical conditions that the patient may have.

Medication orders must also specify:

- *The exact dosage form of the drug* (i.e., solution, suspension, tincture, etc., instead of just "liquid")

The dosage form ordered should be appropriate to the patient's medical condition; a vomiting patient would not be prescribed an oral medication, for example, but would receive the medication in suppository form or by injection. If there is only one dosage form or strength of the prescribed medication, it is not specified.

- The dosage strength
- Directions for use, where appropriate

PHYSICIAN'S ORDER SHEET   546876543   **Rm 345-A**

(Use pen – press firmly, you are making 4 copies)   James, William 5/23/43
                                                            Dr. P. Capelss

                                                            Pt. addressograph

Date	Time	Orders
4/22	0700	CBC, UA
		Regular diet
		Tylenol 5gr 1-2 po q6h prn headache
		Furosemide 20mg qam
		KCl 10mEq bid
		Cefprozil Susp 250mg q12h
		Vicodin 1-2 po q4h prn pain
4/22	2100	D/C Tylenol, start Ibuprofen 400mg q8h PRN
4/23	0700	Increase furosemide 40mg qam
		Physical therapy consult
		Training Ointment to affected area bid

Delmar/Cengage Learning

Figure 1-3: Physician's Order Sheet

In the hospital setting, the **route of administration** of the drug must be specified (e.g., an order for morphine gr 1/4 could be given orally, intravenously, or intramuscularly). This assists the technician in preparing the drug for administration.

Often, patient medications must be prepared for injection in a certain way. The medication order may contain instructions for the proper dilution of a drug and the **diluent** (the liquid that the drug is to be dissolved in) to be used. These should be transcribed onto the MAR.

Total Parenteral Nutrition Solutions (TPNs)

Frequently, a patient who is undernourished, vomiting, or has severe diarrhea may require intravenous feeding, and **total parenteral nutrition** solutions (TPNs) may be ordered. These medications contain a balanced mixture of sugars, proteins, and fats to be administered intravenously. The exact mixture depends on the patient's needs, so *instructions for compounding* (how to make the solution) are also stamped or written on the medication order.

The Generation and Organization of the Medication Administration Record

The medication administration record (MAR) is generated by the pharmacy and serves as a record of medication administration by nursing staff. It contains a list of the drugs dispensed from the pharmacy, the time of dispensing, and the initials of the person dispensing the medication, as well as dosages and times of administration.

Instead of giving a set of dosage instructions with each drug (the SIG), the MAR puts the medication order within a specific **dosage schedule**. This schedule tells when the medications are to be given to the patient and is normally determined by the institution. Most hospitals have set times when "routine" medication is delivered, in order to decrease confusion and minimize the possibility of dosage errors.

The Dosage Schedule

Drug dosages have to be scheduled relative to each other, and medications are usually administered according to the hospital work shift or during preset medication administration times for the hospital. Therefore, the MAR usually contains a dosage schedule for drug administration. For example, the times of administration may be listed across the top of the MAR according to a 24-hour clock. The nurse administering the medication may place a mark in the block underneath the time that the medication was administered to the patient. Next to the time of administration, there may be blank spaces for the pharmacy technician to note the time that the drug was dispensed and his or her initials. The nurse also initials as to the actual time of administration. In this way, an accurate record is kept of when the drug was dispensed and how long the drug was stored before it was given. The MAR also serves as a record that the drug actually was administered, by whom, and the actual time of administration (this is particularly important with narcotic drugs).

The hospital order includes information such as:

- Drugs to be administered, doses and routes of administration, and reason for use
- Date of drug order
- The date that the therapy is started and the date that it is to be discontinued
- The prescriber's name for each drug
- Designation of drugs for which generic substitutions allowed/disallowed
- Drug dosages and schedule for administration
- Dosage instructions
- Instructions for compounding of medications

In a hospital setting, the patient receives several drugs at one time, so dosages must be scheduled relative to each other to avoid medication errors.

The MAR also serves as documentation of the drugs actually administered to the patient, which facilitates accurate patient billing.

Filling the Medication Order

In a hospital setting, the medication order (physician's order) is transmitted to the pharmacy, either directly or by computer. Computerized transmission is preferable, as it decreases the probability of transcription errors. Once in the pharmacy, it is the responsibility of the pharmacist to review the order and evaluate the suitability of the drugs prescribed, with regard to the patient and his or her existing drug and dosage regimen. Once reviewed, the order is passed to the technician for filling. The technician then fills the order. A technician or the nurse then transcribes the information onto the MAR.

Rather than filling an order for an individual drug and sending it up to the floor at the appropriate time for administration, the *unit dose* system is used.

The Unit Dose

A **unit dose** is defined to be the amount of drug needed for a single dose. The dose of drug is calculated, the order is filled with the drug stock available in the pharmacy, and the drug packaged as an individual (unit) dose.

> **EXAMPLE**
>
> An order is for 80 mg tablets of Lasix po bid. The pharmacy has only 40 mg tablets in stock. A unit dose would be the amount of drug needed for a single dose, so two of the 40 mg tablets would be packaged together.

The Unit Dose System

In the unit dose system, all of the drug doses for an individual patient that will be required for an entire day are prepared at one time and distributed to the patient floors.

The individual drugs are read off the medication order, with dosage strength, form, and instructions. The technician is responsible for assessing the instructions for dosage of the drug (e.g., one tablet bid, qid, etc.) and calculating the amount of drug (the number of tablets, number of milliliters, etc.) that will be given to the patient in the course of one day. The technician then prepares the proper amount and places it in a properly labeled container (cassette/drawer) for insertion into the medication cart.

Proper labeling of the cassette should include:

- The patient's name
- The hospital identification number

- The attending physician's name
- The location of the patient (e.g., room 222, bed 1)

The Medication Cart

Modern pharmacies now use medication carts, which are located on the individual patient floors. These carts are free-standing, computerized cabinets containing the daily medications for all patients on a particular floor or wing within a hospital or nursing home. The technician delivers the unit dose cassettes to the patient floor and files the medications within the drawers of the medication cart, so that enough drugs for a particular patient is sent up for an entire day at one time. Normally, the drugs for an individual patient are filed by patient identification number. Unused medications, if the package has not been opened, may be returned to the pharmacy for restocking and patient credit (i.e., medications intended for dosing "as needed," for example, and are not used, or medication assigned to a discharged patient).

Comparison of Medication Orders in Retail and Institutional Settings

The two types of medication orders discussed in this chapter have many things in common: the name of the patient and other identifying information, the prescriber's name and title, and drugs prescribed. The major difference is in the amount of detail presented.

The institutional medication order gives a *detailed schedule of administration*. The retail order gives only instructions to be followed by the patient, because the medication is self-administered. There is *more identifying information* present on the institutional medication order as well, to ensure that the medication is administered to the right patient.

The amount of information included on the order differs also. This information may include *diagnosis, laboratory tests, height and weight,* and *other information about the patient* as well.

Prescription of Controlled Substances

In an institutional setting, the prescription of controlled substances does not require a special form; they are just included on the order. Since prescribers may use the DEA number assigned to the hospital, *there are no prescriber DEA numbers on the order* (which may also have several different prescribers).

Delivery of the controlled substances to the hospital floor or unit may require special documentation, however, including signatures of the technician delivering the medication and the head nurse in the patient care area, documenting transfer of the drug (and responsibility for the drug) from the pharmacy to the patient care area.

In a retail setting, a prescription for a controlled substance (specifically a Schedule II drug, such as morphine or Demerol) requires a **triplicate form** in many states, which must be filed separately from the other prescription forms, with copies sent to the prescriber and the DEA.

Chapter Review Questions

1. Which of the following would be found on an institutional medication order, but not on a retail pharmacy prescription?
   a. patient name
   b. the patient's diagnosis
   c. drug dosage schedule
   d. both b and c

2. Which of the following must be present on the prescription at the time of acceptance?
   a. the prescriber's signature
   b. the exact name, strength, and form of the drug
   c. the age of the patient
   d. both a and b

3. Which of the following may the technician **not** perform?
   a. accept refill requests by telephone
   b. refill authorizations
   c. accept prescriptions by electronic means
   d. both b and c

4. Which of the following is required on a retail prescription but not on a hospital order?
   a. the generic name of the drug dispensed
   b. the strength of the drug dispensed
   c. the DEA number of the prescriber
   d. the name of the prescriber

5. You receive a prescription written by a Dr. Smith. The DEA number is AU1234567. You should take the following action:
   a. fill the prescription
   b. call Dr. Smith's office
   c. alert the pharmacist
   d. give the prescription back to the patient, as it is invalid

6. Prescriptions in the pharmacy may be received:
   a. from a patient, directly
   b. by fax
   c. by e-mail
   d. all of the above

7. Prescriptions received by electronic means:
   a. may be filled directly
   b. may be taken by the technician
   c. must be transferred to paper (a hard copy) before being filled
   d. prescriptions are not taken by electronic means

8. You receive a prescription for secobarbital (a C–II), which was written two weeks ago and appears to be altered. You should:
   a. fill the prescription
   b. consult the pharmacist
   c. refuse to fill the prescription and give it back to the patient
   d. call the prescriber for authorization

9. You receive a prescription for a drug that is available only by brand name. The prescriber has written the generic name on the prescription. You should:
   a. call to see if a generic is available
   b. fill the prescription and consult the pharmacist
   c. tell the patient that the prescription cannot be filled
   d. call the prescriber for authorization to dispense the brand-name drug

10. You receive a prescription for Roxicet. You may enter the following data on the prescription form:
    a. the address of the patient
    b. the age of the patient
    c. all of the above
    d. none of the above

CHAPTER 2

Processing the Medication Order

Quick Study

I. Dosage forms and applications

    A. Solid dosage form (tablet, capsule)
    B. Liquid dosage form (syrup, tincture, solution for injection)
    C. Semisolid dosage form (cream, suppository)
    D. Specific applications for the various types of dosage forms
    E. Use and handling of drugs in suspension

II. Routes of administration

    A. Oral
    B. Sublingual—administration of medication to be dissolved under the tongue
    C. Buccal—administration of medication between the cheeks
    D. Parenteral—administration of medication directly into the body (e.g., into the bloodstream, into the muscle, or under the skin)
    E. Intrathecal—administration of medication into the space between the spinal cord and spinal meninges
    F. Intracardiac—administration of medication directly into the heart

III. Interpreting the written order in the retail setting

    A. Information required on the prescription form, and its use
      • Drug name, strength, dosage form, and amount of drug prescribed
      • Instructions for the patient that correctly interpret written instructions and verify that they are within appropriate guidelines
      • Signature of prescriber and authorization to substitute

- Refills
- Prescriptions for regular prescription drugs versus prescriptions for narcotics and controlled substances and other Schedule II (C-II) drugs

Information to be entered on the prescription form by the technician at the time of acceptance
- Patient's address, phone number, age, and date of birth
- Drug allergies
- Concurrent medications
- Medical history and existing medical conditions
- Insurance provider information

B. Dosage instructions—drug doses and half-life

C. Information to be entered on the form at time of dispensing—use of information (why is it required?) and legality issues
- Identifying information
- Age and gender
- Concurrent medications (including over-the-counter medications)

D. Interpretation of abbreviations

IV. Dispensing the correct medication—in order to prevent medication errors, it is critical to carefully compare the information on the manufacturer's label to information on the prescription, including

- Drug name, dosage form, and strength
- Proper route of administration
- Recommended and safe dosages

V. Interpreting the written order in the institutional setting in comparison to the retail prescription

The Dosage Form

To correctly process a written medication order, it is necessary to know some basic terminology. When the drug is prescribed, it is usually prescribed in a specific **dosage form**. The form in which the drug is used depends on the condition of the patient. Most drugs are taken in tablet form orally (by mouth), but others must be used in a suppository form (e.g., for a vomiting patient), topically, in the eye, systemically, on the skin (for a rash or skin condition), or in oral liquid form (for a child). Some drugs may also be administered through the skin, via the *transdermal patch*.

Since different dosage forms are packaged and used differently, it is important to know which dosage form the drug must be in. In addition, the instructions written by the prescriber on the prescription form are abbreviated, and the technician must be familiar with these abbreviations to accurately convey the instructions to the patient. (See Table 2-1 and Appendix B.)

Table 2-1   Abbreviations Used on Prescription Forms

Abbreviations may appear in either uppercase or lowercase lettering. There is no special meaning attached to capitalization in this case. Periods may also appear after the letters.

When		Where	
cc	with meals	po	by mouth
ac	before meals	od	right eye
pc	after meals	os	left eye
hs	at bedtime (before sleep)	ou	both eyes
qd	once a day (or every day)	ad	right ear
bid	twice a day	as	left ear
tid	three times a day	au	both ears
qid	four times a day	IM	intramuscularly
qod	every other day	IV	into the vein: bolus or drip
q wk	once a week	SC	under the skin
prn	as needed	ID	into the skin
ut dict	as directed	IA	into the artery
atc	around the clock	IT	intrathecal
qh	every hour	IC	intracardiac
w or $\overline{C}$	with	SL	sublingual (under the tongue)
wo or $\overline{S}$	without	PR	rectally, in the rectum

How much		Drug form	
cc	cubic centimeter (same as mL)	tab	tablet
fl	fluid	cap	capsule
g, gm	gram	pul	pulvule
gr	grain	syr	syrup
gtt	drop	susp	suspension
mg	milligram	elix	elixir
mcg	microgram (µg)	ext	extract
aa	of each	tinct	tincture
tsp	teaspoon	ung or oint	ointment
tbsp	tablespoon		

Solid Dosage Forms

Solid dosage forms are those that can be picked up and handled. These include the oral dosage forms of **tablet**, **capsule**, and **enteric-coated tablet** (Figure 2-1).

The Tablet

A tablet is made of pressed powder. How hard the powder is pressed determines how the tablet can be used. For example, a **sublingual tablet** is made to dissolve quickly, under the tongue, and therefore cannot be pressed hard into a dense tablet. (Since the tablet is so soft, it must be handled very carefully to avoid turning it into a pile of powder.) An example of a sublingual tablet would be a nitroglycerin tablet, which is made to dissolve quickly so that the drug may be rapidly absorbed into the system.

Most tablets are lightly coated with a protective coating (a "film" coating) to protect the drug. This is does not affect the absorption or dissolution of the medication. An *enteric* tablet is coated with a hard-shell coating, designed to protect the drug from acid in the stomach. The drugs contained in enteric tablets are normally best absorbed in the basic pH of the duodenum. An exception is enteric-coated aspirin, which is coated so that it will not dissolve in the stomach and subject the stomach lining to its effects. Enteric-coated tablets should not be split or crushed.

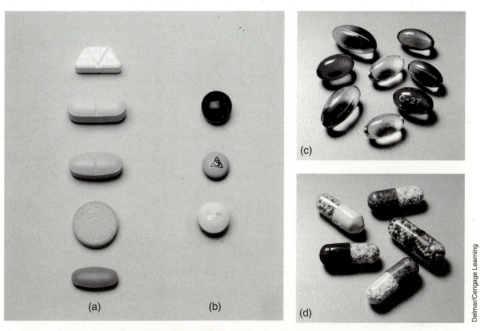

Figure 2-1: Oral Drug Forms. Tablets and capsules vary in size, shape, and color.
(a) Tablets, scored and unscored; (b) Enteric-coated tablets; (c) Gelatin capsule;
(d) Timed-release capsules

Table 2-2	Drugs Available in Lozenge Form

- morphine sulfate
- lorazepam
- haloperidol
- clotrimazole
- nystatin
- diphenhydramine
- metoclopramide
- dexamethasone
- benztropine mesylate

The Capsule

A capsule is a gelatin "container" filled with powdered drug, drug granules, a liquid drug formulation, or an oil. Examples would be antibiotics capsules, liquid vitamins (e.g., A, D, or E), and many over-the-counter cold remedies.

Other Solid Dosage Forms

Other dosage forms, which are less frequently prescribed and solid in nature, include:

- The lozenge: a hard tablet or molded shape containing drug in a sweetened, flavored base. The lozenge is designed to be held in the mouth while it slowly releases drug for oral absorption. This dosage form is particularly useful for administration of pain medication for chronic pain and for the relief of nausea during cancer chemotherapy. Drugs available in lozenge form are listed in Table 2-2.

- Drug powders for inhalation: In this dosage form, a very fine crystalline form of the drug (a microcrystalline powder) is mixed with an inert sugar (e.g., lactose) and packaged into a single-dose "blister." The blister is then inserted into a special apparatus called a "diskhaler," which pierces the blister, aerosolizes the drug, and allows the patient to inhale the medication.

Liquid Dosage Forms

> Liquid dosage forms include syrup, elixir, extract, tincture, solution, and suspension.

The liquid dosage forms for oral use include syrup, elixir, and extract.

- **Syrup** is a sweetened liquid that contains the drug, sugar, and flavoring.
- **Elixir** is similar to a syrup but contains a relatively high percentage of alcohol.
- **Extract** is the oil or active portion of a plant or herb that is usually removed, or extracted, with alcohol (e.g., an oil of peppermint or wintergreen).

Solutions and Suspensions

> Drugs in suspension need to be handled carefully, as drug particles may settle to the bottom of the container while the dose is being withdrawn!

If the drug dissolves completely into the liquid (e.g., syrup, elixir), it is called a **solution**. Another oral dosage form is the drug **suspension**, which is composed of water and drug particles that do not dissolve but remain *suspended* in the water. Suspensions need to be handled carefully, as the drug particles tend to sink to the bottom very quickly. Mixing and drawing the dose can be tricky—the withdrawal of the drug dose must be done immediately after mixing, before the drug particles have a chance to settle. If the suspension is not properly mixed or the dose is not drawn immediately, the wrong dose of drug may be dispensed. If the dose is taken from the top of the container, it may contain too much water and not enough drug. If it is taken from the bottom, the drug solution may be too concentrated because the drug particles tend to sink. In addition to mixing the suspension thoroughly, *how* the dose is withdrawn matters, as well. The dose must be drawn up quickly, as the drug particles may settle while the dose is being drawn.

Tincture

Tincture is another liquid dosage form. In modern times, it is only used topically. The tincture is an alcohol-based drug form, such as tincture of merthiolate, and is normally dispensed in a dropper bottle. These drugs are not to be taken internally.

Semisolid Dosage Forms

The *semisolid* dosage forms include creams, lotions, ointments, and suppositories.

- Creams and lotions are nothing more than emulsions (oil droplets suspended in water), where the drug is usually dissolved in the oil. Creams are thicker, as they contain less water than lotions.

- Ointments may vary from a thick emulsion to a drug suspended in a waxy base, like petrolatum (which is like petroleum jelly, only much stiffer and thicker). These preparations are usually used topically (on the skin or mucous membranes, such as those in the mouth, inside the nose, or rectum) and are normally dispensed in a tube or jar.

- Suppositories are made of wax and oils, and contain the drug that is meant to be released slowly, and in a particular place. They are normally inserted into body cavities, such as the rectum or vagina, where they adhere to the cavity wall and release medication to the immediate area. Rectal suppositories are also used to medicate patients who cannot take medication orally (e.g., a vomiting patient), as the medication, if properly prepared, can be absorbed through the rectal wall into the bloodstream. Suppositories are normally large, and, being primarily made of soft wax, will melt at body temperature. They should be stored in a cool room or refrigerated (depending on the drug), and handling should be kept to a minimum.

Storing Emulsions

Care must be taken when storing emulsions. Freezing the emulsion or exposing it to excessive heat (near a heat source, for example, or storage in a warm room for a long time) will cause the cream to separate into oil and water. Emulsions should not be stored in the refrigerator and especially should never be frozen, as the rapid change in temperature will cause the product to separate faster.

> Emulsions should never be frozen or exposed to heat!

Administering the Drug—The Route of Administration

The route of administration defines how the drug gets into the body. Drugs to be administered by different routes are prepared in different ways. The most common route of administration is by mouth (oral, or po). These drugs are given as a tablet or oral solution. Sublingual tablets (SL) are made to dissolve under the tongue; the underside of the tongue and the floor of the mouth contain large amounts of blood vessels near the surface, which allow the drug to be absorbed into the system very quickly. These tablets are very soft and dissolve easily. Sublingual preparations are also marketed in a spray formulation, which are sprayed under the tongue.

Routes of administration include the following:

- *Intranasal*: a drug in drop or spray form is used
- *Transdermal*: a drug "patch" is used, which slowly releases drug into the skin, where it is picked up by surface blood vessels and absorbed into the body
- *Inhalants*: drugs may be used in powder or liquid form, in combination with an inhalant apparatus, to be taken directly into the lungs (e.g., drugs used for asthma)
- *Administration through body cavities*: drugs may be used in cream or suppository form. They are inserted into body cavities, such as the vagina or rectum, and used for local administration (e.g., for a yeast infection or a case of hemorrhoids, respectively). Rectal administration is also very useful for administration of drugs to a patient who cannot take medications orally, as the drug is absorbed through vessels in the rectal wall.

Drugs may also be administered through the lining of the cheek. This is termed **buccal** (bYOUcahl) administration. The dosage form, in a lozenge or buccal tablet, is inserted between the cheek and the gum.

Medicating the Eye and Ear

Drugs for the eye (ophthalmics) or ear (otics) are administered by drop (gtt). The dropper or dropper container is calibrated to give a drop of the particular size needed to give an accurate dose of drug.

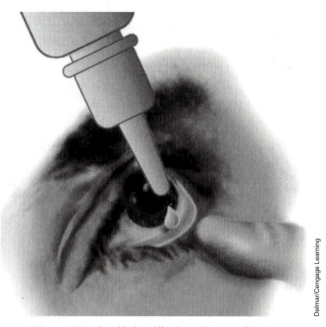

Figure 2-2: Sterile instillation of eye medication

Ophthalmic *ointments* may also be used (e.g., antibiotic ointments) and are applied to the inside of the eyelid (usually at the bottom of the eye). The tip of the ointment tube should never touch the eye.

Parenteral Drug Administration

> Intravenous injections are seen in three forms—the IV bolus, IV drip, and "piggyback" IV.

Any drug that is not given through the digestive system is given parenterally (*para* means "around" and *enteral* refers to the digestive system). In normal medical terms, however, parenteral administration refers to drugs administered by injection. The three most common types of injections are the **intravenous**, **intramuscular**, and **subcutaneous** injections. Other types of injections include the **intra-arterial**, **intracardiac**, **intrathecal**, and **intradermal** injections.

Injectable Drugs

Injections vary according to type. Intravenous injections are prepared in three ways:

- The **bolus**: a one-time single-dose injection
- The **IV drip**: a bag or bottle of liquid that allows drug to be infused over a long period of time (Figure 2-3)
- The **"piggyback" IV**: a solution contained in a smaller IV bag that is infused along with the primary intravenous drip, usually through the same tubing (Figure 2-4)

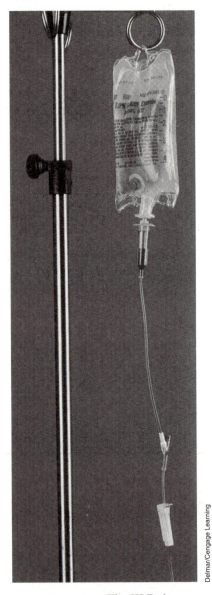

Figure 2-3: The IV Drip

Intramuscular Injections

Intramuscular injections are placed into skeletal muscle. This allows the drug to enter the bloodstream more slowly. This type of injection must first diffuse through muscle tissue before entering the bloodstream, so it requires a large-bore needle in order to penetrate the muscle.

The advantage to this type of injection is that the slow release of drug into the system minimizes shock to the system, allowing it to gradually acclimate to the effects of the drug.

> When preparing an intramuscular injection, a large-bore needle should be attached, as a small needle will not easily penetrate muscle tissue.

Subcutaneous and Intradermal Injections

Injections into or under the skin include subcutaneous and intradermal injections. Subcutaneous injections are placed under the skin, which allows for a slow

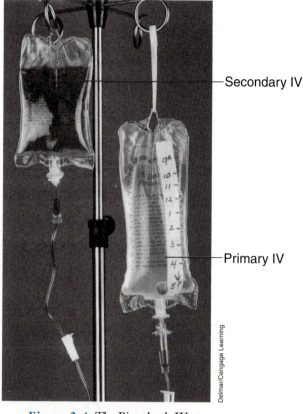

Delmar/Cengage Learning

Figure 2-4: The Piggyback IV

> Intramuscular and subcutaneous injections provide for a slow rate of delivery of drug to the system.

absorption of drug into the bloodstream. Intradermal (ID) injections, which are less common, are placed within the skin layers. Both of these types of injections must be dispensed with a very fine needle (25–31 gauge) on the syringe.

Specialized Injections

Intra-arterial Injections. Occasionally, drugs need to be administered directly into an artery, in order to have the best effect. These are called *intra-arterial* injections. Arteries are very muscular and the blood within them is under very high pressure, so these injections require a somewhat larger bore needle.

Intrathecal and Intracardiac Injections. Intrathecal and intracardiac injections are specialized injection forms. Intrathecal injections are placed into the space between the spinal cord and spinal meninges (e.g., an epidural anesthetic during childbirth), and intracardiac injections are placed directly into the heart. These types of injections allow fast action of a drug by placing the drug at the site of the organ itself.

Interpreting the Prescription Order

Before filling the prescription order, you must first check the prescription form to make sure that the order is genuine, legal, and complete. Certain information must be on the prescription form when it is received, and other information may be filled in by the technician, unless the prescription is for a controlled substance. In this case, no information is to be added, deleted, or corrected on the prescription form.

Table 2-1 lists abbreviations commonly used on the prescription form by the prescriber. These abbreviations must be interpreted accurately to ensure that the correct medication is dispensed and that accurate instructions are provided to the patient for the use of the medication. Additional abbreviations may be found in Appendix A. You may be asked about any of these, even abbreviations seldom used, on the exam, so it is wise to be familiar with them.

Figure 2-5 represents the prescription form that would be received at the pharmacy window. Information required to correctly fill this order is found in the body of the prescription. Review the information required to appear on the prescription:

- *The drug name*: This can be generic (the actual name of the drug) or a brand (proprietary) name. This prescription specifies the exact drug to select for dispensing. This prescription was written for a brand name, Lasix, although the prescriber did sign on the "May Substitute" line, so generic substitution is permissible.

Drugs are dispensed in different dosage forms for different needs.

- *The strength and dosage form of the drug*: Drugs come in different strengths and forms for different needs. The strength and form must be specified, unless the drug comes in only one form or strength. For example, some combination drugs such as trimethoprim with sulfamethoxazole combination or acetaminophen with codeine (Tylenol #3, etc.) are dispensed in a specific dosage and proportion. Mannitol is dispensed only in a solution for injection. The proportions and forms of these drugs do not need to be specified on the prescription form. In contrast, Lasix tablets come in 20 mg, 40 mg, and 80 mg strengths, as well as in oral solution and solution for injection. The dosage strength

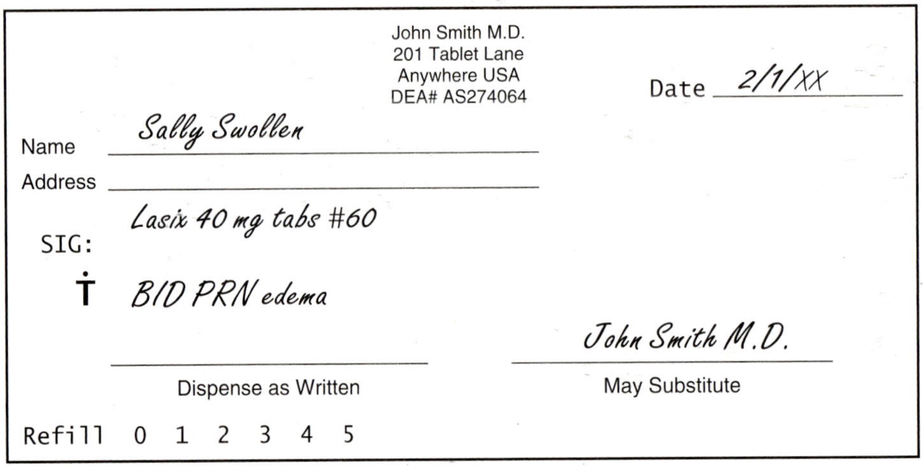
John Smith M.D.
201 Tablet Lane
Anywhere USA
DEA# AS274064

Date 2/1/XX

Name Sally Swollen

Address

Lasix 40 mg tabs #60

SIG:

ṫ BID PRN edema

John Smith M.D.

Dispense as Written | May Substitute

Refill 0 1 2 3 4 5

Delmar/Cengage Learning

Figure 2-5: Sample Completed Prescription Form

and form *did* need to be specified in the sample prescription shown in Figure 2-5.

- *The amount of drug prescribed*: A prescription for tablets, such as that in Figure 2-1, must specify the *number* of tablets to be dispensed. For other dosage forms, however, this may not be the case. For example, a prescription for a liquid dosage form may be specified in more than one way. Either the volume may be specified, or the drug dose may be specified in mg, g, and so on.

> A drug dose may be specified by volume or by equivalent weight of drug.

EXAMPLE

The prescription order is for 500 mL of 10% calcium gluconate solution. Since the volume was given, the specified amount of solution (500 mL) would be dispensed.

EXAMPLE

The prescription order is for 200 mg of Minocin IV. Minocin comes in a sterile solution of 20 mg/mL. In this case, the volume of solution to be dispensed for a 200 mg dose would have to be calculated (e.g., 200 mg divided by 20 mg = 10 mL).

- *Instructions for the patient (the SIG)*: This is where knowledge of the abbreviations in Table 2-1 comes in. Since the instructions must be written out for the patient, the technician must be able to accurately read the SIG. The prescription in Figure 2-5 states that one tablet (designated by a horizontal bar with one vertical bar and one dot) is to be taken twice a day (bid, or *bis in deum*), as needed (prn) for edema. The amount of medication to be taken, and limitations on when or how often it is to be taken, must be included on the prescription form.

> The half-life of a drug is the amount of time taken for half of the serum concentration of drug to be eliminated from the body. It is used to establish accurate dosage intervals.

The spacing of the doses, or dosage interval, is extremely important, as the space between doses is based on the half-life ($T_{1/2}$) of the drug. The $T_{1/2}$ is a measure of how rapidly a drug is cleared from the body, and gives an estimate of how quickly the effects of the drug will be terminated. (There are many ways in which the actions of a drug may be terminated, but the half-life is generally considered to be the main index of the length of a drug's effects.)

The half-life can be used to predict the dosage interval for a drug. To keep the serum levels of a drug relatively constant, the drug should be replaced as it is cleared from the body. Thus, dosage intervals are very important, and the instructions for taking the drug *must* be communicated effectively to the patient. It is also important to communicate to the patient the *proper use* of the drug (e.g., proper insertion of a suppository, instillation of an ophthalmic preparation, etc.).

> **EXAMPLE**
>
> The time it takes a drug to be eliminated from the body is around 5–7 half-lifes. If a drug has a 6-hour half-life, then it would take 30–42 hours to be eliminated. (6 hrs $\times$ 5 = 30; 6 hrs $\times$ 7 = 42.)

- *Signature of the prescriber and authorization to substitute*: The signature must be handwritten *in ink*. The authorization to dispense a generic drug may be indicated in a box on the prescription form, in which the letters "DAW" ("dispense as written") are written (indicating that the exact proprietary label must be dispensed) or absent (indicating that a substitution is permissible). Depending on the state, the prescription form may contain this box or may have a duplicate set of signature lines bearing a designation such as "may substitute" or "no substitution permissible." If the prescriber designates "no substitution permissible," the drug must be dispensed *exactly* as written, in the correct form, strength, and under the specified proprietary label.

> The "may substitute" option gives the patient and pharmacy the option to choose a less expensive generic brand or another proprietary label, as long as the drug, strength, and form remain the same.

Information is normally entered on the prescription form by the technician and then transferred to the patient profile. Information to be gathered includes the following:

- *The patient's address and telephone number*: This information identifies the patient (there may be more than one patient with the same name). It also provides a means of contact with the patient, in case of a problem with a prescription or drug recall.

- *The age or date of birth of the patient*: This information is very important, as it serves to identify the patient (e.g., to distinguish between a father and son with the same name) and assures that the drug dosage prescribed is appropriate for the age of the patient (drug dosage may be reduced in a child or elderly person, for example, as organ functions are less efficient).

- *Drug allergies*: Many drugs are very similar in chemical structure and action. Thus, if a patient is allergic to one drug (e.g., penicillin), he or she may well be allergic to similar drugs, such as amoxicillin or even cephalexin. A history of drug allergies is critical to the care of the patient, as it may help prevent an uncomfortable or even fatal allergic reaction.

> Many drugs interact with each other to produce adverse effects. A particular drug may also greatly increase the therapeutic effects of another drug, which would require an adjustment to the patient's dosage.

- *Concurrent medications*: These are medications already being taken by the patient. A history of concurrent medications should include not only other prescription medications but also those purchased over the counter (e.g., cold remedies), and herbal remedies as well. (The first drugs were little more than pulverized plants, or plant extracts, after all. We have done little more than refine them, in many cases.) *Herbal preparations* can have very potent *drug actions* and interactions and *must be recorded in the patient profile*.

Dispensing the Correct Medication

Once the drug, dosage form, and strength have been established, the correct medication is selected. This medication should be *exactly* what appears on the prescription form.

Verifying the Medication—Use of the Manufacturer's Label

Many drug names look alike and sound alike, so the manufacturer labels must be compared carefully to the prescription order.

> **EXAMPLE**
>
> Extra letters may be present in the drug name on the label (e.g., Adalat CC instead of Adalat). This may mean the drug is a different formulation of the brand-name drug (in this case an extended-release form) or may be a different drug altogether (e.g., quinine and quinidine). Some of those abbreviations can be found in Table 2-3. If the name of the drug does not match exactly, the drug should not be dispensed.

Verifying the Proper Dosage Strength

The choice of dosage strength is less critical than other information. If the dosage strength does not match, it may be possible to convert dosages (see Chapters 4 and 14). If the dosage *form* is incorrect, however, the drug cannot be dispensed by the technician without consulting the pharmacist.

> **EXAMPLE**
>
> The drug order is for 250 mg amoxicillin tablets. There are no tablets in stock, but the pharmacy does have amoxicillin suspension in stock for oral administration. Both dosage forms are for oral administration, so the suspension could be substituted, with proper calculations and patient instruction (this would require the approval of the pharmacist).

Table 2-3	Extended-release Formulations
LA	long acting
SA	sustained acting
SR	sustained release
TR	timed release
ER	extended release

> **EXAMPLE**
>
> The drug order is for Compazine suppositories. You have Compazine solution for oral administration in stock, but no suppositories. The order cannot be filled, as the dosage forms do not match (suppositories are normally prescribed for patients who cannot take medications orally).

Automated Unit Dose Delivery Systems

There are several automated dispensing systems presently marketed for institutional use. One popular and innovative automated unit dose delivery system coming into widespread use in institutional pharmacy is the Pyxis R$_x$ System. The Pyxis system is essentially a computerized cabinet that is located on a hospital floor (unit). The cabinet is stocked with drugs, which are appropriate to the particular hospital unit where it is located. Like the med cart, drugs are filed in locked drawers within the cabinet, and the units are maintained and stocked by pharmacy personnel. The computer within the Pyxis unit is on a local area network, which interfaces with the main hospital computer. Thus, the unit actually charts patient medications as they are withdrawn from the cart by hospital personnel.

Processing of Medication Orders Using the Pyxis System

The Pyxis system streamlines the dispensing of medication. Medication orders are received as usual from physicians in the pharmacy. The pharmacy technician then enters the orders into the main hospital computer system. The orders are then checked by the pharmacist to ensure that the medications and doses are appropriate for the age, weight, and diagnosis of the patient, and that therapeutic duplications and drug-drug interactions are not present. The order is then sent to the Pyxis system. Once the order has been verified and is present in the system, the floor nurse can enter appropriate information into the system when it is time for a patient's medication. The system then allows the withdrawal of the proper unit doses of medication for administration to the patient. Identification of the nurse, by thumbprint or code, must be received by the unit for the medication drawers to unlock and the medication to be withdrawn.

Advantages to the Use of Automated Unit Dosing Systems

The advantages to this system are many: Medication errors are reduced, as the medication dispensed comes directly from the *original* medication order (i.e., not faxed, transcribed, or photocopied); drug-drug interactions are reduced; and patients receive their medications in a more timely manner, allowing more effective dosing. In addition, input from the pharmacist is almost instantaneous. Blood analysis of drug levels can also be included in the computerized information, allowing dosages to be adjusted almost instantaneously. This provides better control over patient medication. Also, as patients are transferred from room to room and floor to floor, their information remains centralized with less chance of record loss. Documentation of drug dispensing and administration is generated automatically with the system, and can be printed out at any time, should a hard copy be needed.

Comparison of Drug Dispensing in Retail and Institutional Settings

Dispensing a prescription in an institutional setting is similar to the retail setting, with a few exceptions. Several drugs are usually prescribed at once (see Chapter 1) using the hospital order; these doses may be sent up to the patient individually (e.g., a medication needed quickly, for an emergency [STAT], or a medication prescribed for pain, emesis, etc., which is not part of the usual routine of drugs), or placed into a **unit dose cart**. Unit dose carts contain the daily medications of the patients on a particular hospital floor. They are prepared daily by technicians and then checked by pharmacists. These computerized carts contain the individual medications of patients on the floor, normally enough to last for one day. The carts are filled daily, from the physician's orders for the various patients on the floor, making it easier for nurses to properly administer medications to patients. Narcotics prescribed "as needed" may not be dispensed in a unit dose cart.

Chapter Review Questions

1. You receive a shipment of lotion that appears to have separated into two layers, within the bottle. The shipment has probably:
   a. always been this way
   b. been exposed to extreme heat
   c. been frozen and allowed to thaw out, perhaps more than once
   d. either b or c could be correct

2. A prescription for a Timoptic reads "1 gtt ou bid." The instructions would be:
   a. take one drop twice a day
   b. take 1 mL twice a day
   c. insert one drop in each ear twice a day
   d. place one drop in each eye twice a day

3. Which of the following is not a solid dosage form?
   a. an indomethacin capsule
   b. a Ceclor pulvule
   c. an antibiotic cream
   d. a Ticlid tablet

4. In an institutional setting, medications are normally filled:
   a. using a unit dose cart, filled daily
   b. by individual dose, as needed
   c. in bulk, so that the nurses can help themselves
   d. by prescription

5. You receive a prescription for Procardia, ordered "Dispense as Written." You check the stock and find Procardia XL. You:
   a. fill the prescription with the available stock
   b. fill the prescription, but adjust the dosage according to the label on the bottle
   c. tell the patient that the prescription cannot be filled
   d. fill the prescription with Adalat, as it is the same thing

6. An enteric-coated tablet protects the drug from:
   a. the basic pH of the duodenum
   b. the acid in the stomach
   c. the lining of the colon
   d. none of the above

7. Elixirs generally contain:
   a. high sugar content
   b. oils or active plant portions
   c. high percentage of alcohol
   d. suspended drug particles

8. SQ injections must be given:
   a. with a very fine needle
   b. with a very large needle
   c. deep into a muscle
   d. through an IV line

9. Drug half-life is used to determine:
   a. how often a drug is given
   b. when a drug expires
   c. when refills are needed
   d. if an allergy is present

10. Dispense as written (DAW) means:
    a. you can dispense whatever is available
    b. you must dispense the brand requested
    c. you only have to use that brand if you stock it
    d. none of the above

CHAPTER 3

Preparation and Utilization of the Patient Profile

Quick Study

I. The patient profile

The patient profile serves to
- Identify the patient
- Maintain a record of medications dispensed to the patient
- Protect the patient against drugs or procedures that could potentially be harmful

A. Information contained in the outpatient profile
- Identifying information: name, date of birth, and contact information
- A record of medications dispensed to the patient: This helps to identify potential drug interactions as new prescriptions are added.
- Drug allergies and adverse reactions: This helps to protect the patient against misprescribed drugs.
- Concurrent medications: This helps to prevent drug interactions and therapeutic duplication.
- Medical history: This helps to prevent a potentially lethal aggravation of existing conditions by prescribed drugs.
- Mental conditions or physical handicaps: This helps to predict the degree of supervision needed with the drug therapy. Physical handicaps such as arthritis may dictate the need for a special cap on the dispensing bottle, or poor eyesight may require large-print labeling, and so forth.
- Insurance information

B. Information contained in the institutional patient profile
  - Height, weight, diagnosis, therapies, laboratory tests, and results: Height and weight may be required to calculate accurate drug dosage. Also, hospital patients may need to be weighed to determine correct drug dosage or weight lost or gained. Diagnosis, concurrent therapies, and test results may help the pharmacist check for accurate therapeutic prescribing.

II. Comparison of the patient profile in the institutional and retail settings

  - More details are included on the order within the institutional setting: goals of therapy, special diet, diagnosis, tests, billing information, billing number, etc.
  - Differences in the type of information included: Refill information and concurrent medications are not applicable to the institutional profile.

The Patient Profile

The **patient profile** has several functions. It serves as a means of distinguishing and identifying patients, serves as a legal record of medications dispensed, and, most importantly, serves as a resource of information that could protect the patient against potentially harmful drugs or procedures. The profiles in an outpatient and institutional setting contain similar information; however, the information contained in a patient profile within an institutional setting (e.g., hospital or nursing home) tends to be more detailed.

The Outpatient Profile

The following are included in an outpatient profile (Figure 3-1):

  - *Identifying information*: This includes the patient's name, address, telephone number, and date of birth.
  - *Drug allergies and adverse reactions* (negative effects caused by a drug): Many times, when a patient is allergic or sensitive to one type of drug, the allergy will extend to similar drugs as well. Rarely, food allergies will cause problems in the tolerance of a drug (e.g., porcine or bovine insulin) or drug "carrier" (a substance that the drug is put into in order to give it enough volume to swallow or inject). For example, dextrose would not be used for a diabetic patient.
  - *Concurrent medications* (use of more than one medication at the same time): Many drugs interact with each other. They may produce similar therapeutic (or toxic) effects that will be additive with each other or may amplify each other's effects (synergism). They might also *reduce* the effectiveness of each other (**antagonism**). Depending on the drugs, concurrent therapy may also alter blood levels of other drugs, requiring

Patient: John Q. Public

Gender: Male

Date of Birth: 11/28/1936

Address: 2218 E. Hagman Way, Tucson AZ, 85710

Telephone: (520) 721-0000

Concurrent Medications and Drug Allergies

Allergies: codeine, sulfa, penicillin

Concurrent: aspirin (PRN), pseudoephedrine (PRN), carbamazepine (200 mg QID)

Medical History: Mitral valve replacement 1995, family history of diabetes.

Insurance: Self-pay

Rx #	Date	Drug Dispensed	Strength	Dosage	Refills	Prescriber	init
1234567	11/2/XX	Lasix	80 mg tab #30	i BID	5	J. Morrow	SBA
1258999	11/15/XX	Ambien	2 mg tab #20	i h.s.	3	S. Norman	BGT
1260001	12/15/XX	Ceclor	250 mg cap #30	i TID	0	J. Morrow	SBA

Delmar/Cengage Learning

Figure 3-1: Patient Profile

a change in the dosage of the drug(s). An accurate listing of concurrent medications is very important. Because many drugs sold over-the-counter are the same (or very similar) to those sold by prescription, *all medications taken, including herbal preparations, must be recorded.*

Another reason that we need to determine concurrent patient medication is to see if any of the drugs prescribed are the same (**drug duplication**) or have the same therapeutic function (**therapeutic duplication**). This applies to the over-the-counter medications as well, which may contain a lower dosage of a prescription drug.

For example, the patient is prescribed a drug by one prescriber, and also receives a prescription for a combination drug from a second prescriber that contains the same drug (or is the same drug under a different brand name).

- *Medical history*: This includes any medical conditions that the patient may have and may also include those of the patient's immediate family. (Certain medical conditions will be aggravated by some drugs, which should be avoided.) If the patient's family members have inherited

If two prescriptions contain the same drugs, an evaluation of the prescriptions must be made by the pharmacist to ensure safety. This also applies to concurrent use of over-the-counter and herbal drugs.

> **EXAMPLE**
>
> A patient is prescribed Vicodin and Tylenol. Both medications contain acetaminophen. This is a drug duplication.

> **EXAMPLE**
>
> A patient comes to the pharmacy window with a prescription for Pen-V-K, an oral antibiotic. You check the patient's profile and see that he has already been prescribed Ceclor, another oral antibiotic, for an ear infection. You should alert the pharmacist, as this is a therapeutic duplication.

> Certain medical conditions will be adversely affected by some drugs. These must be avoided!

medical conditions that have not yet developed in the patient, it is reasonable to assume that these conditions could develop at any time; therefore, the possibility exists that certain drugs or procedures could be harmful, even though the condition has not yet developed.

- *A history of drug abuse*: This may indicate that the patient is not competent to use the medication properly. In an outpatient setting, this may mean that the patient must be supervised more closely and that the amount of medication given out at one time may be more strictly regulated.

> A history of drug abuse may indicate that the patient may not use the medication properly and must be supervised.

- *Special considerations*: Any physical, mental, or cultural handicaps should be addressed. For example, a patient with limited vision may need large-print labels on the dispensing container; another patient with a hearing deficit may need special attention during drug counseling by the pharmacist. A person with arthritis may need to have easy-open caps on dispensing bottles. Also, patients from other cultures may need special consideration due to language or to cultural and religious beliefs.

> Insurance eligibility and type of coverage must be verified at the time of dispensing!

- *Insurance information*: This includes determination of insurance eligibility, the type of third-party payment (co-pay or self-pay, etc.), and the coverage of prescribed drugs. This coverage varies widely among the various insurance plans. Many plans will no longer pay for certain drugs, due to price. Some will authorize only payment for generic drugs, and others will authorize payment for proprietary label drugs only under certain circumstances (i.e., if no other drug is available or the drug is needed for a life-threatening condition).

- *Current prescriptions and refill information*: The outpatient profile will show the status of the patient's various prescriptions, so that the amount dispensed and the amount available on the prescription remain current. This information needs to be updated with each prescription refill.

The Institutional Patient Profile

Patients who are new to the pharmacy must be interviewed to obtain information and create the patient profile. The profile should be updated with each prescription refill.

The institutional patient profile may also include the patient's height, weight, diagnosis, treatment, therapy, diet plans, blood tests, and lab results, as well as the name of the primary physician. However, the institutional profile would *not* include information that is not applicable to institutional policy, such as refill information and concurrent medications other than those prescribed within the institution.

The technician creates a computerized profile for every patient receiving medications from the pharmacy. Normally the format for the profile is contained in the pharmacy computer program, and the information is entered into the program. Patients who are new to the pharmacy must be asked to obtain the information that is necessary for creation of the profile.

The institutional patient profile may include extra information such as height, weight, and laboratory tests. Information on drug refills and concurrent medications are unnecessary to institutional policy and thus are not present.

The profiles of patients with existing profiles (repeat patients) need to be updated with each visit. If any information has changed, such as allergies, concurrent medications, insurance information, or address and telephone number, for example, this information needs to be changed in the profile to reflect the correct information. This may require an additional patient questionnaire if the changes are lengthy; each time the patient comes to the pharmacy, he or she should be asked if the personal information is current and if he or she is taking any new drugs or has experienced any problems with the medication. In addition, the pharmacist may require that the patient be asked about changes in his or her medical condition. The reason for updating the patient profile is to make sure the pharmacist has the most recent information to take into consideration when counseling the patient, so that appropriate advice will be given.

Release of Patient Information

The patient profile must be kept current to ensure that the pharmacist has the most current information to consider when counseling the patient.

In accordance with recent HIPAA revisions, information contained in the patient profile is not to be released, with the exception of nonidentifiable information and information communicated within the various departments of an institution or appropriate business affiliates. In addition, the new regulations mandate that the patient is allowed to request a copy of his or her patient profile. The pharmacy is allowed to charge a fee for this service. (See Chapter 32.)

Comparison of Patient Profiles in Institutional and Retail Settings

Similar Features between Profiles

In general, the profiles in the institutional setting are more detailed than those in the retail or outpatient setting. Factors common to profiles in both settings include:

- information used to locate and identify the patient (e.g., address and phone number in the outpatient setting, and room and bed number in the institutional setting)
- insurance information
- date of birth
- medications prescribed

Profiles in both settings also include the prescriber's name and the date that the medication was prescribed and dispensed.

The Institutional Profile

In the institutional setting, the profile also includes the date and time of day that the medication was dispensed and administered, billing information, and more detailed information such as diagnosis, therapeutic goals, and diagnostic tests.

Major Differences between Profiles in Retail Settings

Some major differences between the profiles in the retail and institutional settings include the following:

- Institutional (hospital) profiles may include diagnosis, a statement of the goals of the therapy, special diet (if any), medical tests that the patient has undergone, and the results of those tests. Since the profile may serve as a document for billing the patient, billing information may also be included. Also included is the hospital billing number assigned to the patient, which gives the billing department access to all insurance information. Retail pharmacy profiles do not contain this information.

- The retail profile does contain a *list of concurrent medications,* since the patient may be taking many drugs concurrently. This is not the case in the hospital profile, as drugs of any kind are discouraged, other than those dispensed by the hospital pharmacy.

- *Refill information* is included in an outpatient (retail pharmacy) profile but would not be appropriate in a hospital or institutional profile.

Chapter Review Questions

1. The following would be found on a patient profile, under "concurrent medications":
   a. prescription drugs
   b. nonprescription drugs, such as Tylenol and aspirin
   c. herbal medications, such as herbal diuretics and goldenseal
   d. all of the above

2. A patient profile would be created for:
   a. a hospital inpatient
   b. a new patient to a pharmacy
   c. a regular pharmacy customer
   d. anyone who receives prescription medications from any pharmacy

3. A former patient comes to the pharmacy with a prescription. His address has changed. You should:
   a. take the new information and update his patient profile
   b. advise the pharmacist
   c. put him in as a new patient and create a new profile
   d. ignore the information, as the address is not important

4. The patient in question 3 comes back with a new prescription and has a rash from the prescription that he had filled a few days ago. You should:
   a. note the rash in the "allergies" section of his patient profile
   b. alert the pharmacist
   c. fill the new prescription
   d. both a and b

5. The following would be found on a patient profile in the retail setting but not the hospital setting:
   a. patient identification
   b. diagnosis and lab test results
   c. concurrent medications
   d. drug allergies

6. An example of medication duplication would be:
   a. a prescription for trimethoprim and another for sulfisoxazole
   b. a prescription for Tylenol #3, when the patient is taking acetaminophen capsules
   c. a prescription for generic digoxin and for Digibind
   d. a prescription for an antihistamine given to a patient taking aspirin

7. Identifying information includes:
   a. hair and eye color of the patient
   b. weight and height of the patient
   c. name and address of the patient
   d. name of both parents

8. Insurance information should include:
   a. co-pay or self-pay information
   b. patient monthly premium payments
   c. dietary considerations
   d. none of the above

9. Retail profiles include:
   a. lab tests and diagnosis
   b. blood tests and diagnosis
   c. treatment and physical therapy
   d. date of birth and telephone number

10. The use of multiple medications at one time is called:
    a. concomitant medications
    b. concurrent medications
    c. effective therapy
    d. polypharmaceutical therapy

CHAPTER 4

Handling Medications

Quick Study

I.   Obtaining the correct medication from inventory

    A.   Interpretation of the manufacturer's label
    B.   Dosage conversions

II.   Choosing the proper container

- Containers vary according to the intended use of the drug (for example, a cream or ointment is placed in a tube, a liquid is placed in a small-necked bottle, a solid dosage form is placed into a large-mouthed plastic container).
- Containers must be sized appropriately for the amount of drug dispensed.
- Containers must be appropriate to the product being dispensed (e.g., a drug that is light-sensitive should be packaged in an amber container).

III.   Properly labeling the container. The label should contain the following:

- The name, address, and phone number of the pharmacy
- The name of the patient to whom the drug is prescribed
- The name of the prescriber
- The date of dispensing
- The name of the drug
- The strength of the drug
- The quantity dispensed
- Dosage instructions
- Refill information

IV. Dispensing liquid medications

A. Measuring liquids for oral dosage: Liquids are usually dispensed into a bottle with markings on the side to determine the volume of drug left in the container as well as determining the approximate amount dispensed. These markings are *not* to be used for patient medication administration (e.g., accurate measurement of the drug).

B. Compounding: the preparation of a solution or medication from a standardized written procedure

C. Proper preparation of parenteral drugs. A laminar flow hood should be used when preparing parenteral products to ensure sterility.
- Intramuscular injections slowly release the drug from the muscle into the blood.
- Subcutaneous injections release a small volume of drug through an injection just under the skin; the drug is slowly absorbed into the bloodstream.
- Intravenous injections allow large volumes of dilute solutions of drugs to be released directly into the bloodstream.
- IV bolus allows a single dose of a drug.
- Intravenous admixtures are medications mixed into a large-volume IV for slow release in the blood.

V. Labeling intravenous solutions: The label should be placed near the top of the IV bag so that any contaminants that may have settled to the bottom are clearly visible.

VI. Working with hazardous drugs: Some drugs may put the handler at risk. Proper personal protective equipment should be worn, which may include the following:

- Clothing that covers the body
- Lab coat
- Goggles with splash guards, if necessary
- Hat, mask, gloves, and shoe covers, if necessary
- *Never* touch the face, mouth, or eyes with your hands when handling drugs

Obtaining the Correct Medication from Inventory

Interpretation of the Manufacturer's Label

After the prescription form has been received and processed, the next step is to obtain the correct medication from inventory. When selecting the medication, you must look closely at the manufacturer's label. Is the name of the drug, the strength, the form, and the manufacturer of the drug exactly the same as what was ordered? All of the information on the drug label must match the order, with the exception of the dosage strength. If the dosage strength is not appropriate for the order, calculations may be done to determine if the dosage strength can be converted to what is needed. Let's say that the order asks for a dose of 100 mg po, and the tablets in stock are 200 mg. If the tablets are scored (a groove runs across the tablet) so that we can accurately break them in half, we can put instructions on the label for the patient to take one-half tablet per dose (100 mg). This is called **dosage conversion** and is perfectly acceptable as long as the calculated dose is accurate.

Figure 4-1 shows a label for Vistaril, a solution for intramuscular injection. The following information should appear on a drug label:

1. The **NDC number**: This number contains codes that denote the generic name of the drug, manufacturer, proprietary label, dosage form, strength, and type of packaging.

2. The amount of drug in each tablet or unit of volume (drug solution or suspension): For a drug in solution or suspension, the concentration is either given in mg or mg/mL or may be easily calculated.

3. The proprietary name and generic name: The generic name always appears on the label, either alone (generic label) or beneath the trade name (proprietary label).

4. The dosage form (e.g., tablet, capsule, suspension, solution)

5. The drug manufacturer

6. The Federal Legend or R_x

Additionally, the manufacturer's label may contain information regarding recommended dosages and safe dosages, instructions on preparation for administration (e.g., rehydration, dilution), and optimum storage conditions. A lot or control number corresponding to the drug manufacturer should be present, as well as the expiration date for the drug. A code designating the drug, manufacturer, and dosage form (the NDC number) should also appear, usually at the top of the label.

> All information on the manufacturer's label must match that of the order, with the exception of the dosage strength. This may be converted to match the order, using a dosage conversion calculation.

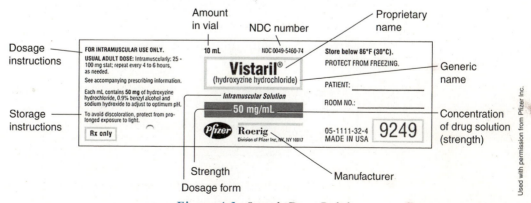

Figure 4-1: *Sample Drug Label*

The National Drug Code (NDC) Number

The NDC number is an 11-digit number, containing three distinct segments (separated by hyphens). The use of NDC numbers allows for rapid and accurate entry of product and labeler information, for use in the national drug quality surveillance program.

Segment 1—The Manufacturer's Identification Code

The first segment identifies the manufacturer or repackager of the drug. All manufacturers and repackaging agencies are required to register with the FDA and receive a unique identifier number, which must be present on the labels of their products. This first segment is five digits long.

Segments 2 and 3—Drug Product Identification and Manufacturer's Packaging

Each drug company is allowed to establish its own codes for the identification of its particular drugs, and the various types of packaging in which they are sold (e.g., dose packs, 500 count bottle, etc.). These codes are registered with the DEA, and make up the second and third segments of the NDC number. The second segment identifies the drug product and is four digits long. The third segment of numbers identifies the packaging of the product. This segment is two digits long.

The NDC number will always be 11 digits long. Its format looks like this:

$$12345\text{-}6789\text{-}01$$

Sometimes an NDC number may appear to be missing numbers. The manufacturer may only print four digits in the first segment or three digits in the second segment. This NDC number still has 11 digits; they have just excluded the leading zeros on the packaging.

EXAMPLE

A drug has the NDC number 04321-0876-02. The manufacturer has the option of printing it as follows:

04321-0876-02

4321-0876-02

04321-876-02

4321-876-02

All are correct and all represent the manufacturer, drug, and packaging filed with the FDA and DEA.

Measuring the Drug for Dispensing

Once the amount of drug to be dispensed has been calculated, the drug is measured for dispensing. An order for almost any amount of drug can be filled, as long as the amount dispensed is accurate and appropriate to the route of administration. Solid dosage forms are easily dispensed accurately. We simply count out the tablets or capsules, using a tablet counter, in a sanitary, accurate manner. Liquids, however, must be measured out using properly calibrated equipment and correct procedures.

Conversion of Solid Dosage Forms

The solid dosage form that can be most accurately converted is the tablet. A capsule or pulvule cannot be accurately divided, so an order for these dosage forms must be filled as written. In other words, if the order is for 250 mg capsules of Cefaclor, and you have 500 mg capsules in stock, the 500 mg capsules cannot accurately be divided, so the order cannot be filled.

Tablets may be accurately divided, but only if they are **scored** tablets (i.e., they have a groove dividing the tablet into halves or fourths). These may be broken at the groove, using a **tablet splitter**, or even by hand.

> **EXAMPLE**
>
> Your order is for 50 mg of phenobarbital, taken orally. You have 100 mg tablets in stock, which are scored in halves. You can fill the order by breaking the tablets at the groove. It is best to break them for the patient to ensure accurate dosing. Otherwise, sending them with a tablet splitter is the next best option.

> **EXAMPLE**
>
> Your order is for 30 mg of phenobarbital, taken orally. Since the 100 mg tablets that you have in stock are scored in halves, and not thirds, you cannot accurately determine what portion of the tablet is 30 mg, and you cannot fill the order. An option would be to use a liquid dosage form but would require a phone call to the physician by the pharmacist.

Dispensing Liquid Dosage Forms

Unlike solid dosage forms, liquid dosage forms must be accurately measured in an appropriately calibrated measuring device. The concentration of drug in the solution or suspension may be found on the manufacturer's label. This concentration is used to determine the proper amount of solution or suspension to dispense for the order. An order of almost any amount can be filled *as long as the amount dispensed is appropriate.*

> ### EXAMPLE
>
> Your order is for 40 mEq of potassium to be administered orally. Your available stock of potassium is a solution of 20 mEq/mL. Upon calculation, you find that the required amount to be drawn up for the order would be 2 mL, which is an appropriate amount to be added to a cup of juice for administration.

> ### EXAMPLE
>
> Your order is for 250,000 units of penicillin to be administered intramuscularly. Your available stock of penicillin is a solution of 25,000 units/mL. Upon calculation, you find that the required amount to be drawn up for the order would be 10 mL, which is too large an amount to be administered as an IM injection. The order cannot be filled with the available stock.

Packaging of Liquid Medications

> An institutional pharmacy might dispense liquids for either oral, topical, or parenteral use, whereas a retail pharmacy would dispense mainly oral and topical formulations.

Drugs in liquid form are usually dispensed in containers specific for the intended use. For example, ophthalmic drugs intended for use in the eye or preparations for use in the ear may be prepackaged in a sterile bottle with a dropper tip. For topical use, solutions may be packaged in a dropper bottle (with a dropper in the cap). The majority of liquids, however, are dispensed for either oral use (by mouth) or parenteral use (by injection). An institutional pharmacy would dispense liquids for either oral, topical, or parenteral use, while a retail pharmacy would dispense mainly solutions for oral or topical dosage.

Measuring Liquids for Oral Dosage

> The markings on a liquid dispensing bottle are not to be used for accurate measurement! They are a guide for the patient to determine approximate volume.

Liquids for oral dosage are normally dispensed in plastic dispensing bottles that have markings on the side for milliliters, drams, ounces, or all three. (For a review of dispensing units, see Chapter 10.) *The markings on a dispensing bottle or dosage cup are not accurate for measurement!* They are a guide for the patient to determine approximately how much is left in the bottle. Never measure a solution or suspension by these markings. Solutions and suspensions must be measured at room temperature, using accurate devices—like graduated cylinders (see Chapter 10).

Parenteral drugs are rarely dispensed from a retail pharmacy; however, it is wise to be familiar with them, as questions on parenteral drug dispensing and related calculations will appear on the exam.

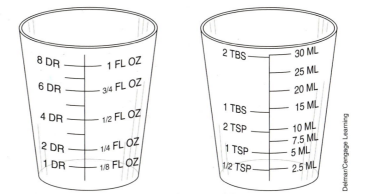

Determining the Amount of Drug to Dispense

Orders for solid dosage forms are usually straightforward; each tablet or capsule contains a specified amount of drug. Dispensing liquid formulations may be a bit more complicated. Orders for liquid formulations are normally given in milligrams, just as those for solid dosage forms are. To accurately dispense the amount ordered, the concentration of the drug solution must be known. This is normally stated on the manufacturer's label. If it is not, it may be calculated from the information that *is* given on the label.

EXAMPLE

Say that you need to draw up a 15 mg dose of methotrexate. The manufacturer's label does not list the concentration of the solution. You, as an astute pharmacy technician, notice that the total amount of drug in the bottle is listed as 250 mg, and the label states that the total volume is 10 mL. A simple division is all that is necessary to obtain the concentration: 250 mg divided by 10 mL = 25 mg/mL.

Choosing the Proper Container for Dispensing

The type of dispensing container varies according to the form and intended use of the drug. Liquid dosage forms for oral administration are placed into bottles suitable for pouring, and creams into jars or tubes, for example.

Once the drug has been accurately measured, it should be placed into an appropriate container and labeled. The type of container used varies according to the intended use of the drug:

- a topical solution may be placed into a bottle with a dropper cap
- a cream or ointment is placed in an ointment tube or jar
- a liquid for oral dosing should be placed into an appropriate bottle, usually with a small neck that is suitable for slow pouring
- solid dosage forms (e.g., tablets) are placed into a large-mouthed dispensing container

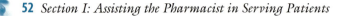

Choosing the Size of Dispensing Container

> The size of the dispensing container should be appropriate to the amount of drug product dispensed. For example, a small volume should be placed into a small bottle.

Care must be taken to ensure that the size of the dispensing container is appropriate for the amount of medication being dispensed. A container that is too large will allow the medication too much freedom to move, which may result in damaged capsules or tablets. In addition, the general appearance would be sloppy and the patient may have trouble retrieving the medication from the container. A container that is too small may crush tablets or force a liquid or cream out of the package.

Sealing the Dispensing Container

All dispensing bottles should be sealed with child-proof caps, according to the Poison Prevention and Packaging Act. An "easy-open" cap may be placed on the bottle if the patient signs a waiver form indicating that this type of cap is requested. This releases the pharmacy from liability should accidental poisoning occur due to unsecured packaging.

In addition to being the proper size and shape, the dispensing container must be appropriate to the drug product being dispensed, as well. For example, many drugs are sensitive to light, which is why drugs are packaged in amber-colored containers. Others are sensitive to humidity and must have caps that seal tightly. Still others (e.g., nitroglycerin) react with most forms of plastic and should be packaged in glass bottles.

Properly Labeling the Container

> If a prescription was filled by generic substitution, the label must contain the name of the generic brand, not the proprietary label originally prescribed!

Once the drug has been packaged, it must be labeled appropriately. Information that is required to be on a label (unless omissions are requested by the prescriber) is as follows:

- *The name, address, and phone number of the pharmacy* (usually preprinted on the label)
- *The name of the patient for whom the drug is prescribed* (or the name of the owner, if the drug is for an animal)
- *The name of the prescriber*
- *Date of dispensing*
- *The name of the drug.* This means the drug that was *actually dispensed*. If the prescription was for a proprietary label (brand name) and the generic drug was dispensed, the generic name and manufacturer should appear on the label.

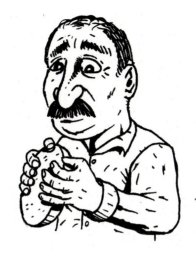

The label on Mr. Greene's suppository prescription reads, "Take one suppository twice daily."

Delmar/Cengage Learning

> **EXAMPLE**
>
> The prescription order is for furosemide, but the patient requests the brand name Lasix. The label must read Lasix, even though the prescription was for furosemide, the generic name may be listed also, but if a brand name is dispensed, it must be on the label.

- *The strength of the medication* (e.g., 40 mg tabs, 5% solution, etc.). If the drug is only available in one strength or is a combination drug, this information may be omitted (depending on your state's regulations).
- *The quantity of drug dispensed* (number of tablets, number of milliliters, etc.)
- *Directions for dosage.* These should be clear, understandable, and appropriate to the user. For example, if the prescription is for a child, the label should read "Give [the drug]." If the drug is for oral dosage, instructions would be "Take. . . ." For rectal or vaginal use, instructions would be "Insert," and so on.

Additionally, the label may contain refill information, and usually the initials of the person dispensing the drug will appear by the date of filling.

Auxiliary Labels

Once an outpatient prescription has been filled and labeled, it is helpful to place reminders on the prescription bottle as to how to use the medication (since the medication will be dosed directly by the patient) and to note any activities that should be avoided while using it. These adhesive labels are called **auxiliary labels**. The auxiliary label reminds the patient of the best way to use the drug for maximum effect, and emphasizes things to avoid. For example, certain activities may be hazardous, such as drinking alcoholic beverages (which may chemically or physically react with the drug) or operating machinery. Many computer systems will print these directly on the dispensing label. These special labels can be purchased with the self-adhesive auxiliary labels already attached.

Once the drug has been dispensed and received by the patient, it now should be entered into the patient profile (Chapter 3).

Compounding of Prescriptions

Preparing a solution, ointment, or powder from a written procedure is often performed by the technician. Legally, these dosage forms must be prepared by the technician according to a standardized, written procedure. The procedure may involve combining the components by weight or by percentages.

Extemporaneous Compounding

Extemporaneous compounding is the preparation of a dosage form for drug delivery that is customized for a particular patient. This requires a degree of professional judgment, and therefore must legally be performed by the pharmacist. If the pharmacist generates a *written protocol* for the preparation of the dosage form, it may be prepared by the technician. *Once the protocol for preparation of the drug is in written form, it is considered an extemporaneous compound suitable for technicians to prepare.*

Preparing Sterile Solutions for Injection Using Aseptic Technique

A solution for injection must be prepared using the aseptic technique. Organisms abound in the air and on the skin, and will proliferate and become virulent if injected directly into the bloodstream.

If a sterile solution is being prepared, such as a drug for injection or a solution for use in surgical irrigation, the technician must prepare the drug dose or solution using **aseptic technique**. Drugs that go directly into the blood do not go through the digestive system. Any bacteria present in the parenteral solution can survive and multiply very quickly in the bloodstream. Bacteria produce toxins, which "poison" the blood (hence the name "blood poisoning"). Cleaning the skin and under the fingernails will not necessarily remove all of these organisms from the skin. Therefore, it is important to wear gloves when preparing these products. Introduction of these organisms directly into the blood can cause **sepsis**. Sepsis is an extremely serious condition that is fatal to the patient if not treated in the early stages, before excessive bacterial growth has occurred. Because of this potentially serious danger, these preparations must be free of viruses, yeast, and particularly bacteria. Thus, when preparing a parenteral dosage form:

- Perform all procedures inside a sterile **laminar flow hood**, with clean, disinfected hands and with hair tied back or covered.

- Disinfect the withdrawal site on the drug vial (the **septum**, or **rubber stopper**) with alcohol, immediately before withdrawal of the drug.

- Both the syringe and needle must be kept sterile. When inside the sterile packaging, the syringe and needle are guaranteed by the manufacturer to be sterile. When the packaging of the syringe is opened, it should be opened from the end that will attach to the needle, and care should be taken not to touch either the syringe or the needle. The protective cap should be left on the needle at all times, unless the needle is being used to withdraw or inject the drug. Note that wearing latex gloves when working in the hood does not guarantee sterility, as they have been exposed to an unsterile environment.

The following should be observed when withdrawing a drug for injection:

- The needle should be placed on the septum, beveled side up, and should pierce the septum at a 45-degree angle, going into the vial. This prevents fragments of the rubber septum from entering the needle and thus the medication (this is known as **coring**).

- When the medication is withdrawn the needle should be at 90 degrees, and care should be taken to *avoid touching the plunger* with the fingers as it leaves the barrel of the syringe. Any organisms deposited on the plunger from contact with your skin will go directly into the patient when the medication is injected.

- Once the medication is withdrawn into the syringe, the protective cap should immediately be placed onto the needle before removal from the hood. This prevents accidental contamination. If the medication is being sent to the nursing floor, the needle should be removed and replaced with a protective plastic or rubber cap. The label should be placed over the plunger end of the syringe barrel as soon as possible to minimize the possibility of dispensing errors.

> The sterile laminar flow hood is a piece of equipment that surrounds the workspace and creates a barrier between the drug and the surroundings, using forced air currents.

The sterile hood laminar flow hood is a piece of equipment that surrounds the workspace and forms a barrier between the user/surroundings and the workspace. It electronically draws filtered room air across the workspace from the back of the hood to the front ("horizontal flow") or pushes it from the top of the hood down over the workspace and out the bottom or front of the hood ("vertical flow"). This creates a barrier from the workspace to the ceiling of the hood to keep organisms in the air away from the workspace. Passing air currents can still force organisms into the hood, however, so it should be located away from traffic in the pharmacy. In the same way, the technician should not "challenge" the efficiency of the sterile hood by talking into it, coughing, or sneezing, as this can cause contaminating organisms to be forced over the air currents and into the sterile workplace.

The following procedures should be followed:

- The manufacturer's container, especially the site where the drug is to be withdrawn (or injected, as in the case of an admixture), must be disinfected with alcohol.

- Should the needle come in contact with clothing, skin, or any surface within the hood during the filling process, the entire syringe assembly should be discarded, to eliminate the risk of contamination.

Working with Hazardous Drugs

Additional safety measures must be taken if the drug is hazardous. Many injectable drugs, such as cancer chemotherapeutics and steroid drugs, can be harmful to the person handling them. So, in addition to keeping the drug sterile, as described above, the technician must wear protective clothing.

Protective Clothing

Protective clothing includes clothing that completely covers the body: No shorts, short-sleeved shirts, or skirts should be worn. In addition, a long protective coat (sterile gown) should be worn to protect the clothing and skin, and safety glasses or goggles may be worn to protect the eyes. The safety glasses should have splash guards on the sides, because when a drug is diluted within a vial the pressure within the vial may buildup, causing the drug to splash out if the vial is opened. Vented needles or venting pins may be used to prevent drug splash.

Additional Safeguards

These coverings are for the protection of the technician, not the drug; they do not help to keep the drug sterile. If the drug is hazardous, the technician may also wear additional disposable body coverings such as a hat, head covering or wig, mask, gloves, and shoe covers. This not only helps to prevent accidental spillage of the drug from touching the skin, but also helps prevent contaminating the other parts of the pharmacy with the drug. The coverings can be removed at the door of the IV room and discarded.

Accidental Drug Exposure

Touching the face, eyes, or mouth while preparing a drug product is not only a source of contamination, it may also be hazardous to the health of the technician. Rubbing the eye or mouth can lead to the introduction of comparatively large amounts of drug into the body.

When working with a sterile drug, particularly one that is hazardous, *care should be taken to keep hands at least six inches inside of the hood,* away from other parts of the body. Whether the drug is hazardous or not, touching the face or rubbing the eye is a source of contamination. This becomes even worse with a hazardous drug, as any contact with the face, particularly the mucous membranes of the eye and mouth, can introduce concentrated drug into the body in doses much larger than the patient would ever get. This can be extremely toxic. Caution should also be observed if the technician is allergic to the drug being prepared. It is best if the task is given to someone who is not allergic to the drug.

> Touching the face, eyes, or mouth while preparing a drug product is not only a source of contamination, it may also be hazardous to the health of the technician. Rubbing the eye or mouth can lead to comparatively large amounts of drug being introduced into the body.

Intravenous Admixtures and Injections

Various sites may be used for drug injection, and each type of injection must be prepared in a different way. The major routes of parenteral administration are intravenous (IV), intramuscular (IM), and subcutaneous (SC), although intradermal, intrathecal, epidural, intracardiac, and intra-arterial injections are also seen.

Intravenous Injections

Intravenous injections may be of small or large volume, as they go directly into the blood. The large-volume injectables are the intravenous drips (IV drips). These are large plastic bags or glass bottles of solution, which may be used alone (for a dehydrated patient, for example) or with an **admixture**.

Intramuscular Injections

Intramuscular injections are designed to be released slowly from the muscle into the blood. This lessens the physiological shock to the body, caused by rapid administration of a drug, and may also increase the length of the drug's effects. Intramuscular injections have a limited volume (less than 3 mL), as there is not much room within the muscle for the drug to go. They require a large needle (19–21 gauge), as the muscle is tough and hard to inject.

Subcutaneous Injections

Subcutaneous injections are also designed for slow release of drug into the system. Since the space under the skin is limited, these injections are also limited in volume (1 mL or less).

Intravenous Admixture

> Intravenous admixtures may be mixed directly into a bulk solution, or administered using separate "piggyback" IV feeding into the IV line.

An IV admixture is a drug that is added to a large-volume parenteral. This is done so that the drug is released slowly into the blood and is less of a shock to the body than a large "all-at-once" dose (a bolus injection). Admixtures are done in two ways. The drug to be administered may be mixed directly into a bulk solution (e.g., D_5W or normal saline), or administered using a separate, very small IV bag (a piggyback IV) that is designed to release the drug slowly into the tubing with the IV drip.

If the drug is mixed in directly with the bulk solution, the resulting drug solution must be labeled appropriately with the name of the solution, the name of the drug, the amount of drug added, and the patient designation.

Proper Labeling of Bulk Intravenous Solutions

When a sterile product, such as an IV bag or admixture, is labeled, the label should be placed toward the top of the container. This is so that any contamination present in the solution, which will tend to sink to the bottom of the container, can easily be seen. The contaminated product can then be discarded before it is administered to the patient.

Proper Labeling of a Bolus Injection

Labels on a syringe should be as narrow as possible and should be placed at the top of the syringe, crosswise, so as not to cover the markings on the syringe (Figure 4-2).

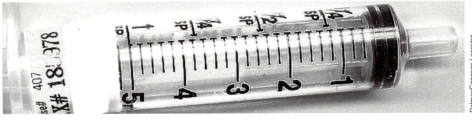

Figure 4-2: A Properly Labeled Syringe

Chapter Review Questions

1. A prescription for Timoptic includes the instructions "i gtt qd ou." What auxiliary label might be chosen to be affixed to the dispensing container?
   a. take with food
   b. drink with plenty of water
   c. may cause drowsiness
   d. for the eye

2. A prescription is to be filled with a refrigerated liquid medication. What should the technician do before filling this prescription?
   a. no meds are stored in the refrigerator
   b. allow the medication to come to room temperature before measuring
   c. refuse to fill it
   d. have the pharmacist fill it because you are not allowed to fill liquid medications

3. An order is received for phenobarbital 50 mg po. The pharmacy has 100 mg tablets in stock. The order can only be filled if:
   a. the tablets are crushed
   b. the tablets are scored
   c. the tablets are scored in half
   d. the order cannot be filled, as the drug strengths do not match

4. The dosage strength of the medication dispensed may not appear on the label if:
   a. the strength is below 10 mg
   b. the drug is a combination drug with only one strength combination
   c. the drug only comes in one strength
   d. both b and c are correct

5. Which of the following are involved in the practice of aseptic technique?
   a. clean hands
   b. use of a laminar flow hood
   c. alcohol disinfection
   d. all of the above

6. Aseptic technique is used for parenteral injections because:
   a. sterility is more important in drugs that are injected directly into the body
   b. any of the thousands of bacteria and fungus around us could cause serious infections if allowed into the bloodstream
   c. bacteria and other organisms multiply rapidly once in the bloodstream and could cause death to the patient, and these organisms are destroyed by the digestive system
   d. all of the above are true

7. Intramuscular (IM) injections require a larger needle because:
   a. muscle tissue is tough and hard to inject
   b. IM injections are given just under the skin
   c. IM injections are usually a thick suspension
   d. they must be given rapidly

8. Protective clothing might include:
   a. glasses, earrings, and a hat
   b. sterile gown/coat, safety glasses, and a mask
   c. boots, sterile gown/coat, and a hard hat
   d. earrings, necklace, and bracelets

9. To prevent coring, you should:
   a. pierce the septum at a 90-degree angle, with the bevel down
   b. pierce the septum at a 45-degree angle, with the bevel down
   c. pierce the septum at a 45-degree angle, with the bevel up
   d. pierce the septum at a 90-degree angle, with the bevel up

10. The NDC number identifies:
    a. manufacturer, drug, and packaging
    b. manufacturer, patient, and date
    c. manufacturer, DEA number, and drug
    d. patient, drug, and DEA number

CHAPTER 5

Proper Storage and Delivery of Drug Products

Quick Study

I. Drug stability and potency

    A. Effects of the environment—humidity and air
    B. Relationship of dosage form to stability
    C. Effects of temperature and light on drug formulations
    D. Use of the manufacturer's label to determine proper handling
    E. Importance of proper packaging and packaging materials

II. Handling the drug to be dispensed

    A. Importance of cleanliness in handling drug products
    B. Drug allergies and sensitivities
    C. Cross-contamination

III. Unit dosing

    A. Preparation of unit doses
    B. Use and care of floor stock: role of the technician and pharmacy
       • Inspection for cleanliness
       • Record-keeping
       • Drug transfer and legal issues

Proper Storage of Drug Products

Part of delivering an effective drug is related to the way the drug is stored in the warehouse and on the pharmacy shelf. Proper storage conditions for drug products are important, and the technician would be wise to be familiar

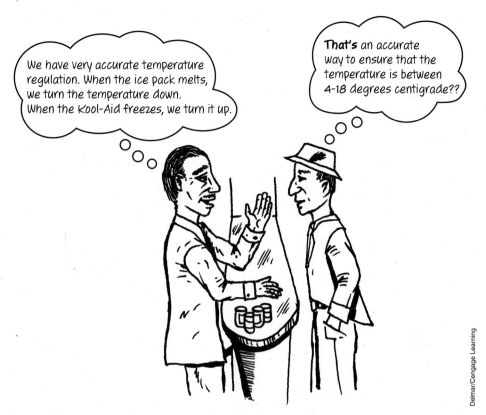

The Sloppy Pharmacy gets an inspection from the State Board of Pharmacy.

with accepted guidelines. The storage conditions of drug products in the pharmacy are subject to spot inspections by the State Board of Pharmacy at any time. Accepted temperature guidelines for storage areas are as follows:

- Refrigerated areas are to be kept within a range of 2–8°C (36–46°F), as measured by a calibrated thermometer (which should be in place in case of an inspection).

- Room temperature is to be kept between 15–30°C (59–86°F).

Remember that drugs are chemicals—some are sensitive to light, others to heat, humidity, or oxygen in the air. Some drugs actually react chemically with their packaging; for example, nitroglycerin will react with most forms of plastic and should be packaged in glass.

> Drugs may be sensitive to heat, light, humidity, and oxygen and should be stored appropriately!

Dosage Forms and Drug Stability

The form of the drug also contributes to stability. The stability of a drug (how well it retains its potency and form) is affected, as mentioned above, by things like water and air (e.g., an injectable drug). A drug that is packaged dry on the shelf may retain its potency longer than if it is reconstituted

> The presence of water may accelerate the breakdown of a drug and severely shorten its shelf life.

with water. The presence of water accelerates the breakdown of the drug and severely shortens its shelf life.

The stability of a drug is greatly increased when it is in tablet form, as compared to other dosage forms (e.g., powder, solution).

Tablets and Other Solid Dosage Drugs

A drug tablet carries most of the drug inside of the dosage form, protected from air and moisture. Thus, the tablet form may retain potency longer than a loose, powdered form of the same drug, simply because less of the drug is exposed. Various storage conditions may also help to protect the drug from breakdown. These include:

Opaque glass or plastic packaging. Since the energy from light rays tends to speed up the breakdown (degradation) of most drug products, drugs are routinely packaged and dispensed in opaque bottles or bottles made of brown plastic or glass. Drugs should be kept out of direct sunlight, and care must also be taken to be sure that the container lid forms a tight seal against humidity and oxygen, which can also destroy the drug.

> The shelf life and potency of a drug may be extended by the use of opaque packaging, refrigeration, and dehydration.

Refrigeration. Colder temperatures tend to slow down any chemical reaction, so storage of drug products in a cool, dry place will help to retard chemical breakdown and retain potency. Refrigerated storage may also be utilized, but this may not be appropriate for all drugs; the manufacturer's label should be consulted prior to refrigerating a drug. Cooler temperatures also decrease the rate of growth of microorganisms, so storing sterile products in a cool environment will increase their shelf life accordingly.

Dehydration. Drugs in solution tend to break down faster than those in powder form. Some drugs are received in powder form for this reason (i.e., a longer shelf life) and are reconstituted just before use. If the drug is stored in solution form (hydrated), its shelf life is limited and, depending on the rate of use, much of it may degrade and have to be discarded.

Determining the Proper Storage Conditions for a Drug

The manufacturer's label on the stock bottle should be consulted to determine the proper storage conditions for a drug. The manufacturer's label, in addition to allowing us to accurately calculate the amount of drug dispensed per dose, gives additional information that is necessary for the proper handling of the drug.

The label contains information about the temperature at which the drug should be stored and also states any storage conditions that should be avoided (e.g., cold, light, or humidity). For example, if the label states "protect from light," this means that the drug is light-sensitive and should be stored appropriately (e.g., packaged in amber glass or plastic). If the label states "keep container tightly closed," this means the drug is sensitive to the oxygen or humidity in the air. Many drugs will absorb water out of the air, which decreases their potency. If there are no storage instructions, the drug should be stored at room temperature, away from bright light and heat.

The label shown in Figure 5-1 is that of Pfizerpen, an injectable form of penicillin. The drug is received in a dry state within the vial and is to be reconstituted before use, according to instructions on the label. The label also gives instructions as to proper storage temperature for the drug, both before and after hydration. The instructions state that the hydrated suspension may be kept for one week in the refrigerator.

The label may specify a specific temperature or range of temperatures at which the drug should be stored. The technician must be familiar with what these temperatures mean, in terms of where in the pharmacy the drug should be stored. Table 5-1* should be committed to memory.

> If no instructions for storage appear on the manufacturer's label, the drug should be stored at room temperature on the pharmacy shelf.

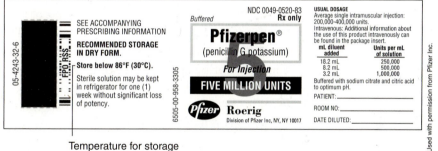

Temperature for storage

Figure 5-1: The Manufacturer's Label, Showing Proper Storage Conditions (used with permission from Pfizer Inc.)

Table 5-1   Temperatures for Proper Drug Storage

Storage Designation	Storage Temperature
Freezer	Not to exceed 2°C (36°F)
Cold (refrigerator)	Between 2° and 8°C (36–46°F)
Cool	Between 8 and 15°C (46–59°F)
Room temperature	Between 15 and 30°C (59–86°F)
Warm	Between 30 and 40°C (86–104°F)
Excessive Heat	Above 40°C (104°F)

If the label states a storage temperature of:

- 8–15°C, the drug should be refrigerated. Some common items would include:
  - Vaccines
  - Suppositories
  - Famotidine injection
  - Succinylcholine
  - Insulin
- below 0°C, it refers to storage in the freezer. (Usually, this is a warning as to how the drug should not be stored—many drugs are sensitive to extreme cold.)
- 25°C (75°F), this is normal room temperature. The drug may be stored on the pharmacy shelf.

Label warnings might include the following:

- 30°C or 85°F (a "warm" room). Drugs will lose potency when exposed to heat.
- above 35°C or 95°F ("extreme heat"). This is too high a temperature for drug products.
- freezer storage [0°C (32°F) or less]. Drugs are sensitive to extreme cold.

Importance of Proper Packaging and Labeling

The volume of drug solution stated on the manufacturer's label allows accurate calculation of the number of doses available. This information may assist in accurate calculation of the drug concentration.

The label may provide an indication of how the drug should be packaged. The type of drug packaging is important. For example, many drugs are light-sensitive and are packaged in opaque or amber plastics. Some drugs react chemically with plastic, so they will carry a warning to use only glass packaging. The label also provides information for proper handling (e.g., shake well before using).

The dosage form is clearly stated on the label (e.g., a suspension). (What does that mean in terms of handling the drug and drawing up the dose? Review Chapter 3.) The label also states the amount (volume) of suspension in the bottle. This is useful in two ways. First, it tells us how many doses we can draw out of the bottle. Second, and very importantly, if the concentration of the drug suspension or solution is not given on the bottle, it can be calculated by dividing the total amount of drug in the bottle by the total volume of drug suspension or solution in the bottle. Then the proper amount needed for dispensing can be calculated.

Importance of Cleanliness and Sanitation During Storage

In addition to following the manufacturer's instructions when handling a drug, care must be taken to keep the drug clean and sanitary during storage. Dust on the bottle or shelves can contain molds, fungi, or bacteria that can enter the bottle when it is opened and contaminate the drug.

Proper Sanitation of Tablet Counters and Other Measuring Devices

When a tablet counter or other measuring device is used, it is important to clean the device before and after each use to avoid **cross-contamination** of drugs. This may include washing with detergent and water, or simply wiping the counter down thoroughly with an alcohol wipe. Equipment for liquid measure should be washed with soap and water and thoroughly dried before use.

Avoiding Cross-Contamination of Drugs Due to Improper Sanitation

When more than one drug is handled at once, some residual drug may remain on the measuring device and will contaminate the second drug with another medication that may be harmful to the patient (even a trace of drug remaining on a counting tray could cause a severe allergic reaction should the patient happen to be allergic to it). At the very least, the patient may receive trace amounts of a drug that is not appropriate for his or her condition.

> Cleanliness of measuring devices is extremely important to prevent cross-contamination of drugs!

Patients who are allergic to penicillin may suffer serious consequences if exposed to even the tiniest trace of the drug. These may include life-threatening anaphylactic reactions characterized by severe shock and an inability to breathe. Because of the serious nature of penicillin allergies and the potential for life-threatening reactions in allergic patients, separate tablet counters and other equipment may be reserved for the measurement of penicillin.

Preparation of Unit Doses

> A unit dose is the amount of drug needed for one dose.

In an institution, it is more efficient to dispense an entire day's worth of medication at one time, to be administered by the floor staff, rather than order each individual dose from the pharmacy. This dose is calculated, dispensed, and, usually, delivered to the patient care area by the technician once a day. A *unit dosing system* is used in an institutional pharmacy. Simply stated, it is the daily preparation and delivery of enough drug to last for the entire day. A unit dose is simply enough drug for one dose in a prepackaged container (e.g., one 500 mg capsule or two 250 mg capsules of amoxicillin for a prescribed dose of 500 mg). Unit doses are stored in a medication cart and are filed under a patient's name or hospital identification number (see Chapter 1).

Calculating a Daily Dose

A daily dose is calculated from the physician's order. The amount of medication per dose is multiplied by the number of doses per day (a 24-hour period). For example, if an order is for "cimetidine 300 mg tid ac," the calculation would be:

$$\frac{1 \text{ tablet}}{\text{dose}} \times \frac{3 \text{ doses}}{\text{day}} = 3 \text{ tablets per day}$$

This amount would be packaged appropriately and labeled with the patient's name, location, and hospital number as well as the drug name, strength, and form, if appropriate. Tablets may be packaged in blister packs or other appropriate packaging to keep the drug sanitary and separate from other drugs. Injectable medications, other than controlled substances, may be sent in a prefilled syringe, vial, or dosette.

Exceptions to Unit Dosing

> Exceptions to unit dosing include medications that cannot be measured accurately for a unit dose, such as creams and lotions, and liquids for oral dosage.

Exceptions to unit dosing include those medications that cannot be accurately measured for a unit dose, such as creams and ointments, and liquids for oral medication. These medications are sent to the patient floor in bulk, packaged in a tube, jar, or bottle, as appropriate. When the exchange of medications takes place each day (unused medications are picked up and new doses delivered), these bulk medications are not replaced, but simply transferred from the previous day's medications to the current medications. With this system, the patient is charged only for the medication that is used. Unused drugs are picked up and returned to the pharmacy for credit.

In the past, narcotics and other Schedule drugs were not included in the daily dose system of dispensing. This is no longer the case, as most institutions now have computerized carts that require the nurse or pharmacy technician to enter a specific code, assigned only to them, in order to unlock the drawers within the cart. In addition, when withdrawing drugs, the nurse must enter information into the computer, such as the name of the patient for whom the drugs are intended, as well as such information as the drug to be administered, its dosage form, and amount withdrawn. This keeps an accurate, computerized record of who withdrew the drugs from the cart, how much was withdrawn, and to whom it was administered, making the storage of controlled substances more secure. This computerized system can also record the wastage due to partial dosing or contamination.

Use of Pharmacy Inventory as Floor Stock

> Drugs that are used on a routine basis may be kept on the patient floor as floor stock, which is maintained by the medical staff and supervised by the pharmacy.

To further decrease the workload of the pharmacy and increase the availability of medication to the patient floors, the pharmacy may send drugs to individual patient floors to use as **floor stock**. In this case, the nurses' station or emergency room staff would be responsible for keeping a supply of the drugs and drug products on hand that are normally needed on a routine basis. Drugs would then be inventoried by the floor staff and ordered in quantities from the pharmacy. If an item is used often, it might be ordered daily. If it is not used often, it would be ordered less frequently. Even though the storage and inventory are done by the floor staff, the pharmacy staff is still responsible for ensuring that the drugs are properly stored and dispensed. Periodic checks must be made to ensure that the following criteria are met:

- *Proper storage conditions:* All drugs must be stored at the proper temperature. Pharmacy personnel may measure the temperature of storage areas, such as refrigerators, and must ensure that all drugs are stored appropriately and in a sanitary manner, according to the instructions on the manufacturers' labels. This may include checking to see if drugs that are supposed to be refrigerated are being left on the counter when not in use, or if caps are being left off of the bottles when not in use. (If this happens, the drug potency may be reduced and contamination may occur.)

- *Proper dispensing conditions:* Drugs must be dispensed in a clean, sanitary manner that is appropriate to the particular drug, and the dispensing area and utensils must be clean and sanitary. In addition, sloppy handling may lead to contamination and caps may be left off of the stock bottles, exposing the drug to air, light, and humidity, which would lower the drug potency. Improper handling may also expose the drug to dust and microorganisms in the air, such as bacteria, fungi, and viruses.

- *Proper sanitation of dispensing areas:* Inspections may be conducted to ensure that the general environment of the dispensing area is clean and sanitary. This includes inspections of equipment used for measuring drugs for dispensing to ensure that they are clean and being properly used. No dirt, clutter, used syringes or needles, or contaminated materials should be present in the dispensing area (e.g., urine or blood specimens, or other laboratory specimens), nor should any food or drink be present.

- *Proper record-keeping:* Proper records must be kept of disposition of drugs, just as in the pharmacy. A current inventory of floor stock, records of drugs dispensed to patients, and records of drugs ordered and received must all match. *This is especially important with controlled substances*, particularly Schedule II drugs. Any discrepancies must be reported immediately to the pharmacist and supervising professional (e.g., head nurse) on the floor.

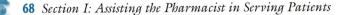

Documenting Drug Transfer from the Pharmacy to Floor Stock Areas

> When delivering drugs to patient care areas, the technician must obtain an authorized signature upon delivery and provide a complete inventory of drugs delivered. The signature of the supervising nurse or medical professional is required for delivery of controlled substances.

Proper Record-Keeping

Accurate records must be kept of the transfer of drugs from the control of the pharmacy to the control of the patient care area. When requested drugs are delivered to patient care areas, the technician must receive a signature of the person accepting the drugs and must provide a complete inventory of drugs delivered.

Information and Signatures Required for Transfer of Controlled Substances

If the delivery to the patient care area contains controlled substances, additional paperwork is required that specifies the exact amount of drug to be transferred and includes all information about the drug: the generic name, proprietary name, dosage and dosage form, manufacturer, lot number, and expiration date. The signature of the head nurse or supervising medical professional is required for delivery of any controlled substance (particularly Schedule II drugs) to be used as floor stock outside of the main pharmacy, unless the drugs are placed into a locked, secure area (e.g., a computerized medication cart). A signature by any other person is not acceptable. The receipt of the drug(s) by the patient care area is acknowledged by this signature, and responsibility for the drugs' disposition and appropriate records are transferred at this time.

Chapter Review Questions

1. The best way to determine the storage conditions for a particular drug is to:
   a. ask the pharmacist
   b. refer to the *United States Pharmacopoeia*
   c. try different ways of storage
   d. refer to the manufacturer's label

2. The stability of a drug refers to:
   a. how it reacts with plastic
   b. how it is stored on the pharmacy shelf
   c. how long it remains potent
   d. how it should be dispensed

3. A reconstituted drug in suspension:
   a. is more stable than a dry powder
   b. is normally stored on the pharmacy shelf
   c. will generally remain potent longer if it is refrigerated
   d. should not be shaken

4. You have a bottle of drug in solution. The label does not state the concentration of the drug in the solution, but the amount of drug and the volume of liquid in the container both appear on the label. To dispense 30 mg of this drug, you can:
   a. obtain further information from the *United States Pharmacopoeia*
   b. estimate the amount of drug to be dispensed by the volume needed for injection
   c. calculate the concentration from the information given on the label
   d. The order cannot be filled

5. Contamination of dispensed drugs may occur from:
   a. dust clinging to the bottle and cap falling into the medication
   b. residual drug clinging to a measuring device that has not been properly cleaned
   c. unfiltered room air
   d. not using a laminar flow hood when dispensing the medication

6. Drugs in nursing floor inventories that are "slow movers" should be:
   a. ordered less frequently
   b. removed from inventory
   c. reduced in price
   d. put in a special area

7. You receive an order for "cefaclor 250 mg ii bid." The drug is available in 250 mg capsules. A daily dose for this patient would be:
   a. two capsules
   b. three capsules
   c. four capsules
   d. This drug could not be dispensed as a unit dose

8. Which of the following would not be dispensed as a commercially available unit dose package?
   a. cimetidine tablets
   b. verapamil tablets
   c. phenergan syrup
   d. compazine suppositories

9. A drug label says to store the drug between 15–25°C. The drug should be stored:
   a. in a warm room
   b. on the pharmacy shelf
   c. in the refrigerator
   d. in a cool room

10. The care of drugs stored on the nursing floors, or anywhere in the hospital, are the responsibility of:
    a. nurses aides
    b. pharmacy
    c. physicians
    d. patients

CHAPTER 6

Receiving Payment for Goods and Services

Quick Study

I. Receipt of payment for pharmacy services

   A. Self-pay

   B. Third-party payment: Benefits and exclusions
- The pharmacy is paid by the insurance provider (co-pay).
- The patient pays and is reimbursed by the provider (out-of-pocket).

   C. Institutional pharmacy billing
- Charges are billed to the patient account based upon information from the medication administration record (MAR).

II. Profit and markup: calculation of selling price and net profit

Receipt of Payment for Pharmacy Services

There are basically two ways in which the pharmacy can receive payment for services. One is **self-pay**, in which the patient pays the pharmacy directly. The second is payment by a **third-party payer**. The third-party payer can be used in two ways:

1. The patient can pay the pharmacy and be reimbursed (**out-of-pocket**), in which case the pharmacist must fill out an **insurance affidavit** stating the drugs received, price, and other information required by the insurance company.

2. The patient can pay a small amount (**co-payment** or **co-pay**) and the pharmacy bills the insurance company for the balance of the charge.

Third-Party Payers—Health Plan Benefits and Exclusions

> The technician must be familiar with the various insurance plans and what they cover.

The technician needs to be familiar with the billing of third-party payers. These payers may include:

- traditional insurance companies, such as those received under an employee benefit package
- government plans such as Medicare and Medicaid
- private insurance companies

> Each health care plan has specific benefits and may exclude certain drugs, or limit quantities dispensed.

Each health care plan has specific benefits and may or may not include payments for medications. Those plans that cover prescription medications may limit coverage in various ways, such as exclusion of outpatient prescriptions, limitation of outpatient coverage to oral dosage forms, exclusion of proprietary drugs, or limitations on quantity. Some health care plans have a "closed" formulary. This means that they will only pay for specific drugs for specific diagnoses. Exceptions may be considered, but often the patient ends up paying the difference between the cost of what they (health care plan) would cover and the exception drug requested.

Insurance coverage must be verified at the time the prescription is received. Specific coverage information may be contained in the pharmacy's computer database. It should be noted that some insurance plans allow only generic drugs to be dispensed. If the patient or prescriber requests a brand name (proprietary label), the patient would have to pay the difference in price. Exceptions to plan policy may be made by the insurance company under certain circumstances (e.g., the condition is life-threatening or there is no generic brand marketed).

Once the insurance coverage or method of payment has been established, the forms to be submitted to the insurance company must be identified and completed and the price of the medication calculated.

Institutional Pharmacy Billing—Role of the Medication Administration Record

> In an institutional setting, charges for medications are billed to the patient's account as the medication is dispensed.

In an institutional pharmacy setting, charges are billed to the patient's account based on information from the medication administration record (MAR). Normally, charges are billed to the patient's account at the time the medication is dispensed, which simplifies the billing process and improves billing accuracy. Medications that are dispensed but not administered are returned to the pharmacy and appropriate credit issued to the patient's account.

Insurance coverage verification and billing in a hospital setting are normally done by a separate billing or accounting department within the institution.

Calculation of the Price of the Medication

The selling price of a medication begins with the cost of the medication to the pharmacy (**cost price**). This is then increased by a certain percentage or dollar amount to the *selling price*.

The Dispensing Fee

All medications dispensed by prescription will also include a **dispensing fee**, This may be either a percentage of the price or a flat fee added to the cost of the prescription.

Profit and Markup

The **markup** rate or percentage of a drug is normally expressed as a percentage of the cost. For example, a markup of 100% would mean that the increase in price would be equal to the cost. (Since 100% is the same as multiplying a number by one, the markup is the same as the cost.)

> **EXAMPLE**
>
> The cost of a drug is $10. The markup is 100%, so $10 × 1 = $10. $10 (cost) + $10 (markup) = $20.
>   The cost of a drug is $10. The markup is 50%, so $10 × 0.5 = $5. $10 (cost) + $5 (markup) = $15.

The markup of a drug is not the same as the net profit that is made on the drug, as the cost of storing, inventory, and general overhead expenses must be taken into account when calculating the actual profit made. A discussion of the calculation of profit and markup may be found in Chapter 19.

Chapter Review Questions

1. The two types of third-party pay plans are:
   a. co-pay and self-pay
   b. co-pay and out-of-pocket
   c. reimbursement and self-pay
   d. third-party billing and reimbursement

2. The insurance affidavit:
   a. is a sworn contract to pay charges
   b. is a document that is filled out so that the pharmacy gets paid
   c. must be completed by the pharmacist
   d. is completed by the patient and sent to the insurance company

3. Which of the following is not an example of a third-party payor?
   a. Medicare
   b. Medicaid
   c. a man ordered to pay medical expenses as a result of a lawsuit
   d. a major insurance company

4. The selling price of a medication is based on the:
   a. patient's income
   b. amount the insurance will pay
   c. cost price to the pharmacy
   d. dispensing fee

5. Insurance companies that only pay for a defined list of drugs has a/an
   a. open formulary
   b. small budget
   c. high markup
   d. closed formulary

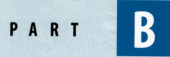
Pharmaceutical Calculations

CHAPTER 7

Fractions, Decimals, and Algebra Review

Quick Study

I.   Using fractions

   A.   Writing fractions
- Proper fraction—Written correctly, the numerator (top) is smaller than the denominator (bottom).
- Improper fraction—The numerator is greater than the denominator.

   B.   Adding and subtracting fractions—Find the common denominator and perform the calculation:

$$\frac{1}{4} + \frac{1}{2} = \frac{1}{4} + \frac{2}{4} = \frac{3}{4}$$

$$\frac{1}{2} - \frac{1}{4} = \frac{2}{4} - \frac{1}{4} = \frac{1}{4}$$

   C.   Multiplication of fractions—Multiply the numerators, then multiply the denominators. Reduce the fraction, if necessary:

$$\frac{4}{16} \times \frac{1}{2} = \frac{4}{32} = \frac{1}{8}$$

   D.   Division of fractions—Divide the numerators and then divide the denominators. Flip over (invert) the second fraction or divisor and multiply:

$$\frac{3}{4} \div \frac{1}{2} = \frac{3}{4} \times \frac{2}{1} = \frac{6}{4} = \frac{3}{2} \text{ or } 1\frac{1}{2}$$

E. Converting fractions to decimals—Decimals are fractions expressed in terms of tenths:

$$\frac{1}{10} = 0.1, \ \frac{1}{100} = 0.01, \ \frac{1}{1000} = 0.001$$

F. Calculating a decimal from a fraction—Divide the numerator of a fraction by the denominator and express as a decimal:

$$\frac{3}{4} = 3 \div 4 = 0.75$$

Always place the zero in front of the decimal point so that the number is not misinterpreted; .75 may look like a decimal, but the "point" could be a spot on the paper!

G. Calculations with decimals
- Addition and subtraction
- Multiplication and division by a factor of ten
    1. Dividing by ten moves the decimal one place left.
    2. Multiplying by ten moves the decimal one place right.

II. Use of cross-multiplication

- Used if the ratio between two quantities is known

III. Rounding numbers

- Based on one digit following the place where the number should be rounded

IV. Using Roman numerals

- Add the incremental values as they are written from left to right.
- If a smaller value precedes a number of larger value, subtract the smaller from the larger.

Using Fractions

A fraction is nothing more than a part of a whole thing. It is expressed as a comparison (ratio) of the number of parts needed to the total number of parts in a whole (e.g., one part in a total of four = $\frac{1}{4}$). See Figure 7-1.

> **EXAMPLE**
>
> An order is for 10 mg of drug. 40 mg scored tablets are available.
>
> $$\frac{\text{Amount Needed} = 1\cancel{0}\text{mg}}{\text{Whole Tablet} = 4\cancel{0}\text{mg}} = \frac{1}{4} \text{tablet is needed}$$
>
> *Note:* If you think of fractions as parts of a whole thing, pharmaceutical calculations will be much easier.

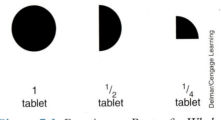

| 1 tablet | ¹/₂ tablet | ¹/₄ tablet |

Figure 7-1: Fractions as Parts of a Whole

Writing Fractions

The correct way to write a fraction is with the top number smaller than the bottom (e.g., $\frac{1}{2}$). If the top number is larger than the bottom number, it is called an **improper fraction**, and the value is more than one. So (to be "proper"), we should write this number as a whole number with a fraction (e.g., $1\frac{3}{4}$). This is called a **mixed fraction**.

Adding and Subtracting Fractions

Finding the Common Denominator

The **common denominator** is simply a number that is divisible by the denominators of both fractions involved. For example, if the fractions that we wish to add are $\frac{1}{4}$ and $\frac{1}{2}$, the common denominator would be 2×2, or 4. If the fractions are more complex, such as $\frac{1}{3}$ and $\frac{1}{8}$, the common denominator would be 3×8, or 24.

- For ease of calculation, you should be careful to choose the smallest common denominator possible. For example, when adding $\frac{3}{8}$ and $\frac{5}{6}$ the common denominator should be 24, rather than 48, which is obtained by simply multiplying the 6 and 8 together.

  Once the fractions have a common denominator, we can add the top parts together, reduce, and get the answer.

> Whatever is done to the numerator of the fraction must also be done to the denominator. In this way, the fraction stays the same, as we are really just multiplying by one (e.g., $\frac{2}{2}$).

EXAMPLE

$$\frac{1}{4} + \frac{1}{2}$$

Step 1. *Find the common denominator.* $2 \times 2 = 4$, so the common denominator is 4, and $\frac{1}{2}$ becomes:

$$\frac{1}{2} \times \frac{2}{2} = \frac{2}{4}$$

Delmar/Cengage Learning

The problem then becomes:

$$\frac{1}{4} + \frac{2}{4} = ?$$

Step 2. We can now add the numerators of the fractions and obtain:

$$\frac{(1+2)}{4} = \frac{3}{4}$$

Subtraction of fractions is done in a similar way, except that instead of adding the top numbers, we subtract them.

> **EXAMPLE**
>
> $$\frac{2}{3} - \frac{1}{2} = ?$$
>
> Step 1. *Find the common denominator.* The smallest number divisible by both two and three is six, so the fractions now become
>
> $$\frac{2}{3} \times \frac{2}{2} \ (\text{or} \ \frac{4}{6}) \ \text{and} \ \frac{1}{2} \times \frac{3}{3} \ (\text{or} \ \frac{3}{6}).$$
>
> Step 2. *Rewrite the problem:*
>
> $$\frac{4}{6} - \frac{3}{6} = \frac{(4-3)}{6} = \frac{1}{6}$$

Rewriting the problem with each step is a great way to keep the calculation organized and decrease the possibility of errors!

It is important to get in the habit of rewriting the problem at each step. Memory is faulty, and this way the problem is organized and clear in your mind as well as on paper. You are less likely to make a mistake.

Multiplication and Division of Fractions

In the majority of actual pharmaceutical calculations, we use fractions in problems involving multiplication and division. These calculations are simpler, as we do not have to have a common denominator.

Multiplying Fractions

> **EXAMPLE**
>
> $$\frac{3}{8} \times \frac{1}{3} = ?$$

Step 1. Multiply the numerators ($3 \times 1 = 3$)

Step 2. Multiply the denominators ($8 \times 3 = 24$)

Step 3. Divide and reduce:

$$\frac{\overset{1}{3}}{\underset{8}{24}} = \frac{1}{8}$$

Division of Fractions

The easiest way to divide a fraction by a fraction is to flip the fraction on the bottom over (invert) and multiply the two.

Problem:
$$\frac{1}{4} \div \frac{1}{2} = ?$$

To divide, we invert the $\frac{1}{2}$ and rewrite the problem as:

$$\frac{1}{4} \times \frac{2}{1} = ?$$

Multiply the two fractions as follows:

$$\frac{1 \times 2}{4 \times 1} = \frac{2}{4}$$

Now, reduce the fraction:

$$\frac{2 \div 2}{4 \div 2} = \frac{1}{2} \quad \text{and the answer is } \frac{1}{2}$$

> By simplifying as much as possible before doing a calculation, you reduce the possibility of errors and make the calculation easier!

Converting Fractions to Decimals

The modern equivalent of the fraction is the decimal. Converting fractions to decimals can make calculation easier. Decimals are commonly used with orders given in the metric system (see Chapter 11). To convert a fraction to a decimal, we simply divide the top number by the bottom number and insert a point, or period, where the whole numbers end and partial numbers begin.

EXAMPLE

Convert $1\frac{1}{2}$ to decimal form.

In this problem we have a whole number as well as a fraction. Place the whole number to the left and then calculate the decimal from the fraction, as we did above. A decimal point is placed between the two to differentiate between the whole number and the fraction:

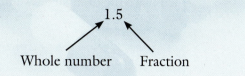

1.5

Whole number   Fraction

> Decimals are based on fractions of ten:
>
> $\dfrac{1}{1} = 1.0$
>
> $\dfrac{1}{10} = 0.1$
>
> $\dfrac{1}{100} = 0.01$
>
> $\dfrac{1}{1000} = 0.001$, etc.

Decimals are based on fractions of ten. A whole number such as 1 (think of it as $1) would be expressed as $1.00 (100 pennies). $\frac{1}{100}$ of a dollar is one cent, or $0.01. Ten cents is $\frac{1}{10}$ of a dollar, or $0.10. $\frac{1}{1000}$ of $1, if there was such a thing, would be $\frac{1}{2}$ of a cent, or $0.001.

EXAMPLE

Convert $\frac{1}{4}$ to a decimal.

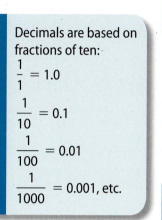

The 0 before the .25 is a placeholder that tells you there are no whole numbers. The decimal point separates the whole numbers from the fraction (decimal), which is 25 hundredths.

Properly Writing Decimals

> If a number is less than one, it is important to place a zero to the left of the decimal point.

Use of the 0 (placeholder) before the decimal is very important. If it is not used and the number is just written .25, there can be big problems in interpretation. The dot you see on the drug order before the 25 could be just a speck of dirt on the order or computer screen or a flaw in the paper! The order could be for 25 mg instead of 0.25 mg! Depending on the drug, that's a difference big enough to cost a patient's life. The placeholder makes it clear that the number is a decimal and not a whole number.

Calculations with Decimals

> The placeholder makes it clear that the number is a decimal and not a whole number.

Adding and Subtracting Decimals
Decimals are added and subtracted like regular numbers:

$$\begin{array}{r} 0.10 \\ +0.05 \\ \hline 0.15 \end{array} \quad \text{or} \quad \begin{array}{r} 0.10 \\ -0.05 \\ \hline 0.05 \end{array}$$

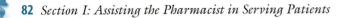

Multiplying and Dividing Decimals

To multiply or divide decimals, do the calculation as if no decimal were present, then place the decimal back into the answer.

EXAMPLE

$$1.2 \times 2.5$$

Step 1. Multiply as usual, disregarding decimal points. By multiplying 12×25, we obtain 300.

Step 2. Now, insert the decimal point:

Since there is one decimal place in the 1.2 and one also in the 2.5 (a total of two), we need to move the decimal place attached to the 300 over two places from the right.

$$300. \longrightarrow 3.00$$

The answer to the problem is then 3.00—round to 3. Trailing zeros could be problematic also. The 3.00 could be read as 300 if the decimal was not noticed. Always round the decimals to the whole number if they are zeros.

Division of decimals is done in a similar way. Using the previous example, let's *divide* the decimals:

EXAMPLE

$$\frac{2.5}{1.2} = ?$$

Step 1. Multiply both numbers by 10 to remove the decimal. Now, the 1.2 becomes 12, and the 2.5 becomes 25.

Step 2. Divide normally:

$$\frac{25}{12} = 2.08$$

Note: Remember that each time we move the decimal over one place, we are multiplying or dividing by 10. Moving the decimal one place to the *left* of the number means *dividing* by 10, while moving it one place to the *right* means *multiplying* by 10.

Use of Algebra in Pharmaceutical Calculations

Knowledge of simple algebra is extremely useful in calculations, especially when using the **ratio-proportion** method to calculate dosage (see Chapters 14–17). Of particular use is **cross-multiplication**.

Using Cross-Multiplication

If we know the relationship between two quantities (e.g., milliliters and teaspoons), we can calculate another quantity that we might need. For example, say we have 100 mL of cough syrup and want to know how many one-teaspoon doses are in the bottle. We set up a problem where we set the two relationships equal and go from there:

Problem: You have 100 mL of cough syrup. The order is for one teaspoon BID. Given that there are 5 mL in one teaspoon, how many doses are in the bottle?

Solution:
1. First, recognize that the question is really asking how many 5 mL doses are in the 100 mL bottle. All other information is irrelevant to the calculation.

2. Set up the formula:

$$\frac{5 \text{ mL}}{100 \text{ mL}} = \frac{1 \text{ tsp}}{? \text{ tsp doses}}$$

3. Cross-multiply and set the two multiplication products equal: use "X" for the amount to be calculated. This gives us the following equation:

$$\frac{5 \text{ mL}}{100 \text{ mL}} \diagdown \frac{1 \text{ tsp}}{? \text{ tsp dose}} = X$$

4. This gives us the following equation:

$$5 \text{ mL} \times X \text{ tsp doses} = 100 \text{ mL} \times 1 \text{ tsp}$$

5. Divide both sides of the equation by 5 mL to get "X" by itself on one side:

$$X \text{ tsp doses} = \frac{100 \text{ mL} \times 1 \text{ tsp}}{5 \text{ mL}}$$

then cancel:

$$X \text{ tsp doses} = \frac{\overset{20}{\cancel{100}} \text{ mL} \times 1 \text{tsp}}{\underset{1}{\cancel{5}} \text{ mL}} = 20 \text{ tsp doses}$$

Rounding Numbers

When a calculation produces a number that is very long and cumbersome, it is necessary to round off the number. This becomes particularly important when a calculated dose comes out to be more precise than the calibrations on your measuring device. To round a number accurately, first locate the first digit following the number where it should be rounded (e.g., 3.5<u>8</u>). If the digit is greater than five, round up. If it is less than 5, round down. If the number is equal to 5, then we must look at the number immediately to the left of the 5 to determine which way to round (see second example below). If this number is even (e.g., 2, 4, 6, 8), round the number down; if it is odd, round up.

EXAMPLE

You calculate the amount to be drawn up for an injection to be 1.1265 mL. The syringe is only accurate to 0.01 mL, so you need to round to two decimal places.

Looking at the amount to be rounded, 1.1265, find the second decimal place (the 2) and look at the numbers immediately following it. In this case, it is 6. Since 6 is greater than 5, you will round the number up from 1.12 to 1.13.

EXAMPLE

The amount to be drawn up is calculated to be 1.1250 mL. In this case, the last digit is **equal** to 5. Now, the decision to round up or down is determined by the number that precedes the last digit. This is 2, which is an even number. Thus, we round *down* to 1.12. If the number had been an odd number (for example, 3), we would have rounded *up*.

Using Roman Numerals

A knowledge of Roman numerals, both uppercase and lowercase, is necessary for the exam. In modern use, prescribers may use lowercase Roman numerals to specify the number of units of medication per dose on a written prescription. In addition, specification of amounts of drugs measured in apothecary units also requires the use of Roman numerals.

Calculating with Roman Numerals

Roman numerals are based on a series of letters. A number, in this system, is made up of individual Roman numerals that are written from left to right in descending order of value (e.g., MCVII). To convert the number into the traditional Arabic numbering system, the individual values of the numerals are added. See Table 7-1 for commonly used Roman numerals and their values.

EXAMPLE

$$M\ (1000) + C\ (100) + I\ (1) + I\ (1) = 1{,}102$$

The order (placement) of the individual numbers is important—numerals written from left to right in order of *descending* value are *added*, whereas a smaller numeral placed to the left of a larger numeral is *subtracted*. For example, MC = 1,000 + 100, but CM = 1,000 – 100!

Problem: Convert MCXXIII to an Arabic number.

Solution: The individual numerals should first be separated, then added:

$$M = 1{,}000$$

$$C = 100$$

$$X = 10$$

$$X = 10$$

$$III = 3\ (1 + 1 + 1)$$

Table 7-1		Commonly Used Roman Numerals and Their Values
ss	=	$\frac{1}{2}$
I (i)	=	1
V (v)	=	5
X (x)	=	10
L (l)	=	50
C (c)	=	100
D (d)	=	500
M (m)	=	1,000

Note: Numerals may be expressed as capital letters or lowercase letters. The values do not change whether lower- or uppercase.

Then add the numerical values to obtain the value of the number.

$$1,000 + 100 + 10 + 10 + 3 = 1,123$$

EXAMPLE

Convert the number MCMXCVII to an Arabic number.

Solution: First, separate the numbers:

$$M = 1,000$$

$$CM = 900 \ (1000 - 100)$$

$$XC = 90 \ (100 - 10)$$

$$VII = 5 + 1 + 1 = 7$$

Then add the numerical values to obtain the value of the number:

$$\text{Total: } 1,000 + 900 + 90 + 7 = 1,997$$

Chapter Review Questions

Compute the following:

1. 0.01×50

2. 0.1×25

3. 10×0.25

4. 100×0.002

5. $\dfrac{1}{4} + \dfrac{1}{2}$

6. $\dfrac{3}{4} \div \dfrac{1}{2}$

7. xxi + xiv

8. LXXX + XIX

Round the following to two decimal places:

9. 1.0035

10. 0.0255

11. 0.1550

12. 0.1450

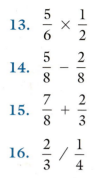

Compute the following:

13. $\dfrac{5}{6} \times \dfrac{1}{2}$

14. $\dfrac{5}{8} - \dfrac{2}{8}$

15. $\dfrac{7}{8} + \dfrac{2}{3}$

16. $\dfrac{2}{3} \big/ \dfrac{1}{4}$

Convert to Arabic numbers:

17. CDLX

18. MMCVII

Convert to Roman numerals:

19. 2010

20. 678

CHAPTER 8

Systems of Measurement

Quick Study

I. Common systems of measurement

    A. The household system: teaspoons, tablespoons, cups, pints, quarts, gallons, ounces, pounds

    B. The metric system: liters, milliliters, microliters, kilograms, grams, milligrams, micrograms

    C. The apothecary system: grains, drams, scruples, minims

II. International units and milliequivalents

    A. International units (IU or U): An arbitrary conversion to the metric system that varies with a particular drug. Used to describe dosage of drugs such as insulin, penicillin, etc.

    B. Milliequivalents (mEq): These terms refer to the number of positively charged ions per liter of a salt solution: the molecular weight of a salt or ion ÷ ionic charge = 1 Equivalent (Eq). 1/1000 Eq 1mEq.

III. Converting units between systems of measurement

    A. Use of conversion factors to change between systems of measurement (see Table 8-1)

    B. Determining the amount to dispense—converting between units of measure:

$$\text{Units on head} \times \frac{\text{units of order}}{\text{units on head}}$$

C. Converting between units of liquid measure:
  • Percent (*%w/w, %w/v, %v/v*)
  • Ratio (e.g., 1:100, 1:1,000)
D. Temperature conversions: degrees Fahrenheit (°F) = degrees Celsius (°C) × 9/5 (+ 32)

Common Systems of Measurement

There are three basic systems of measurement that are commonly used in the pharmacy. These are the household system, the **metric system**, and the **apothecary system**. Of these, the metric system is the most commonly used both on the order and on the manufacturer's label.

The Household (or Avoirdupois) System

This is the system that the average patient would use at home. It includes *teaspoons, tablespoons, cups, pints, quarts,* and *gallons* for liquid measure, and *ounces* or *pounds* for measuring weight. The physician's order and dosage instructions may be given in the metric system and should be translated into this system of measurement when possible, so the patient can understand and use it.

The Metric System

This is the system used in European countries and in all disciplines of science and medicine. Here volume is measured in *liters*: 1/1,000 of a liter is a *milliliter* (mL), and 1/1,000 of a milliliter is a *microliter* (mcL or μL). Less commonly used are *centiliters* (1/100 of a liter) and *deciliters* (1/10 of a liter). Weight is measured in *grams, milligrams,* and *micrograms* as well as the larger *kilogram*, which is 1,000 grams (kilograms are used in calculating per weight dosages; see Chapter 13).

The Apothecary System

The apothecary system is an archaic system that is seldom used in the United States. However, a few drugs are still prescribed using apothecary weights and volumes, and you will see these measurements on the exam. In this system, volume is measured in drams and weight in grains (see Table 8-1).

Table 8-1	Common Conversion Factors		
Unit of Measure	**Abbreviation**	**Conversion**	
grains	gr i	= 60 mg–65 mg	
1 pound household	lb	= 454 g;	= 16 oz
fluid ounce	℥ i oz	= 30 mL;	= 8 drams (6–8)
drams	ℨ i	= 4 mL; (5 mL)*	= 3 scruples
1 minim	ℳ i	= approximately 1 gtt	
teaspoon	1 tsp	= 5 mL	
tablespoon	1 tbsp	= 15 mL	
1 pint	1 pt	= 16 fl. oz	
1 quart	1 qt	= 2 pints;	≅ 1 L (960 mL actual)
1 gallon	1 gal	= 4 quarts	

*For calculating purposes, the dram is often converted to 5 mL.

International Units and Milliequivalents

There are two other types of measurement that the technician should be familiar with. These are the international unit (IU) and the milliequivalent (mEq). These expressions of drug concentration are used frequently in hospital pharmacy practice and will appear on the certification exam. You will be expected to understand and use these measurements in calculations.

The International Units

> Examples of drugs that are measured in units are insulin, heparin, and penicillin G.

The **international unit** system measures the amount of drug in units (IU or U). The milligram amount of drug per unit varies with the drug, so unless the conversion factor is given on the manufacturer's label or referenced, conversion from units to mg is not done. The international is used just like any other unit of measurement in calculations (e.g., mg, mL, g, etc.), so do not be intimidated by it.

Milliequivalents and Equivalents

A **milliequivalent** (**mEq**) refers to the number of positively charged ions per liter of salt solution. It is normally seen on solutions of salts, such as potassium chloride (KCl). One equivalent (Eq) is 1,000 mEq and is calculated by dividing the molecular weight of the element by the charge or valence. We determine both the molecular weight and charge from the periodic table of the elements.

We normally use *milli*equivalents rather than equivalents, and it will be stated on the drug label. Most labels will already have the milligram conversion listed. *Note:* It is not necessary to memorize molecular weights for the exam. They will be provided.

Converting between Systems of Measurement

A knowledge of conversion factors is necessary when receiving and dispensing orders. If an order is for "morphine gr iss," one must be able to quickly calculate that $1\frac{1}{2}$ grains is 90 mg, as the concentration of the morphine in stock will be expressed in the more modern metric system. Additionally, one must be able to interpret the order and place instructions on the label that the patient will be able to follow. For example, if an order is dispensed with the instructions "take 5 mL bid," the technician must be able to translate this into "take **1** teaspoonful twice a day," unless a calibrated spoon or dropper is dispensed with the medication, which allows the patient to measure the dose in milliliters.

Converting between systems is just a matter of memorizing conversion factors and using them. Since it is easier to calculate and dispense amounts using the metric system, conversions are usually done to and from the metric system (i.e., not from apothecary to avoirdupois, etc.). The conversion factors in Table 8-1 should be committed to memory.

Note that there are minor differences between the various systems. For example, 1 lb = 12 oz in the apothecary system but 16 oz in avoirdupois. And an ounce may vary from 28.6 g to 30 g depending on the system of measurement. This is of relatively minor importance in the actual practice of pharmacy; however, various conversions may appear on the exam. If the system is not stated, assume 16 oz in a pound and an ounce is 30 g (weight) or 30 mL (volume).

Do not confuse grains and grams. An old-fashioned way of abbreviating grams is gr. However, this is actually the abbreviation for grains. Grams should be abbreviated g or gm, not gr. The abbreviation gm is seldom used today because it can also be confused for grains (gr). Also note that when using the apothecary system, numbers go after the unit and are expressed in Roman numerals, unless the amount is less than $\frac{1}{2}$. If using Arabic numbers, the number appears before the unit. *For example:* gr v and gr ss are written correctly, but gr 5 and gr $\frac{1}{2}$ or v gr and ss gr are not correct.

> Do not confuse grains and grams! Grams should be noted as "g," not "gr."

Converting between Units of Measure

To calculate the amount of medication to dispense, the first thing one should do, before attempting the calculation, is *convert* the order into the metric system. Since this system is so simple to use, attempting the calculation using any other system would be much more difficult.

The technician should memorize the following metric conversions:

$$1 \text{ kilogram} = 1{,}000 \text{ grams}$$

$$1 \text{ gram} = 1{,}000 \text{ milligrams}$$

$$1 \text{ milligram} = 1{,}000 \text{ micrograms}$$

The conversion formula is as follows:

$$\text{Strength of units that you have} \times \frac{\text{Number of units thats you want}}{\text{Units that you have}}$$

For example, say the order is for 0.5 g of drug and our stock is in milligrams. We would set up the conversion, using the values in the list above, like this:

$$0.5 \cancel{g} \times \frac{1{,}000 \text{ mg}}{\cancel{g}} = 500 \text{ mg.}$$ Now we can continue with the calculation.

We can do the same when converting between systems. Say our order is in grains and we need to convert to milligrams. Table 8-1 tells us that there are 60 mg/gr. So,

> If 60 mg conversion does not produce the answer provided, or a number that makes sense, then recalculate using 65 mg for the conversion factor.

$$\text{gr i} \times \frac{60 \text{ mg}}{\cancel{\text{gr}}} = 60 \text{ mg}$$

Now that the order and stock are in the same units, our calculation can proceed.

Problem: We have an order for cough syrup, and the SIG reads: 10 mL po bid. What instructions should be put on the label for the patient?

Solution: The patient will probably use a teaspoon for measure. We need to convert the instructions into teaspoons. There are 5 mL per teaspoon, so:

$$10 \cancel{\text{mL}} \times \frac{1 \text{ tsp}}{5 \cancel{\text{mL}}} = 2 \text{ tsp}$$

The label should read, "Take two teaspoons of the syrup twice a day."

Problem: How many milligrams are in $1\frac{1}{2}$ grains?

1 gr = 60 mg, so using ratio proportion method you would get the following:

$$1 \text{ gr}/60 \text{ mg} = 1.5 \text{ gr}/\text{"X"}$$

$$1X = 60 \times 1.5 \ (90)$$

$$X = 90 \text{ mg}$$

So, $1\frac{1}{2}$ grains = 90 mg.

The key to conversion is to make sure that the units match and cancel properly. If we are looking for milligrams and have grains, for example, the grains would all have to cancel out (see above), leaving only milligrams. *The units that you do want should be the only ones left, and all the others should cancel out.*

EXAMPLE

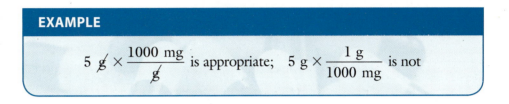

$$5\ \cancel{g} \times \frac{1000\ \text{mg}}{\cancel{g}} \text{ is appropriate;} \quad 5\ g \times \frac{1\ g}{1000\ \text{mg}} \text{ is not}$$

Units of Liquid Measure

There are different ways to describe a drug concentration in a specified amount of drug solution. The two most common ways to express a concentration are *percent* and *ratio*. Salt solutions are often expressed in percent: either weight/volume (*%w/v*), volume/volume (*%v/v*), or weight/weight (*%w/w*) percentages. The most common expression is weight per volume. (See Chapter 9 for a discussion of percentages.) Drugs such as epinephrine may be expressed in a ratio form.

Percentages

Percentages are expressed as parts per 100. These may be expressed as weight per volume (e.g., grams/100 mL), as volume per volume (mL/100 mL), or as a weight per weight percentage (g/100 g).

Converting Ratios

In a ratio, the number on the left is always grams, and the number on the right is milliliters (liquids), or grams (solids). For example, 1:1,000 is 1 g in 1,000 mL or 1 g in 1000 g!

The concentration of some drugs (e.g., epinephrine) is expressed in the form of a ratio. This may be 1:10, 1:100, or, most commonly, 1:1,000. The number on the left of the colon always means grams, and the number to the right is milliliters. Thus, 1:1,000 means 1 g/1,000 mL. Similarly, 1:100 = 1 g/ 100 mL (think—what is this in percent?) and 1:10 = 1 g/10 mL. Once the ratio is written out in grams per volume, it can be used in a calculation.

Temperature Conversions

The temperature scales used in pharmacy are the Fahrenheit (°F) and the centigrade or Celsius (°C) scales. Traditional temperature measurements (the household scale) are in °F, and in the scientific field (and in Europe), temperature is measured in °C. Conversion may be done as follows:

$$°C = (°F - 32) \times \left(\frac{5}{9}\right)$$

$$°F = °C \times \left(\frac{9}{5}\right) + 32$$

Remember that 0°C (32°F) is the freezing point of water. Thus, the temperature on the Fahrenheit scale is automatically 32° more than the Celsius scale (0° + 32°). Thus, when we convert between the Fahrenheit and Celsius scales, we must add or subtract that 32° difference. When converting from Fahrenheit to Celsius, we subtract 32° right away before doing the actual conversion to the Celsius scale. When converting the other way (from Celsius to Fahrenheit), we add the 32° *after* converting.

Remember, °F > °C! A temperature on the Fahrenheit scale is larger than that on the Celsius scale, even without the 32°. You will always wind up with a smaller number when converting °F to °C and a larger number when converting °C to °F.

Problem: If 25°C is room temperature, what is the room temperature in °F?

Solution: To obtain the temperature in degrees Fahrenheit, we must first multiply by the conversion factor and then *add 32*, as the freezing point of water is 32° Fahrenheit (0° Celsius). Thus:

$$25°C \times \left(\frac{9}{5}\right) + 32 = 77°F$$

Shortcut: Multiply 25°C by 9, divide by 5 + then add 32.

Chapter Review Questions

1. gr $\frac{1}{4}$ = _____ mg

2. 5 g = _____ mg

3. 100 mcg = _____ mg

4. 1 g = _____ mcg

5. gr i ss = _____ mg

6. gr i = _____ g

7. 1 t = _____ mL

8. 5 t = _____ mL

9. 10 g = _____ kg

10. 0.5 L = _____ mL

11. gr v = _____ mg

12. How many milliliters are in 3 drams?

13. How many microliters are in 0.5 L?

14. How many teaspoons are in one tablespoon?

15. How many milliliters are in 12 ounces?

16. How many drams are in 12 ounces?

17. 100 mcg = _____ g

18. 5°C = _____ °F

19. 86°F = _____ °C

20. −5°C = _____ °F

CHAPTER 9

Using Percentages and Ratios

Quick Study

I. The percentage as a unit of measure: A percentage is an amount divided by 100.
    - *Weight per volume* (*w/v*) = g/100 mL
    - *Weight per weight* (*w/w*) = g/100 g
    - *Volume per volume* (*v/v*) = mL/100 mL
    A. Converting from percent to milligrams when filling the order
    B. Using alligation to combine solutions when a specific percentage is desired

II. Using drug concentrations expressed as ratios: converting ratios to percentages and milligram amounts to fill an order. The following ratios should be memorized:
    - 1:1,000 = 1 mg/mL
    - 1:100 = 10 mg/mL
    - 1:10 = 100 mg/mL
    A. Converting from a percentage to a ratio: parts per 100, place parts on the left side of the ratio (e.g., 1% = 1:100)

Percentage: A Unit of Measure Expressed in Parts per 100

Before we begin working with percentages, we must define what a percent is. A percent is something divided by 100. This can mean one of three things:

- g of drug/100 mL of solution: This is called a weight per volume solution (*w/v*).
- g of drug/100 g of solid dosage form (e.g., cream, suppository): This is called a weight per weight (*w/w*). This type of percentage might be used to make a cream or ointment.
- mL/100 mL: This is called a volume per volume (*v/v*) percentage and is used in mixing two solutions.

When you see a % sign, always think amount per 100. The principle is the same for all percents, so we will concentrate here on the most commonly used: *w/v* percent. Whenever you have a fraction or ratio that you are trying to convert to a percent, you need to convert the top number to grams and get 100 mL on the bottom. Then you have a *w/v* percent.

> When you see a percent sign, think amount/100!

EXAMPLE

You have a solution of drug that contains 10 mg/mL. What is the percentage of drug in the solution?
Solution:

Step 1. A *w/v* percentage is always in **g** per 100 mL, so we must first convert the 10 milligrams to grams by moving the decimal place over three places to the left. Then rewrite 10 mg/mL as 0.01 g/mL.

Step 2. The denominator of the fraction must be 100 mL, so multiply both numerator and denominator by 100:

$$\frac{0.01 \text{ g}}{1 \text{ mL}} \times \frac{100}{100} = \frac{1 \text{ g}}{100 \text{ mL}} \text{ or } 1\%$$

Now we have converted 10 mg/mL into 1 g/100 mL, which is 1%.

When changing a fraction to a w/v percent, always think g/100. To change a percent to a fraction, do the opposite—express the percent as grams per 100 and simplify (2% = 2 g/100 mL).

EXAMPLE

You have 1 g of drug in 50 mL of solution. What is the percent of the solution?
Solution: Your ratio is 1 g/50 mL. You want g/100 mL. You have grams on the top of the ratio already, so leave that. You now need to have 100 mL on the bottom to get a percent. So you multiply the 50 mL on the bottom by 2. You must now multiply the top number by 2 (you are actually multiplying the whole fraction by 2/2, which is 1).

$$\frac{1 \text{ g}}{50 \text{ mL}} \times \frac{2}{2} = \frac{2 \text{ g}}{100 \text{ mL}}$$

Your solution is **2%**.

Converting a Drug Solution from Percent to Milligrams

What happens if the concentration of a drug solution is expressed in percent and the order is in milligrams? You can easily convert a percentage solution into mg/mL in order to fill a prescription.

EXAMPLE

You have a solution of 1% lidocaine. What is the concentration in mg/mL?

Solution: 1% = 1 g/100 mL

We want mg, not grams, so convert 1 g to 1,000 mg. Rewrite:

$$\frac{1,000 \text{ mg}}{100 \text{ mL}}$$

and cancel

$$\frac{1,0\cancel{00} \text{ mg}}{1\cancel{00} \text{ mL}} = \frac{10 \text{ mg}}{\text{mL}}$$

Now that you know the solution is 10 mg/mL, you can accurately draw up an order for 2 milligrams of lidocaine from the ampule (see Chapter 15).

EXAMPLE

How many mg are in 10 mL of the 1% solution?

Solution:

$$1\% = \frac{1g}{100 \text{ mL}} = \frac{1,0\cancel{00} \text{ mg}}{1\cancel{00} \text{ mL}} = \frac{10 \text{ mg}}{\text{mL}}$$

$$10 \text{mg/mL} \times 10 \text{ mL} = 100 \text{ mg}$$

> **Remember:** Concentration of drug × volume of solution = amount of drug

Using Alligation

Now we will address how to make a solution of a certain percentage from two existing solutions (of different concentrations) or solids. For this calculation, we can use a method called **alligation**. Alligation works when mixing two solutions that contain different percentages of drug to make a third solution of intermediate percentage.

EXAMPLE

You have a 20% solution and a 5% solution of calcium gluconate in stock. You need a 10% solution. How can you mix these two solutions together to get the 10% solution?

Solution: First make a chart, as follows:

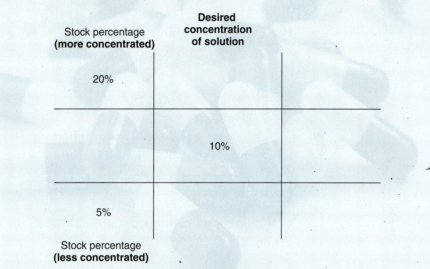

Note that the more-concentrated solution (the 20% stock) is in the upper-left corner and the less-concentrated solution (the 5% stock) is in the lower-left corner. The solution that you are trying to make (10%) goes in the middle. Note that the concentration of the solution that you are trying to make must have a concentration intermediate between the two stock solutions.

To calculate the amounts of each stock solution to mix, simply subtract diagonally and fill in the chart, as shown below:

$$20\% - 10\% = 10 \text{ parts.}$$

Since the 10 parts appears on the same line as the 5% solution, 10 parts of the 5% solution will be needed.

Similarly, $10\% - 5\% = 5$ parts, so five parts of the 20% solution will be needed.

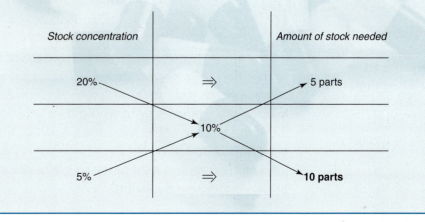

Making the Desired Solution

To make the 10% solution, you need to mix 5 parts of the 20% solution with 10 parts of the 5% solution.

The volume of a part depends on how much of the 10% solution you need to make. For example, in this problem you need to make 150 mL of the 10% solution. From the chart, you need 5 parts of the 20% solution and 10 parts of the 5% solution, which is 15 parts total. Because you need to make 150 mL of solution, the volume of one part would be:

$$\frac{\overset{10}{\cancel{150}} \text{ mL total}}{\underset{1}{\cancel{15}} \text{ parts}} = 10 \text{ mL per part}$$

Therefore, we add 100 mL (10 parts × 10 mL/part) of the 5% solution and 50 mL of the 20% solution (5 parts × 10 mL/part) to make 150 mL of the 10% solution.

To summarize:

- Fill in the alligation chart properly, with the desired concentration in the middle space.

- Subtract the numbers diagonally, placing the resulting numbers in the spaces on the right-hand side of the chart.

- Look across the top and bottom of the chart to determine the relative amounts of each solution to add together (number of parts of each).

- Add the number of parts together to obtain the total number of parts.

- Divide the desired volume of solution that you wish to make by the total number of parts to determine the amount of volume per part.

- Mix the two solutions together in the appropriate volumes.

Using Drug Concentrations Expressed as a Ratio

The Ratio

> A ratio is always expressed as grams per milliliters for liquids, with grams on the left and milliliters on the right:
>
> 1:1,000
> g mL

For the exam, you will need to know how to convert a ratio to a percentage and to convert dosage amounts from a ratio.

A *ratio* is written as two numbers separated by a colon (e.g., 1:10, 1:100, or 1:1,000). *The number on the left of the colon is always in grams, and the number to the right is in milliliters for liquids, and grams for solids.* Thus, a 1:1,000 solution of drug would have a concentration of 1 g of drug per 1,000 mL (1 mg/mL). Similarly, a 1:100 solution would have 1 g of drug per 100 mL, and so on.

Once the ratio is written out as grams per unit of volume, it can be used in the conversion calculation.

Converting from a Ratio Concentration to mg/mL

If you receive an order that is expressed in milligrams and your stock concentration is expressed in ratio configuration, you should first write out the ratio as grams per milliliters (e.g., a 1:100 ratio would be 1 g/100 mL). Then convert to milligrams per milliliter (e.g., 1,000 mg/100 mL), and cancel, as appropriate (e.g., 10 mg/mL). You now have the concentration in milligrams per milliliter and can proceed with the calculation.

To use a stock concentration that is expressed in a ratio to fill an order, first rewrite the ratio as grams/volume in milliliters. Then proceed with the calculation.

It might be helpful for you to memorize the three most commonly encountered ratios in terms of mg/mL. These are as follows:

$$1{:}1{,}000 = 1 \text{ mg/mL}$$

$$1{:}100 = 10 \text{ mg/mL}$$

$$1{:}10 = 100 \text{ mg/mL}$$

Problem: Your order is for 1 mg of epinephrine, and the available stock is a 1:100 solution. What volume is dispensed?

Solution: Step 1: Conversion of units:

Write down both order (1 mg) and stock (1:100 solution). Recall that 1:100 is 1 g/100 mL. The order is in mg, so first convert g to mg:

$$\frac{1\cancel{g} \times 1{,}000 \text{ mg}}{\cancel{g}} = 1{,}000 \text{ mg}$$

The stock concentration of $\dfrac{1g}{100 \text{ mL}}$ now becomes

$$\frac{1{,}0\cancel{0}0 \text{ mg}}{1\cancel{0}0 \text{ mL}} = \frac{10 \text{ mg}}{\text{mL}}$$

Step 2: Calculation:

Calculate the amount dispensed (Use the order ÷ stock method). The ratio-proportion method may also be used.

$$\text{Order: } \frac{1 \text{ mg}}{\text{Stock: } 10 \text{ mg/mL}} = 0.1 \text{ mL dispensed}$$

You dispense 0.1 mL of epinephrine to fill the order.

You may also see a problem on the exam that will ask you to calculate the dose received by the patient. Calculate this as follows:

Problem: You dispense a bolus injection of 0.5 mL of a 1:1,000 solution of epinephrine. Calculate the dose of epinephrine that the patient will receive.

Solution:

Step 1: Convert the stock to mg/mL:

$$\frac{1\,g}{1,000\,mL} = \frac{1,000\,mg}{1,000\,mL} = \frac{1\,mg}{mL}$$

Step 2: Set up the problem so that the units cancel, leaving you with a dose in mg:

$$0.5\,mL \times \frac{1\,mg}{mL} = 0.5\,mg$$

Converting from a Ratio to a Percentage

To convert from a ratio to a percentage, the calculation is easy. Simply convert the ratio into parts per 100.

> **EXAMPLE**
>
> Determine the percentage of drug in a 1:100 solution.
> *Solution:* 1:100 = 1 g per 100 mL. By definition, 1 g/100 mL = **1%**.

Chapter Review Questions

1. Express 1:1,000 in mg/mL.

2. An ophthalmic solution contains 1% drug solution. If a patient uses 0.2 mL of drug per eye, what is the dose of drug being placed in each eye?

3. A bottle contains 5 mL of a 2% solution. The dose is 5 mg. How many doses are contained in the bottle?

4. A suppository contains 5% zinc oxide. How much zinc oxide is contained in a 5 g suppository?

5. You need 80 mL of a 2% solution of boric acid. You have a 1% solution and a 5% solution in stock. How much of each solution do you need?

6. A procedure for making cortisone cream states that the cream contains 200 mg of cortisone per milliliter of cream. What is the percentage of cortisone?

7. You are making lactated Ringer's solution. The procedure calls for 20 g of lactic acid per liter. What is the percentage of lactic acid?

8. 500 mL of cream contains 5 g menthol. What is the percentage of menthol?

9. How many grams of zinc chloride are needed to make 1,500 mL of a 2% solution?

10. How many mg are in 15 mL of a 5% solution?

11. A solution contains 2 g of drug per 25 mL of solution. What is the percentage of drug in the solution?

12. You have 5 g of sodium chloride. How much saline (0.9% NaCl) can you make?

13. What is the concentration in mg/mL of a 7% solution?

14. Express 2% in terms of a ratio.

15. You need to make 100 mL of a 5% solution. You have 60 mL of a 10% solution and 50 mL of a 2% solution. Can you fill the order?

16. How many milligrams of cortisone are in 5 g of a 1% cortisone cream?

17. A solution of drug is 50 mg/mL. What is the percentage of drug in the solution?

18. How many mg of drug are in 5 mL of a 1:100 solution?

19. An order is for 0.50 g of magnesium sulfate, intravenously. The patient is a 55-year-old man, weighing 250 pounds, with a heart condition. The pharmacy has 3 mL and 5 mL syringes on hand, and a 50% solution of magnesium sulfate. Can the order be filled?

20. A procedure for compounding Compazine suppositories yields fifty 10 gram suppositories, each containing 0.25% Compazine. An order is for Compazine 0.25% suppositories BID. What is the dose of Compazine that the patient receives?

CHAPTER 10

Measuring Equipment

Quick Study

I.   Measurement of solutions: There are two types of liquid measurement.

    A. Measurement of small volumes
- Use of a calibrated syringe, dosage cup, or dropper
- Types of syringes
  1. The oral syringe
  2. Syringes for parenteral use
  3. The insulin syringe

    B. Choosing the appropriate measuring device: The size of any measuring container and calibrations should be appropriate to the volume to be measured.

    C. Measurement of larger volumes: Use of the graduated cylinder

II. Measurement of solid materials: Drug compounding

    A. Proper use of the torsion balance

    B. Proper use of the double-pan balance

    C. Proper use of the prescription balance

III. Pitfalls to inaccurate measurement (discussed throughout chapter)

- The effect of temperature on the accuracy of measurement
- Failure to use clean equipment
- Failure to read the volume measurement at the appropriate place (e.g., syringe plunger, meniscus of cylinder)
- Importance of proper size and calibration of measuring equipment

Types of Measurement

There are two types of measurement that we need to be concerned with: measurement of solid materials (which would be used in bulk compounding, for example) and liquid measurement. Because liquid measurement is the most common, we will begin the discussion here.

Liquid Measurement

Solutions and suspensions must be measured using accurate devices. For small volumes (less than 10 mL), a **syringe** or a small graduated cylinder may be used for accurate measure. For larger volumes (more than 10 mL), a **graduated cylinder** of appropriate size should be used.

- *The measuring device selected should be the closest possible size to the volume being measured.*

Choosing the Appropriate Measuring Device

In general, measuring devices for liquids are considered to be accurate to 20% of their volume. Graduations and markings are also less detailed on larger measuring devices, so the accuracy of measurement becomes less.

> **EXAMPLE**
>
> An order calls for 10 mL of solution for oral dosage. You have a graduated cylinder that holds 100 mL and one that holds 10 mL. If possible, the 10 mL cylinder (or a 10 mL syringe) should be used for the greatest accuracy in measurement. If these are not available, the size of device closest to the volume being measured should be chosen (e.g., a 20 mL syringe or 25 mL graduated cylinder).

- *Solutions should be measured all at once.*

Each time a solution is measured in a device, some solution clings to the inside when it is emptied. Syringes have a rubber plunger that fits closely to the sides of the barrel and helps to scrape off any material sticking to the sides, so less drug remains on the plastic. Even so, it is not necessarily a good practice to use any device more than once for measuring.

The Effects of Temperature on Liquid Measurement

Solutions should be measured at room temperature. The temperature of the solution or work area will affect the accuracy of drug measurement.

When liquids are warm, they expand and take up more volume. When cooled, they contract, and less volume will be measured. Thus, if we are in a warm room while measuring, the patient will actually get less drug, as the volume that we measured was deceptively expanded.

> **EXAMPLE**
>
> A drug solution is made in a room that was at 23°C (73°F). The concentration of the solution was 10 mg/mL. Later, the temperature of the room rose to 28°C (82°F), and an order was received for this drug, specifying a dose of 20 mg. The technician withdraws 2 mL of solution, assuming that it contains 20 mg of drug. The patient will not receive the correct dose in this case, as the volume of solution has expanded, while the amount of drug contained in the solution remained the same. The patient will be underdosed.

In the same way, if a solution made at room temperature is taken from the refrigerator, the volume measured will appear smaller. Unless the medication is allowed to warm to room temperature before measuring, the patient will get a solution of drug that is slightly more concentrated than what is desired. Temperature is also important in weight measurements (see below).

Devices for Measuring Liquids

There are essentially two types of measuring devices used in the dispensing of liquids: the graduated cylinder, which is used to measure and dispense liquids intended for oral dosage; and the syringe, which may be used to measure and dispense liquids intended for either oral or parenteral dosage.

Measuring Devices for Patient Use

Devices used by the patient for measuring are the *calibrated dropper, calibrated spoon, oral syringe,* and *dosage cup.* These devices are not used for dispensing but may be sent with the medication to allow the patient or caregiver to more accurately measure the medication. The dispensing of an accurate measuring device along with the prescription helps ensure accurate measurement of the medication and thus accurate dosing. If these calibrated devices are not dispensed, the patient may use a variety of devices for measure, from a household eyedropper, which may measure anywhere from 0.05 mL to 0.1 mL per drop, depending on the size of the dropper orifice; to a teaspoon, which may measure anywhere from 4 mL to 8 mL, depending on the silverware manufacturer. A *calibrated* measuring device, such as a calibrated dropper, has markings to show how much drug solution is actually being given, as opposed to a household eyedropper or teaspoon, which have no calibrations and dispense an unknown amount of drug. Calibrated spoons are often adjustable and can be used with more than one prescription.

The Oral Syringe

The oral syringe and dosage cup are also used for oral dosing. The oral syringe may look like a syringe for parenteral administration, but it has no needle attachment, which precludes the nurse or technician from mistakenly administering an oral medication by injection. An oral syringe also may simply look like a fat plastic syringe with a rubber squeeze bulb at the top, such as the kind commonly sold in drugstores. Again, the calibrations, which are in milliliters, make accurate dosing easier (no conversion is necessary).

The Dosage Cup

The dosage cup is plastic and holds one ounce (30 mL). It normally has markings on the sides for measurement in all three systems: drams, milliliters, and the maximum volume of one ounce. The smallest amount that can be accurately measured in a dosage cup is one dram (4 mL). Note that the measurements on a dosage cup are really not very accurate; they are designed for things like cough syrups, where an overdose or underdose of a milliliter or two is not critical. In fact, none of the calibrated equipment for measuring oral dosages are very accurate. The exception would be an oral syringe designed to dispense oral liquids and suspensions accurately, similar to a syringe for parenteral injections.

> Calibrated equipment for oral dosage is of limited accuracy!

Dispensing Large Volumes of Liquid—The Graduated Cylinder

When dispensing a large volume of a liquid for oral use, a graduated cylinder is normally used. This is a glass or plastic cylinder that has graduations, or markings for measurement, on the sides (see Figure 10-1). When using a plastic cylinder, you may simply fill the cylinder to the appropriate mark and read the correct volume from the marking scale. However, when using a glass cylinder, measurement is a little more complicated. In a plastic cylinder, the top of the liquid appears as a straight line and is easy to read. However, in a glass cylinder, the light from the room refracts off the glass and causes an optical illusion that the surface of the liquid inside the cylinder is curved. This "curved" portion is called the **meniscus**. When reading the correct volume from a glass cylinder, one must look not at the top of the liquid but at the bottom of the curved part (meniscus). Graduated cylinders can be calibrated, if necessary, by filling the cylinder with an amount of water and weighing it (1 mL of water should weigh 1 g at 25°C).

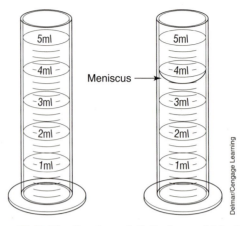

Figure 10-1: The Graduated Cylinder and Meniscus

Accurately Dispensing Small Volumes Using a Syringe

The syringe for injection is made of sterile plastic and is made to accommodate a needle. In contrast, the oral syringe, which is not sterile, does not accommodate a needle. It is made for oral dosing, as discussed previously. The sterile syringe is accurately calibrated. The type of calibrations depend on the size of the syringe.

> **EXAMPLE**
>
> A 0.5 mL syringe is calibrated in increments of 0.005 mL; a 1 mL syringe (tuberculin, or TB syringe) in increments of 0.01 mL; and the larger sizes (3, 5, and 10 mL) in increments of 0.1 mL (see Figure 10-2). *A syringe is only accurate to the smallest calibration on the barrel!*

Accurately Measuring Volumes in a Syringe

When a syringe is used, *the amount of solution drawn up is measured by the first black line* (nearest the plunger tip) made by the side of the plunger, *not the rubber cone* that extends into the solution (see Figure 10-2). Again, solutions should be as close to room temperature as possible (without harming the drug) before measuring to avoid errors in measurement.

Dispensing Insulin

Insulin syringes are to be used for the measurement of insulin only!

Syringes intended for the administration of insulin are used only for that purpose. They are calibrated in **units**. *These units are specific to the concentration of normal (U-100) insulin only.* They may not be used with any other drug that might be measured in units (e.g., heparin, streptomycin, penicillin), as the amount of drug per unit varies with the drug.

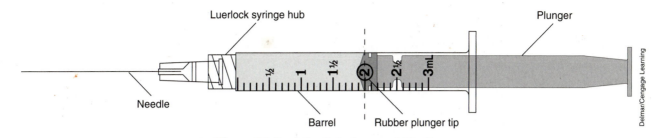

Delmar/Cengage Learning

Figure 10-2: *A 3 mL Syringe and Needle*

The needle on the syringe is permanently attached and is usually a 28–31 gauge needle (abbreviated on the packaging as 31G; you may also see "ga" used, which is an older abbreviation). This needle is very fine and easily bent. (See Chapter 14 for a discussion of needles.)

Using a Tuberculin Syringe to Dispense Insulin

Note that 100 units of normal insulin is equivalent to 1 mL volume. This conversion is important, because, if no insulin syringes are available, a tuberculin (1 mL) syringe may be used as follows: the amount of insulin dispensed can be calculated by dividing the order by 100 units/mL (normal insulin), to obtain the amount to dispense in milliliters. The insulin can then be dispensed in a tuberculin (1 mL) syringe with a 30G needle or, in an emergency, a standard 25G or 27G needle.

> Remember: 1 cc (1 mL) of U-100 insulin 100 units

Measuring Solids

Measuring devices are normally not used to dispense a solid drug (e.g., tablet, capsule) directly. However, if a solution or semisolid dosage form is to be compounded (a procedure that the technician may legally perform if written instructions exist; see Chapter 18), a weight scale may be used. To accurately weigh a gram of material or more, there are several methods. Weighing very small amounts requires a prescription balance.

Weighing Large Quantities

To weigh large quantities of material, such as that required to make a solution, a **solution balance** may be used. This balance has only one weighing pan, which hangs at the end of the scale, and is not very sensitive (thus it could not be used to weigh small quantities).

Another piece of equipment designed for weighing large quantities is the **double-pan balance** (or counterbalance). This is the oldest of the devices used for weighing large quantities (grams and kilograms). This device balances (or hangs) two pans opposite each other and works on the principle of gravity. The material to be weighed is placed on one pan. On the other is

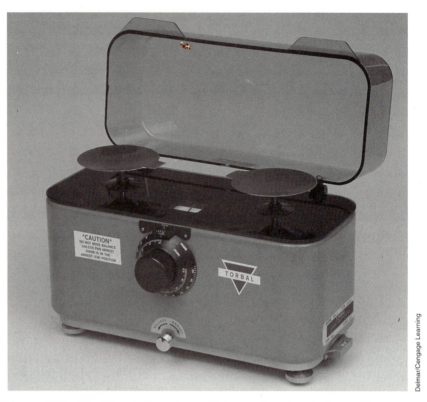

Figure 10-3: The Class A Prescription Balance, Required in Every Pharmacy, Has a Scale Sensitivity of 6 mg to 120 g

placed one or more carefully calibrated counterweights. When the two pans balance, the weight of the material is equal to the weight of the counterweights, and the weight of the material can be determined (each counterweight weighs a specific amount, which is printed on it).

If very small quantities are to be weighed, the **prescription balance** is used (see Figure 10-3). This is a very sensitive instrument, weighing as little as 5 or 6 mg accurately, but it cannot weigh large quantities; the largest amount that can be weighed is about 100–120 g. It is sometimes called a Class A prescription balance.

Factors That Affect the Accuracy of Weight Measurement

When these instruments are used to weigh material, *the positions of the material being weighed and the counterweights on the surface of the weighing pans are critical for accurate measurement.* Both the material to be weighed and the counterweights (if any) must be placed *exactly* in the middle of the weighing pan(s). If they are not, the weight obtained for the material will not be accurate, because the pan will list to one side. Also, when using counterweights, the counterweights should not be touched, as skin oil from the fingers adds weight. Forceps or padded tweezers should always be used to carefully handle the weights.

> Temperature is critical in weight measurements! A difference in temperature between the scale and the material being weighed will cause the formation of air currents, which will result in inaccurate measurement!

The Effect of Temperature on Weight Measurement

As with liquid measurement, *temperature is critical in weight measurements.* With solid measurements, however, the expansion of the material with temperature is not the problem. A difference in the temperature of the material in relation to that of the scale will actually change the weight measurement. If the material to be weighed is warm, it will warm the air around it, creating air currents that surround the material and rise, slightly lifting the material off the pan and causing the weight reading to be lower than it really is. This can make a big difference in the weight measurement. As the material cools, more of the material will rest on the pan and the weight will then appear to increase, so that if it is weighed several times, the weights will vary as the material cools. (If your scale is cold and the material that you are weighing is at room temperature, you may have the same effect.) Weighing any material when warm or cold will result in an inaccurately prepared drug product.

Chapter Review Questions

1. To accurately measure 15 mL of cough syrup, a _____ should be used.
   a. 10 mL graduated cylinder, used twice
   b. 10 mL syringe, used twice
   c. 20 mL graduated cylinder
   d. 50 mL graduated cylinder

2. You dispense 10 mL of a suspension for oral dosing (10 mg/mL at 25°C), directly from the refrigerator. As a result, the patient could:
   a. be overdosed
   b. be underdosed
   c. receive the correct dose
   d. none of the above are true

3. In order to be sure that an accurate amount of ophthalmic solution is placed into the eye, the patient should be provided with:
   a. a dosage cup
   b. an eyedropper
   c. a calibrated eyedropper
   d. a syringe

4. When a graduated cylinder made of glass is used, an accurate reading of the amount of fluid measured would be made by looking at the:
   a. top of the fluid in the cylinder
   b. sides of the meniscus
   c. bottom of the meniscus
   d. marking on the cylinder that is closest to the fluid

5. At 25°C, 1 mL of water weighs:
   a. 10 mg
   b. 5 g
   c. 100 mg
   d. 1 g

6. When a double-pan balance is used to weigh material for compounding, the:
   a. sample and weights should be placed in the middle of their pans
   b. weights should not be touched
   c. the material to be weighed and the balance should both be at room temperature
   d. all of the above are true

7. A cream compounded by the technician that was supposed to contain 2% cortisone was found to contain 2.2% cortisone. A probable explanation might be that:
   a. the technician handled the counterweights when weighing
   b. the cortisone was warmer than the scale
   c. the cortisone was weighed on the wrong type of scale
   d. the technician did not put in enough cortisone

8. A household teaspoon measures:
   a. exactly 5 mL
   b. between 4 mL and 8 mL
   c. more accurately than an oral syringe
   d. exactly 10 mL

9. An insulin syringe is used for:
   a. insulin only
   b. any drug measuring less than 1 mL
   c. skin test antigens
   d. none of the above

10. Class A scales are:
    a. used in all pharmacies
    b. sensitive from 6 mg to 120 g
    c. used by pharmacists only
    d. a and b are correct

CHAPTER 11

Conversion of Solid Dosage Forms

Quick Study

I. Dosage conversion

    - Converting between units, to match the order to the available stock
    - Order stock amount dispensed
    - Using the ratio-proportion method

II. Converting between measurement systems

    - Conversion between the metric, household, and apothecary systems

Dosage Conversion—Solid Dosage Forms

Pharmacies stock only a limited supply of drugs and drug dosage forms, compared to what is available. Perhaps one strength of a particular drug tablet is more commonly prescribed than another, so the pharmacy stocks only the strength that is most commonly ordered. The prescriber does not necessarily have much knowledge of the pharmacy or its formulary, so it is necessary, on occasion, to *convert* the order to match the stock available. This can be done only if the dosage form is appropriate to the conversion— scored tablets, for example. To convert an order, we must follow three steps:

1. Make sure that the units (e.g., mg, g) of both the order and the stock match. If they do not, convert one to match the other. (Which one

is converted really makes no difference. It is preferable to convert the order to match the stock.)

2. Divide the order by the available stock (or use the ratio-proportion method, as discussed below) to obtain the amount dispensed.

3. Make sure that your answer is appropriate for patient administration.

EXAMPLE

You calculate that ten tablets must be dispensed from your stock for one dose to fill a prescription order. A patient is not going to take ten tablets at once, so a higher dosage strength should be used.

Let's do some problems.

Problem: You have an order for Lasix tabs #30, 80 mg bid. The pharmacy has only 40 mg tablets.

Solution: Divide the order by the stock, to get the number of tablets dispensed.

Remember: Order ÷ stock = amount dispensed per dose

Step 1. *Write down the information that you have.* (If you are faced with a "story" problem on the exam, this is especially useful.) You must first ask yourself what the question is asking—what does the examiner want to know? Then think of how you would figure it out, go to the problem, and extract the appropriate information. That way, you will not be confused by extra information that may be given in the problem.

$$\text{order} = 80 \text{ mg tablets}$$

$$\text{stock available} = 40 \text{ mg tablets}$$

Step 2. Divide the order by the stock.

$$\frac{80\,\text{mg}}{\text{dose}} \div \frac{40\,\text{mg}}{\text{tablet}} = 2 \text{ tablets dispensed per dose}$$

Since the order is for 30 of the 80 mg tablets, we dispense 30 × 2, or 60 tablets of the 40 mg strength.

A second and very valuable way to do this type of calculation is by the *ratio-proportion* method. This method is very helpful, particularly for liquid dosage conversions (see Chapters 12 and 14). In this method, we make a *ratio* of the order and a ratio of the stock and set them equal, solving algebraically.

> **When faced with a problem:**
>
> 1. List the information given.
> 2. Determine what the question is asking.
> 3. Determine the best way to find the answer.
> 4. Extract the information needed to solve the problem.

EXAMPLE

Again, the order is for 40 Lasix tablets, 80 mg strength.

Step 1. Tabulate the order and the available stock and set them equal.

$$\frac{80\,mg}{dose} = [order] = \frac{40\,mg}{tablet} = [stock]$$

Step 2. Cross-multiply:

$$80\ mg \times 1\ tablet = 40\ mg \times 1\ dose$$

Divide both sides of the equation to get the number of tablets per dose:

$$\frac{80\ \cancel{mg} \times 1\ tablet}{40\ \cancel{mg} \times 1\ dose} = 2\ \text{tablets per dose}$$

Problem: Your order is for haloperidol tablets, 0.25 mg. You have 0.5 mg tablets in stock.

Solution:

$$\frac{\text{Order}}{\text{Stock}} = \frac{0.25\,mg/dose}{0.5\,mg/tablet} = 1/2\ \text{tablet per dose}$$

Matching Up the Units

As discussed previously, whenever you work with a number problem, you must make sure that the *units* assigned to the numbers (e.g., g, mg, gr, etc.) are the same before attempting to solve the problem. In other words, if your order is in milligrams and your stock is in grams, you must first convert either the stock to milligrams or the order to grams before beginning the calculation. If you encounter international units and you need to convert, the conversion factor (if available) should be on the product label—for instance, 250 mg of penicillin G is 400,000 U. If no conversion factor is available, the dosage conversion cannot be done.

Problem: Your order is for ampicillin, 0.5 g per dose. The pharmacy stocks ampicillin in 250 mg capsules.

Solution: First, recalling that there are 1,000 mg/g, convert the 0.5 g to mg to match the stock.

$$0.5\ \cancel{g} \times \frac{1,000\,mg}{1\ \cancel{g}} = 500\,mg$$

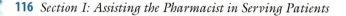

Then, do the calculation:

$$\text{Order} \div \text{stock} = 500 \text{ mg}$$

$$\frac{^{2}5\cancel{00} \text{ mg /dose}}{_{1}250 \text{ mg /capsule}} = 2 \text{ capsules per dose}$$

Be aware, however, that the calculation could not be done the opposite way! Since capsules cannot be accurately broken in half, an order for 250 mg could not be filled if the pharmacy stocked only 500 mg capsules.

Converting between Measurement Systems

Although the apothecary system is rather archaic, you may still receive orders signed in grains or (rarely) drams (scruples and minims are not commonly used in practice; however, they may appear on the exam). Know how to convert between the metric and apothecary systems (see Chapter 8 for review). *Remember:* convert the units first, before continuing with the problem.

Problem: You have an order for thyroid gr $\frac{1}{4}$ po bid prn. You have 30 mg tablets in stock (scored in fourths). What do you dispense?

Solution: One dose is $\frac{1}{4}$ grain. Recall that gr i is 60 mg. First, convert the units. In this case, convert grains to milligrams, since they are easier to work with:

$$1/4 \text{ grain} \times \frac{60 \text{ mg}}{\text{grain}} = 15 \text{ mg ordered}$$

Then, do the calculation:

$$\frac{^{1}\cancel{15} \text{ mg}}{_{2}\cancel{30} \text{ mg/tablet}} = \frac{1}{2} \text{ tablet dispensed}$$

> Do not let the various units confuse you! As long as the units match between order and stock, the calculation can be done.

Problem: You have an order for penicillin G, 200,000 U q4h. You have 400,000 U strength tablets in stock.

Solution:

$$\frac{^{1}2\cancel{00},\cancel{000} \text{ U}}{_{2}4\cancel{00},\cancel{000} \text{ U tablet}} = \frac{1}{2} \text{ tablet}$$

Chapter Review Questions

Calculate the amount of tablets dispensed, per dose, given the following:

1. You have an order for Decadron 1.5 mg po bid. You have 750 mcg tabs in stock.

2. Your order is for prednisolone 0.005 g po q6h. You have 5 mg tabs in stock.

3. Your order is for levothyroxine 125 mcg po qd. Your stock is 0.25 mg tabs, scored in half.

4. Your order is for morphine gr ss. Your stock is 30 mg tabs.

5. Your order is for furosemide 80 mg bid. You have 40 mg Lasix tabs in stock.
   a. Dispense a unit dose.
   b. Dispense a daily dose.

6. Your order is for phenytoin 60 mg tid. You have Dilantin, 30 mg capsules.
   a. Dispense a unit dose.
   b. Dispense a daily dose.

7. Your order is for Orinase, 250 mg. Your stock is 0.5 g tablets (scored).

8. Your order is for penicillin, 600,000 U po. You have 250 mg tabs in stock. The label says that one 250 mg tablet contains 400,000 U. The tablets are scored in half.

9. You have an order for Synthroid 0.1 mg. You have 50 mcg tablets available.

10. Your order is for aspirin gr v. You have 300 mg tablets available.

11. Your order is for morphine gr iss. You have 30 mg tablets in stock.

12. Your order is for KCl, 20 mEq. You have 10 mEq tablets in stock.

13. Your order is for morphine 1gr. You have 30 mg tablets in stock.

14. You have a vial containing 500 mg of morphine. How many doses of gr iss can be filled from the vial?

15. You have an order for 40 mg of isosorbide dinitrate, controlled-release tablets. The pharmacy has 20 mg controlled-release tablets in stock.

CHAPTER 12

Conversion of Liquid Dosage Forms

Quick Study

I. Converting units between liquid and solid dosage forms (e.g., solid to liquid dosages)

- Simplifying the stock concentration: a stock solution expressed in mg/mL is easier to work with
- Use of fractions: multiplication and division of fractions
- Using the ratio/proportion method to convert between liquid and solid dosage forms
- Use of the "order over stock" method

Converting between Liquid and Solid Dosage Forms

In the hospital pharmacy, it may be necessary to convert an order for a drug that is expressed in solid amounts (e.g., grams, grains) to a liquid or suspension. For example, a physician may order furosemide 80 mg po but may ask for the dosage form to be an oral solution instead of a tablet. Instead of counting out one 80 mg tablet, you would have to determine the proper amount of solution to dispense. The same type of calculation would be used to determine the amount of drug to be dispensed for injection as well (see Chapter 15); the difference is that the drug solution or suspension is handled differently.

Hint: You may wish to review fractions covered in Chapter 7 before continuing. The type of calculation used for these problems requires a thorough knowledge of fractions.

Problem: You have an order for 500 mg of cephalexin in suspension. In stock is Keflex suspension, reconstituted to 125 mg/2 mL. How much would you dispense?

Solution: To do the problem by the "order over stock" method, you need to review fractions (see Chapter 7). Fractions are especially useful if the drug concentration is expressed as an amount of drug in a volume of solution that is greater (or less) than 1 mL (for example, 2 mg/5 mL):

$$\frac{\text{Order: } 500\,\text{mg}}{\text{Stock: } 125\,\text{mg}/2\,\text{mL}} = 500\,\text{mg} \times \frac{2\,\text{mL}}{125\,\text{mg}}$$

$$= (500\,\text{mg} \times 2\,\text{mL}) \div 125 = 8\,\text{mL}$$

Ratio/proportion method: $\dfrac{125\,\text{mg}}{2\,\text{mL}} = \dfrac{500\,\text{mg}}{X}$

$$500\,\text{mg} \times 2\,\text{mL} = 125\,\text{mg} \times X$$

$$1000\,\text{mg}/125\,\text{mg} = X$$

$$8\,\text{mL} = X$$

Hint: In general, it is a good idea to simplify as much as possible before starting; it saves a lot of time, effort, and potential mistakes. Let's do a problem that requires conversion.

Problem: You need 50 mg of drug. Your stock is a 5% solution.

Solution: Step 1. Convert the units of measurement so that order and stock match. Calculate the concentration of the stock in mg/mL:

Recall that 5% is 5 g/100 mL.

The order is in milligrams, so we must convert the 5 g to mg: 5 g = 5,000 mg, so the concentration of the stock is

$$\frac{5,000\,\text{mg}}{100\,\text{mL}} = 50\,\text{mg}/\text{mL}$$

Step 2. Do the calculation.

Order = 50 mg, stock = 50 mg/mL

$$\text{Order} \div \text{stock } \frac{\overset{1}{50\,\text{mg}}}{\underset{1}{50\,\text{mg}}/\text{mL}} = 1\,\text{mL to be dispensed}$$

Now, let's try a problem where the concentration is not so easily simplified.

Problem: You have an order for potassium chloride, 30 mEq po qd.

Your stock is KCl 20 mEq/15 mL. Dispense one dose.

Solution: First, simplify as much as possible. The stock concentration can be simplified by dividing both numbers by 5:

$$\frac{^4\cancel{20} \text{ mEq}}{_3\cancel{15} \text{ mL}}$$

The concentration becomes 4 mEq/3 mL.

Now we can do the problem. This can be done in one of two ways: the "order over stock" method, or ratio/proportion. Both will be demonstrated.

The "Order Over Stock" Method

$$\text{Order:} \frac{30\,\text{mEq}}{\text{Stock:} \ 4\,\text{mEq}/3\,\text{mL}} = 30\,\cancel{\text{mEq}} \times \frac{3\,\text{mg}}{4\,\cancel{\text{mEq}}} = 22.5 \text{ mL dispensed}$$

The Ratio/Proportion Method

Here we set the two ratios equal to each other and solve algebraically:

3 mL of stock = 4 mEq

30 mEq ordered = X mL

Step 1. Rewrite the information:
3 mL of stock = 4 mEq
"X" mL ordered = 30 mEq

Step 2. Set the ratios equal:

$$\frac{4 \text{ mEq [stock]}}{3 \text{ mL}} = \frac{30 \text{ mEq [order]}}{\text{X mL dispensed}}$$

The *X* is going to give us the number of milliliters to dispense. We want to get the *X* by itself on one side of the equation with numbers on the other side, so we can figure out the volume to be dispensed.

Step 3. We **cross-multiply** both sides of the equation:

$$\frac{30\,\text{mEq}}{\text{X mL}} \diagdown\diagup \frac{4\,\text{mEq}}{3\,\text{mL}}$$

and

$$30 \text{ mEq} \times 3 \text{ mL} = 4 \text{ mEq} \times (X)$$

Step 4. Divide both sides of the equation by 4 mEq, so that we can get the amount dispensed by itself on one side:

$$\frac{30 \cancel{\text{ mEq}} \times 3 \text{ mL}}{4 \cancel{\text{ mEq}}} = 22.5 \text{ mL dispensed}$$

> **Units are very important. If you do not put in the units and cancel them, you will have no idea if your calculation is correct!**

Note: Notice that the mEq units cancel out, leaving only mL. It is very important that the units you don't want (mEq, in this case) cancel out in the problem, leaving the units that you do want (mL).

Hint: Even if you are really not sure how to set up a calculation on the exam, if you set it up so that the units you don't want cancel and the ones you do want stay in the problem, it will probably be right.

Setting Up the Ratio Properly

It should be noted that, at the beginning of the ratio/proportion calculation, the two ratios were arranged so that the units on the *top* of the ratio on the left side were the same as those on the *top* of the ratio on the right. In the same way, the units on the bottom of the ratio are also the same on both sides of the equal sign. It does not matter where the units are placed (e.g., on the top or bottom of the ratio), as long as the placement is the same on both sides, as shown below.

EXAMPLE

The ratio is written correctly, with the units on the top and bottom matching across:

$$\frac{30 \text{ } mEq}{X \text{ mL}} = \frac{4 \text{ } mEq}{3 \text{ mL}}$$

Writing the ratio as:

$$\frac{X \text{ } mL}{30 \text{ mEq}} = \frac{3 \text{ } mL}{4 \text{ mEq}}$$

would also be correct, since units match across the equal sign.

> **If the ratio is set up properly, the units will cancel when you cross-multiply. If the units do not cancel properly, the ratios have been set up wrong and need to be corrected.**

However, writing the ratio as:

$$\frac{30 \text{ mEq}}{X \text{ } mL} = \frac{3 \text{ } mL}{4 \text{ mEq}}$$

would not be correct.

Chapter Review Questions

Practice solving the problems by both ratio/proportion and "order over stock" methods.

1. Your order is for promethazine syrup 12.5 mg po tid. The stock solution is 6.25 mg/5 mL. What amount is dispensed?

2. Your order is for erythromycin/sulfisoxazole suspension 0.75 g po. You have a solution in stock that is 200 mg/5 mL. What amount is dispensed?

3. Your order is for sulfisoxazole suspension 300 mg po stat. You have a solution in stock that is 250 mg/5 mL. What amount is dispensed?

4. Your order is for cyclosporine 150 mg po. You have a solution in stock that is 100 mg/mL. What amount is dispensed?

5. Your order is for hydrocortisone cypionate suspension 30 mg. You have a solution in stock that is 10 mg/5 mL. What amount is dispensed?

6. Your order is for theophylline 40 mg. You have a solution in stock that is 80 mg/15 mL. What amount is dispensed?

7. Your order is for ampicillin 0.5 g. You have a solution in stock that is 250 mg/5 mL. What amount is dispensed?

8. Your order is for Prozac 10 mg. You have a solution in stock that is 20 mg/5 mL. What amount is dispensed?

9. Your order is for theophylline 120 mg. You have a solution in stock that is 80 mg/5 mL. What amount is dispensed?

10. Your order is for Lasix 40 mg po. You have a solution in stock that is 10 mg/mL. What amount is dispensed?

CHAPTER 13

Pediatric Dosages

Quick Study

I.   Computation of pediatric doses

   A.   Computation of dose by body weight (in pounds or kilograms)
   - mg/kg of body weight
   - (weight of the child adult dose) ÷ 1.7

   B.   Computation of dose by body surface area (BSA)
   - Using a nomogram to determine BSA
   - Body surface area in m² dose in mg/m²

   C.   Young's Rule and Clark's Rule

$$\text{Young's Rule:} \frac{\text{age of child in years}}{(\text{age} + 12)} \times \text{adult dose}$$

$$\text{Clark's Rule:} \frac{\text{weight of child}}{150} \times \text{adult dose}$$

II.   The recommended daily dosage range—calculation of safe doses

   A.   The safe dose and safe dose range
   - Use of the manufacturer's label adult dose

Computation of Doses on the Basis of Body Weight or Surface Area

Computation of Dose by Body Weight

The proper dose of drug to administer to a patient (adult or child) is often calculated based on the patient's body weight. The suggested doses for these drugs are often expressed on the manufacturer's label as a number of milligrams per kilogram of body weight. *A child's dose will always be smaller than the adult dose*—the adult dose may be divided by a factor of 1.7 to obtain the child's dose (see Calculating Child's Dose for examples).

Problem: A child weighs 25 kg. The recommended adult dose is 10 mg/kg. Calculate the dose.

Solution: The weight of the patient is already expressed in kilograms, so no conversion is necessary. Simply multiply the recommended dose in mg/kg by the weight of the patient:

$$25 \text{ kg} \times \frac{10 \text{ mg/kg}}{\text{dose}} = 250 \text{ mg/dose}$$

It is important not to be confused here by the term *dose*. The dose is how much we give the patient *per unit of body weight*. The per-weight dosage is used to calculate how much drug is actually administered to the patient.

Problem: The patient weighs 35 kg. The recommended adult dose for the drug is 2 mg/kg. Calculate the dose for the patient.

Solution: Again, no conversion is necessary. The patient should receive 2 mg for every kg of body weight (35 kg):

$$2 \text{ mg} \times 35 \text{ kg} = 70 \text{ mg/dose}$$

Occasionally, we may need to convert the patient's weight (adult or child) into kilograms before beginning the calculation, if it is expressed in pounds.

Problem: A patient weighs 44 lb and receives a drug with a recommended dose of 10 mg/kg. Calculate the dose.

Solution: This time, we need to first convert the patient's weight into kilograms. Recall that there are *2.2 lb per kilogram* (see Chapter 8):

$$\frac{44 \text{ lb}}{2.2 \text{ lb/kg}} = 20 \text{ kg}$$

Then, calculate the dose:

$$20 \text{ kg} \times \frac{10 \text{ mg}}{\text{kg}} = 200 \text{ mg}$$

Computation of Dose by Body Surface Area (BSA)

In this method, the dose is related to the size of the person rather than the weight. This is the most accurate way to dose medications. The **body surface area (BSA)** is the total area of the surface of the body, as if we were to remove all of the skin and lay it out to be measured. This way, the dose relates to how *large* the person is, rather than how much he or she weighs. This calculation is often used in pediatrics and chemotherapy. Pediatric patients vary in size and weight at similar ages, so this is far more accurate. Chemotherapy is so toxic that it is important to dose as accurately as possible.

Measurement of Body Surface Area

To find a person's body surface area, you could use a **nomogram**. This is a chart that relates the height and weight of a person to his or her body surface area. To use this chart, you will need a ruler. First, determine the height and weight of the patient, making sure that the units are in the same system (i.e., height in meters and weight in kilograms, or height in inches with weight in pounds).

- *Height:* Find the height of the patient on the scale at the left of the chart, making sure to use the scale in the appropriate units.

- *Weight:* Find the weight of the patient on the scale at the right of the chart.

- *BSA:* Lay the ruler between the two points (height and weight) and draw a line between them. The line will intersect a scale in the middle of the chart. Read the number from this scale, and you have the patient's BSA in m^2. (Since a nomogram is presently not included in the PTCB exam, it will not be presented here. However, any pharmacy math text should have a nomogram for practice. Examinees will, however, be expected to perform calculations relating to body surface area, using information provided.)

Thus, the recommended dose is given in mg of drug/m^2. We can use the BSA in the following two ways. Body surface area is measured in square meters (m^2).

- *Computing a dose for an individual patient.* This is accomplished by multiplying the body surface area of the patient in m^2 by the dose in mg/m^2—giving a dose in mg or mL.

- *Checking the prescribed dose for safety.* This is accomplished by dividing the dose by the BSA of the patient, which results in the amount of drug administered. This amount is then compared to the safe-dose range on the manufacturer's label.

Problem: Using a BSA of 0.4 m^2, calculate the dose for a patient prescribed 40 mg/m^2 kanamycin.

Solution: Simply multiply the BSA by the prescribed dose:

$$40 \text{ mg/m}^2 \times 0.4 \text{ m}^2 = 16 \text{ mg}$$

The nomogram is not used much anymore. Formulas are more accurate and most pharmacy computer programs have these formulas in their data banks. There is one formula for patient measures in pounds and inches, and another for patient measures in kilograms and centimeters.

EXAMPLE

A patient weighs 66 pounds and is 42 inches tall.

$$BSA = \sqrt{\frac{pounds \times inches}{3131}} = \sqrt{\frac{66 \times 42}{3131}} = \sqrt{0.8853} = 0.94 \text{ m}^2$$

EXAMPLE

A patient weighs 30 kg and is 106 cm tall.

$$BSA = \sqrt{\frac{kg \times cm}{3600}} = \sqrt{\frac{30 \times 106}{3600}} = \sqrt{0.8833} = 0.94 \text{ m}^2$$

Calculating a Child's Dose (Ages 2–12)

Doses for pediatric patients are calculated differently from adult doses. This is due to the differences in size, weight, and degree of organ development between adults and children. To determine the dose for a child, we divide the adult dose by a conversion factor of 1.7, as described previously.

Problem: The recommended adult dose of a drug is 2 mg/kg. Calculate the dose for a 34 kg child.

Solution: Begin by calculating the adult dose as before:

$$2 \text{ mg/kg} \times 34 \text{ kg} = 68 \text{ mg/dose}$$

Then divide by the conversion factor to determine the child's dose:

$$\frac{68 \text{ mg}}{1.7} = 40 \text{ mg per child's dose}$$

Problem: Using a BSA of 0.4 m², calculate the dose for a child, if the adult dose of kanamycin prescribed is 40 mg/m².

Solution: Simply multiply the BSA by the prescribed dose, to obtain the adult dose:

$$40 \text{ mg/m}^2 \times 0.4 \text{ m}^2 = 16 \text{ mg per dose}$$

Then divide the adult dose by the conversion factor:

$$\frac{16 \text{ mg}}{1.7} = 9.4 \text{ mg}$$

Young's Rule and Clark's Rule

There are two other methods for calculating children's doses: Young's Rule and Clark's Rule.

Young's Rule

Young's Rule is easy to remember, because it calculates the dose by the *age* of the patient (a child is a *young* person).

$$\text{Young's Rule:} \frac{\text{age of child (years)}}{\text{age of child} + 12} \times \text{adult dose} = \text{child's dose}$$

Clark's Rule

Clark's Rule relates the dose to the child's weight (in pounds), as compared to an adult weight of 150 lb.

$$\text{Clark's Rule: adult dose} \times \frac{\text{weight of child}}{150} = \text{child's dose}$$

It would be wise to commit these rules to memory, as they will be on the exam.

> **NOTE**
>
> Calculations performed by these two methods will not always produce identical answers. Therefore, if you are asked to compute a child's dose by Young's Rule and use Clark's Rule instead (or another method, if you can't remember either one), you will not get the correct answer on the exam.

> **EXAMPLE**
>
> A child weighs 30 lb and is four years old. Another child is also four years old but weighs 40 lb. The adult dose of Keflex is 250 mg. Calculate both of the children's doses by (1) Young's Rule and (2) Clark's Rule.
>
> Child 1. *Young's Rule*:
>
> $$\frac{250 \text{ mg}}{\text{dose}} \times \frac{4 \text{ yr}}{4 \text{ yr} + 12} = 62.5 \text{ mg}$$
>
> *Clark's Rule*:
>
> $$\frac{250 \text{ mg}}{\text{dose}} \times \frac{30 \text{ lb}}{150} = 50 \text{ mg}$$
>
> Child 2. *Young's Rule*: This calculation produces the same result as for Child 1: 62.5 mg
>
> Using Clark's Rule, however, produces a different dosage calculation:
>
> $$\frac{250 \text{ mg}}{\text{dose}} \times \frac{40 \text{ lb}}{150} = 66.7 \text{ mg}$$

Safe Dosages

Occasionally, it may be necessary for the technician to check the dosage prescribed to make sure that it is safe. The *manufacturer's label* carries information about dosage, including the recommended adult dose. This sometimes, but not always, includes the recommended child's dose. It also should include the safe dose range.

The Safe Dose Range

The *safe dose range* presents a minimum dose at which the drug is effective, and a maximum dose (at which toxicity may be seen). A range of 0.2–0.8 mg, for example, means that a dose of 0.2 mg, 0.8 mg, or anything in between is acceptable for dosing, but anything below 0.2 mg (which would be ineffective) or above 0.8 mg (which would be toxic) is unacceptable. The technician may need to perform calculations to check the prescribed dose to be sure that it is safe. If the dose prescribed falls outside the safe dose range, the problem should be brought to the attention of the pharmacist.

Problem: The dose of amoxicillin prescribed for a 44 lb child is 250 mg qid. The label gives a safe dose range of 15–50 mg/kg per day. Is the dose safe?

Solution: First, convert the child's weight from pounds to kilograms:

$$\frac{44 \text{ lb}}{2.2 \text{ lb/kg}} = 20 \text{ kg}.$$

Next, divide the 250 mg dose by the child's weight to obtain the mg/kg amount for one dose:

$$\frac{25\emptyset \text{ mg}}{2\emptyset \text{ kg}} = 12.5 \text{ mg/kg per dose}$$

The safe dose range, however, is expressed as a *daily* dose range. The amount prescribed *per day*, however, is four times the dose (qid), or 50 mg/day. This amount falls within the range of 15–50 mg/kg/day. The dose is safe.

Problem: The recommended child's dose of Keflex is 25 mg/kg/day in two divided doses. If a child weighs 22 lb, how much drug would be prescribed per day?

Solution: First, convert pounds to kilograms: 22 lb ÷ 2.2 lb/kg = 10 kg of body weight. Next, multiply the recommended daily dose, which is 25 mg/kg/day for a child, by the body weight in kg, to get the amount of drug actually given:

$$\frac{25 \text{ mg}}{\text{k\!g}} = 10 \text{ k\!g} = 250 \text{ mg/day}$$

Problem: A child, weighing 44 lbs, is prescribed hydroxyzine pamoate 10 mg IM. The pediatric safe dosage is stated to be 1 mg/kg/dose. Is the drug safe?

Solution: First, convert the child's weight to kilograms:

$$44 \text{ lb} \times \frac{1 \text{ kg}}{2.2 \text{ lb}} = 20 \text{ kg}$$

Next, calculate:

$$\frac{10 \text{ mg/dose}}{20 \text{ kg}} = 0.5 \text{ mg/kg/dose}$$

0.5 mg/kg/dose is below the safe dose ceiling of 1 mg/kg/ dose, so **the drug is safe.**

Single Dose Safe Range versus Daily Dose Safe Range

The safe dose and safe daily dose ranges are important, but for different reasons.

A *single dose* of the drug will enter the body, perform a physiological action, and then gradually be eliminated from the blood through the actions of the kidney and liver. When a dose is too high, adverse physiological actions may occur, which may damage organs or even cause death. A *range* of acceptable doses is given because different people (particularly older and very young patients) clear drugs from the system more slowly than others, so one safe dose would not be appropriate for everyone.

A *cumulative* (or daily dose) *range* is given because the drug may have a cumulative effect. For example, if a patient takes one 5 mg dose of drug at 8 a.m. and then another dose four hours later, the first dose of drug may not be completely eliminated, resulting in elevated blood levels. As the patient continues to take another dose every four hours, throughout the day the drug levels may build up to toxic levels. The establishment of a maximum allowable daily dose will prevent this from happening.

Problem: The maximum pediatric dose of a drug is 1 mg/kg. The order is for 10 mg to be given to a five-year-old child, weighing 15 kg. Is the dose safe?

Solution: First, we need to calculate the dose to be given on a per-kilogram basis:

$$\frac{10 \text{ mg}}{15 \text{ kg}} = 0.67 \text{ mg/kg}$$

Since the dose given to the child is 0.67 mg/kg, which is less than the maximum dose of 1 mg/kg, the dose is safe.

Chapter Review Questions

1. You have an order for kanamycin 40 mg/m². A child is 36 inches tall and weighs 30 lb. You calculate the BSA to be 0.6 m². Calculate one dose.

2. A child weighs 66 lb. The order is for cloxacillin 250 mg q6h. The safe dose described on the label is 50 mg/kg/day. Is the dose safe?

3. An adult dose of phenobarbital is 100 mg. Calculate the dose for a child weighing 22 lb.

4. Your order is for ethambutol 15 mg/kg for a child weighing 22 kg. Calculate one dose.

5. An adult dose of Keflin is 1 g. What is the dose for a child weighing 25 lb?

6. Your order is for Narcan neonatal 0.5 mg/kg. The infant weighs 5,500 g. Calculate the correct dose for the infant.

7. Your order is for clindamycin 20 mg/kg. The child weighs 88 lb. Your stock is Cleocin 300 mg/mL. How much do you dispense?

8. Your order is for diazepam 0.25 mg/kg. The child weighs 22 lb. Your stock is a 5 mg vial diluted to 2 mL. What amount is dispensed?

9. A child is 36 inches tall and weighs 50 lbs. What is this child's BSA?

10. A child is eight years old and weighs 50 lb. The adult dose of cephalexin is 250 mg. Use both Clark's Rule and Young's Rule to calculate the child's dose.

CHAPTER 14

Parenteral Dosages

Quick Study

I. Parenteral dosage forms

- Subcutaneous
- Intramuscular
- Intra-arterial
- Intrathecal
- Intracardiac
- Intravenous

II. Preparation and use of the IV bolus and IV drip

III. Drug reconstitution and calculation of drug concentration

    A. Use of the manufacturer's label

IV. Choosing the appropriate syringe and needle for dispensing

    A. The accuracy of syringe calibrations decreases as the syringe size increases
    B. Use a syringe calibrated to the exact amount to be withdrawn
    C. Choosing the appropriate needle for the type of injection

V. Calculation of the correct amount to be dispensed

- Use of percentages and ratios
- Preparation of intramuscular and intravenous injections

Parenteral Dosage Forms

There are two ways to administer medication into the body: **enteral**, which means that the medication goes into the digestive tract and is then absorbed into the blood; and **parenteral**, which means that it bypasses the digestive tract and goes into the blood through a more direct route.

Parenteral dosage forms are normally thought of as anything that is injected intravenously (i.e., the drugs go directly into the blood), but other dosage forms may also be classified as parenteral. Drugs administered by intramuscular and subcutaneous injections, or by transdermal patch, for example, are absorbed directly into the blood from other tissues but just a little more slowly, which minimizes the adverse effects that may be seen with rapid injection.

The following are several examples of parenteral injections. The technician should be familiar with them and their uses:

- *Subcutaneous injections (sub-q, or SC):* Used with drugs such as insulin. In this type of injection, drug is injected under the skin.
- *Intramuscular injections (IM):* In this type of injection, drug is injected into the muscle for slow absorption.
- *Intra-arterial injections (IA):* Drugs are injected directly into an artery.
- *Intrathecal injections (IT):* Drug is injected into the space surrounding the spinal cord.
- *Intracardiac injections (IC):* Drug is injected directly into the heart.
- *Intravenous injections (IV):* These are the most common, along with IM and sub-q. There are two forms of IV injections:
  - The IV bolus (drug is given all at once—a syringe is prepared with the entire dose)
  - The IV drip (given over a long period of time—an IV "bag" or bottle of drug solution is prepared)

Calculation of Parenteral Doses

Parenteral doses are calculated similarly to the oral doses in Chapter 12. However, these doses are prepared under sterile conditions (aseptically) for injection directly into the blood or tissues.

Determining the Concentration of a Drug Solution

As with the oral and liquid doses, drug concentrations ordered may also be expressed as a percentage or ratio, as well as in amount of drug per unit of volume. Drug concentrations should be given on the manufacturer's label. If it is not, it can be easily calculated. For instance, the label may state that the bottle contains 500 mg of drug and the volume is 20 mL. A simple division tells us that the concentration of drug in the bottle is 25 mg/mL.

Drugs for injection are usually stocked in dry form to preserve stability and need to be diluted with the proper solution (e.g., sterile water or saline). The amount of diluent added to the powder determines the final concentration.

The use of ratio/proportion is helpful in calculations involving liquids for injection.

Problem: The order is for atropine sulfate 0.8 mg, and the available stock is 0.4 mg/mL.

Solution: Set the ratios of the order and stock equal:

Step 1. $(\text{order})\dfrac{0.8\ \text{mg}}{\text{mL}} = \dfrac{0.4\ \text{mg}}{X\ \text{mL}}(\text{stock})$

Step 2. Cross-multiply:

$$\dfrac{0.8\ \text{mg}}{X\ \text{mL}} \times \dfrac{0.4\ \text{mg}}{\text{mL}} \rightarrow 0.8\ \text{mg} \times 1\ \text{mL} = 0.4\ \text{mg} \times X$$

Step 3. Divide both sides of the equation by 0.4 mg, and cancel units:

$$\dfrac{\overset{2}{\cancel{0.8}}\ \cancel{\text{mg}} \times 1\ \text{mL}}{\underset{1}{\cancel{0.4}}\ \cancel{\text{mg}}} = X = 2\ \text{mL}$$

The ratio/proportion method is especially useful when we have a drug concentration that does not simplify.

Problem: An order is for phenobarbital gr i IM. Available stock is 200 mg/3 mL.

Solution: First, convert grains to mg: gr i × 60 mg/gr = 60 mg

Next, calculate:

Step 1. $\left(\dfrac{\text{order in mg}}{\text{dose in mL}}\right)\left(\dfrac{60\ \text{mg}}{X}\right)\left(\dfrac{200\ \text{mg}}{3\ \text{mL}}\right)(\text{stock concentration})$

Step 2. Cross-multiply:

$$\dfrac{60\ \text{mg}}{X} \times \dfrac{200\ \text{mg}}{3\ \text{mL}} \rightarrow 60\ \text{mg} \times 3\ \text{mL} = 200\ \text{mg}\ (X)$$

Step 3. Divide by 200 to solve for the dose dispensed:

$$X = 0.9\ \text{mL}$$

Problem: An order is for lidocaine 25 mg intramuscularly. The stock available is a 1% solution.

Solution: First, convert the stock from a percentage into a mg/mL solution:

$$1\% = 1 \text{ g}/100 \text{ mL} = 1{,}000 \text{ mg}/100 \text{ mL} = 10 \text{ mg/mL}$$

Then, do the problem (we will use the order/stock method):

$$\frac{\overset{5}{25 \text{ mg}}}{\underset{2}{10 \text{ mg}/\text{mL}}} = 2.5 \text{ mL}$$

Choosing the Proper Syringe

> The size of the syringe should be as close as possible to the volume measured!

The size of the syringe that is chosen to draw up the medication should be as close as possible to the volume of drug being drawn up, as was discussed in Chapter 10. In other words, if you dispense a 1.5 mL dose, choose a 3 mL—not a 5 mL—syringe. A 1 mL dose should be dispensed in a 1 mL syringe. The reason for this is that the larger the syringe, the less accurate the markings. The accuracy of a syringe is also proportional to its volume, so you should always measure volumes in the size of syringe closest to the volume being measured.

Choosing the Appropriate Needle

Choosing the proper size of needle to attach to the syringe is also important.

- A *large-bore needle:* (16–18 G) will draw up and dispense liquid quickly, so it is used for drug rehydration, dilution, and admixtures. A large-bore needle is also necessary to penetrate dense muscle tissue, so it must be dispensed on a syringe that is to be used for an IM injection.
- A *fine needle:* (25–30 G) is needed for subcutaneous and intradermal injections to penetrate the more delicate tissues of the skin with a minimum of discomfort.
- An *intermediate-bore needle:* (19–22 G) is used for IV injections, to penetrate the smooth muscle layer of the vessel without causing extravasation (leakage) from the vein.

Proper Dilution of Drugs for Injection

The manufacturer's label may contain very useful instructions for dilution and preparation of the drug. For instance, the label on a bottle of penicillin may contain a dilution table that allows you to prepare a specific concentration of drug solution. This enables you to draw up a specific amount of solution for injection that contains the proper amount of drug. (See Figure 14-1.)

Figure 14-1 shows a label for penicillin G potassium. It contains a table for reconstitution. According to the table, the addition of 18.2 mL of diluent

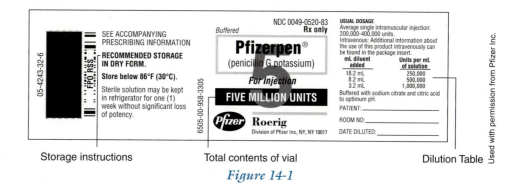

| Storage instructions | Total contents of vial | Dilution Table |

Figure 14-1

gives a final concentration of 250,000 units/mL, while the addition of 8.2 mL of diluent gives a concentration of 500,000 units/mL solution, etc.

> **NOTE**
>
> The dilution table is present on the label to assist in preparation, but you will also have to know how to prepare a dilution on your own, and how to *back-calculate*, to correct an error in dilution. These types of problems are almost certain to be on the exam.

Using the Dilution Table

In order to use the dilution table, the technician must first decide what volume is needed for the order (an IM injection must be no more than 3 mL in volume; 2 mL is preferable) and compute the concentration needed. Then, this concentration is compared to those listed on the chart. You should then identify the concentration listed in the chart that is closest to the concentration that you need, and read across the chart to determine the proper amount of **diluent** (i.e., water, saline, or D_5W that must be added to the drug to make the solution).

Problem: Using the label in Figure 14-1, prepare an order for 800,000 units penicillin IM.

Solution: We would like to have about 2 mL for an IM injection. The order is for 800,000 units.

$$\frac{800,000 \text{ U}}{2 \text{ mL}} = \frac{400,000 \text{ U}}{\text{mL}}$$

This is the concentration of drug that we want. According to the chart, we can get a concentration of 500,000 units/mL by adding 33 mL of diluent to the vial of drug. We reconstitute with 8.2 mL of water and calculate the amount to draw up for the dose:

$$\frac{8\,00,000 \text{ U (needed)}}{5\,00,000 \text{ U/mL (stock)}} = 1.6 \text{ mL}$$

Chapter Review Questions

Calculate the amount dispensed for each of the following:

1. Your order is for Demerol 20 mg IM. Available stock is 50 mg/5 mL.

2. Your order is for morphine gr ss. Available stock is 6 mg/mL.

3. Your order is for heparin 4,000 units SC. Your stock is heparin 10,000 U/5 mL.

4. Your order is for 50 units of U100 insulin. The pharmacy is out of insulin syringes. How much insulin would you dispense (in mL) using a 1 cc syringe?

5. Your order is for 1 mg of epinephrine. Your stock is a 1:1,000 solution.

6. Your order is for aminophylline 50 mg. Available stock is 500 mg/20 mL.

7. Your order is for Tigan 150 mg. Available stock is 100 mg/mL.

8. Your order is for Depo-Provera 0.2 g. Available stock is 500 mg/5 mL vial.

9. Your order is for atropine sulfate 0.2 mg. Available stock is 400 mcg/mL.

10. Your order is for 350,000 units of penicillin IM. Using the manufacturer's label shown in Figure 14-1, calculate the volume you should add. How much do you dispense for an IM bolus of 350,000 units?

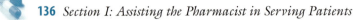

SEE ACCOMPANYING PRESCRIBING INFORMATION	Buffered	NDC 0049-0520-83 Rx only
RECOMMENDED STORAGE IN DRY FORM.	**Pfizerpen®**	
Store below 86°F (30°C).	(penicillin G potassium)	
Sterile solution may be kept in refrigerator for one (1) week without significant loss of potency.	*For Injection* **FIVE MILLION UNITS**	
	Pfizer **Roerig** Division of Pfizer Inc, NY, NY 10017	

USUAL DOSAGE
Average single intramuscular injection: 200,000-400,000 units.
Intravenous: Additional information about the use of this product intravenously can be found in the package insert.

mL diluent added	Units per mL of solution
18.2 mL	250,000
8.2 mL	500,000
3.2 mL	1,000,000

Buffered with sodium citrate and citric acid to optimum pH.

PATIENT: _____

ROOM NO: _____

DATE DILUTED: _____

05-4243-32-6

FPO RSS

6505-00-958-3305

Storage instructions   Total contents of vial   Dilution Table

CHAPTER 15

Intravenous Calculations

Quick Study

I.   Preparing intravenous medication for administration

- Salt solutions (e.g., saline, Ringer's solution)
- Sugar solutions (e.g., dextrose)
- Solutions for irrigation
- Addition of potassium or drug admixtures to IV drip solutions

A.   Calculation of flow rate

- Volume per time (V/T): $\dfrac{drops}{time}$ or $\dfrac{mL}{time}$ is most useful in dose per time
- calculation.
- V/T × drop factor = drops per time

Preparing Intravenous Medication for Administration

Intravenous drugs are administered in two ways: the **bolus**, which is an injection given all at once, and the **IV drip**, which is administered over a long period of time. We discussed the bolus injections in Chapter 14. We will now discuss the IV drip calculations.

Understanding Flow Rate

The first thing that we need to understand, when discussing IVs, is the concept of **flow rate**. When a patient is connected to an IV drip, the fluid flows in at a particular speed. The rate of flow is either determined by a "controller" (a mechanical device) or by an **infusion set**, which consists of a plastic barrel (or drip apparatus) connected to plastic tubing. One end of the barrel is inserted into the bottom of the IV bag or bottle, and the other leads into the tubing that connects the bag to the patient. The IV flows through the tubing and into a needle that is inserted into the patient.

An infusion set is calibrated to deliver a drop of a certain size (expressed as a number of drops *per milliliter*, or **drop factor**). The rate at which the drops flow into the tubing (and thus the patient) is adjusted manually by the nurse.

The Drop Factor

The size of the drop is determined by the **drop factor**. Together, the calibration of the infusion set (the size of the drop), and the rate of flow determine how much of the IV solution goes into the patient per unit of time.

Infusion sets come in *10 gtt/mL, 15 gtt/mL,* (standard), *20 gtt/mL,* and *60 gtt/mL* (microdrip) sizes (see Figure 15-1).

Intravenous (IV) Solutions

Solutions that are commonly infused include:

1. Common salt solutions
   - Normal saline (NS)—0.9% sodium chloride
   - 1/2 normal saline (1/2 NS)—0.45% sodium chloride
   - 1/4 normal saline (1/4 NS)—0.225% sodium chloride

2. Sugar solutions and commonly used mixtures
   - D_5W—5% dextrose (glucose) in water
   - Ringer's solution (or lactated Ringer's)

> **NOTE**
>
> Saline solutions may have potassium chloride added. (These are labeled in red, as potassium overdosage is lethal. Red-print labeling is easy to see and helps to prevent accidental death from potassium overdosage.)

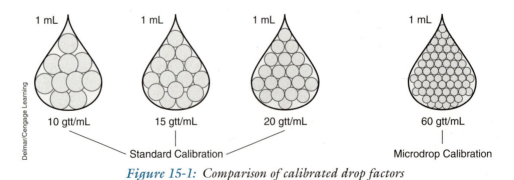

Figure 15-1: Comparison of calibrated drop factors

Saline Solutions

Saline is a salt solution that is made of sodium chloride (i.e., table salt). *Normal saline (NS)* is 0.9% sodium chloride, which is a concentration (or *osmolarity*) similar to that found in blood plasma. Salts, particularly sodium, tend to attract water. If the salt concentration in the blood were to become too high (hyper), water would be drawn out of the cells and tissues and into the blood. Too low a plasma (blood) concentration (hypo) would drive water *into* the cells and out of the blood, which could literally cause them to explode. Since the concentration of saline (0.9% salt) is near that of blood plasma, it will neither draw water from the tissues nor cause water to move into the tissues.

$\frac{1}{2}$ NS and $\frac{1}{4}$ NS are reduced-salt forms of saline that are useful in patients with various conditions. They are also used to make IV admixtures, when the addition of the admixture to normal saline may increase the concentration (osmolarity) of the solution, to the point where it may be detrimental to the patient, in the judgment of the prescriber.

Intravenous Admixtures

Various drugs known as IV admixtures may be added directly to these solutions for slow infusion. Alternatively, a small IV bag (**piggyback IV**) containing a drug solution may be hung with the IV bag, which mixes with the primary intravenous fluid as it is released to the patient. (See Chapter 16.)

Calculation of Flow Rate

Flow rate is volume per time. To determine the flow rate, simply take the volume of fluid that the patient is to receive and divide it by the time of infusion.

> **EXAMPLE**
>
> A patient receives 250 mL of normal saline in two hours. What is the hourly flow rate?
>
> *Solution:* $\dfrac{\text{volume}}{\text{time}} = \dfrac{250 \text{ mL}}{2 \text{ hr}} = 125 \text{ mL/hr.}$

Sometimes the flow rate is needed in minutes rather than hours.

> **EXAMPLE**
>
> A patient is to receive 1 L of heparinized saline in a one-hour infusion. What is the flow rate in mL/minute?
>
> *Solution:* The amount to be infused is 1 L (1,000 mL). The time of infusion is one hour (60 min). Dividing, we have:
>
> $$\frac{100\cancel{0} \text{ mL}}{6\cancel{0} \text{ min}} = 16 \text{ mL/min.}$$

Calculating Flow Rate in Drops per Time Using an Infusion Apparatus

Calculating flow rate by drops requires an extra calculation. Since we are now calculating flow rate by the number of *drops* per time, we need to take the drop factor into account.

The drop-factor calibration of the infusion set (designated by a number printed on the package) allows us to calculate how much volume is contained per drop. For example, an infusion set labeled 10 gtt/mL would produce a drop equal in volume to 1 mL/10 gtt, or 0.1 mL.

The drops are counted as they fall from the barrel of the infusion apparatus. The number of drops falling per minute is the flow rate in gtt/min.

It may be necessary to calculate a flow rate in drops/min, so that the person administering the IV can manually adjust the drop rate to achieve the proper flow rate. To do this, we take the flow rate in milliliters per time and divide by the number of drops in a milliliter (the drop factor) to obtain a flow rate in drops/min, which can be set by the person administering the IV. This calculation is also useful in determining which infusion apparatus to include with the IV. For example, if the flow rate needed is 10 mL/min, that is 600 drops per minute using a microdrip apparatus (60 gtts/mL). This is difficult to accurately count. Using a macrodrip apparatus (10 gtts/mL), only 100 drops per minute would have to be counted.

Calculating Flow Rate in Drops per Time

Remember: (Volume ÷ time) × drop factor = drops per time

Problem: An order states that 100,000 units of penicillin is to be added to a 1 L bag of saline and infused in 5 hours. Your infusion set is labeled 10 gtt/mL. What is the flow rate in gtt/min?

Solution: 1 L of NS is infused in 5 hours. Disregarding the amount of drug, as the entire 1 L bag is to be infused, the flow rate is:

$$\frac{1{,}000\,\text{mL}}{5\,\text{hr}} \quad \text{or} \quad \frac{200\,\text{mL}}{\text{hr}}$$

We need the rate in *minutes* in order to calculate gtt/min. Since there are 60 minutes in 1 hour, this becomes:

$$\frac{20\cancel{0}\,\text{mL}}{6\cancel{0}\,\text{min}} \quad \text{or} \quad \frac{3.33\,\text{mL}}{\text{min}}$$

Multiplying the flow rate in milliliters by the drop factor changes the milliliters to drops:

$$\frac{3.33\,\cancel{\text{mL}}}{\text{min}} \times \frac{10\,\text{gtt}}{\cancel{\text{mL}}} = 33.3\,\text{gtt/min}$$

Note: We cannot have a fraction of a drop, so this becomes just 33 gtt/min.

Converting Drops per Time to Milliliters per Time

If we have the flow rate in drops per time and need to do a calculation, we can easily convert the flow rate back to milliliters per time:

Problem: An IV is running at a rate of 20 gtts/min. The infusion apparatus is a *macrodrip* apparatus (10 gtt/mL). What is the flow rate in mL/hr?

Solution: First, we change drops to milliliters:

$$\frac{20 \text{ gtt/min}}{10 \text{ gtt/mL}} = 2 \text{ mL/min}$$

Note that we *divided* by the drop factor this time.

We *multiplied* to convert milliliters to drops, and we now *divide* to convert drops to milliliters.

$$\text{mL} \rightarrow \text{gtts} = \text{multiplication}$$
$$\text{gtts} \rightarrow \text{mL} = \text{division}$$

Next, calculate the flow rate per hour: 2 mL/min × 60 min/hr = 120 mL/hr

Chapter Review Questions

1. 1 L of saline is administered over 10 hours. Find the flow rate in (a) mL per hour and (b) mL/min.

2. The infusion set used with the IV bag in question 1 states that the drop factor is 15 gtt/mL. Calculate the flow rate in gtt/min.

3. 500 mL of D_5W runs for 4 hours. Calculate the flow rate in mL/hr and mL/min.

4. 1 L of NS runs for 16 hours, 40 min. Calculate the flow rate in mL/hr and mL/min.

5. You have an order for aminophylline 250 mg in 250 mL NS to run for 8 hours. The infusion set is labeled 60 gtt/mL. What is the flow rate in drops per minute?

6. The order is for 150 mL of NS infused over 3 hours. The infusion set is labeled 60 gtt/mL. Calculate the flow rate in gtt/min.

7. 1 L of NS is infused at 100 mL/hr. How long will the infusion go?

8. 300 mL of lactated Ringer's solution is infused in 5 hours. The flow rate is 15 gtt/min. What is the drop factor?

9. 1 L of saline runs for 10 hours at 1,000 gtt/hr. Calculate the drop factor.

10. 600 mL of Ringer's lactate runs for 10 hours. The flow rate is 60 gtt/min. Calculate the drop factor.

11. You have a bag of saline with an infusion apparatus that is labeled 15 gtt/mL. The flow rate is 60 gtt/min. What is the hourly rate of infusion?

12. You have 1 L saline, which is to be infused in 6 hours. Available are 10 gtt/mL and 15 gtt/mL infusion sets. Calculate the flow rate for each in gtt/min.

13. 1 L of saline is infusing at a rate of 100 mL/hr. How much saline does the patient get in 40 minutes?

14. 120 mL of NS is to be administered in 30 minutes using an infusion set labeled 15 gtt/mL. What is the flow rate in gtt/min?

15. 300 mL of D_5W $\frac{1}{2}$ NS is delivered in 90 minutes. Your drop factor is 10 gtt/mL. Calculate the flow rate in gtt/min.

CHAPTER 16

Intravenous Admixtures

Quick Study

I. Infusing medications over time—the IV drip and admixture

    A. Rehydration and reconstitution of drugs
    -   Rehydration is adding water to a dry form of a drug or substance to create a solution.
    -   Reconstitution is the addition of any diluent to a powdered form of substance to create a solution.
    -   To calculate the amount of diluent to add to reach a desired concentration

Infusing Medications Over Time—The IV Drip and Admixture

Occasionally, it may be necessary for the patient to receive a drug or medication slowly over a period of hours. In this case, the technician may be asked to prepare an IV solution that contains the proper dosage of drug to be infused over time. For example, the order might read "Penicillin G-K 100,000 units in 1 L NS" or "heparin sulfate 1,000 units/hr in D_5W." The proper amount of drug to be added must be calculated, withdrawn, and added to the IV.

Rehydration and Reconstitution of Drugs

The choice of solution to be added is important. Many drugs are unstable if mixed with water. Injectable drugs are supplied in powder form and must be rehydrated (reconstituted) before use. Drugs are always supplied in a solution that is **isotonic** to the body. In other words, the concentration of drug and salt particles present in the solution is the same as that in the body fluids. The particles (e.g., salt or sugar) that introduce the drug solution into the body will neither dehydrate nor overhydrate the cells. If the drug is already mixed with the salts necessary to make the solution, the technician need only add water to the dry powder. This is technically called *rehydration*, as we are only giving back the water to the original solution. If the vial contains only the drug or the drug with some extra ingredients to help it work, the instructions may be to add another **diluent** to the powder (e.g., saline, distilled water, or D_5W). This is called **reconstitution**. Once diluted, the drug has a limited shelf life, which may be extended by refrigeration. For simplicity's sake, we will refer to the dilution of a powdered drug as **reconstitution**.

Problem: The order is for penicillin G-K 500,000 units to be delivered over 10 hours. A vial of penicillin contains 10,000,000 units in dry form, which must be reconstituted. You have 1 L bags of saline available. Calculate the amount of penicillin to add to the IV.

Solution: First, note the following regarding the problem:

1. We are ignoring the irrelevant information, such as time of infusion and the size of the IV bag.

2. We are assuming that the entire 1 L of saline will be infused, so the total amount of drug put into the bag will be given to the patient. Therefore, the amount of drug added to the bag should equal the order.

We want to add as small a volume of drug as possible to the bag, so as not to change its volume. About 1–5 mL would be about right. Let us set up a ratio/proportion to calculate the amount of diluent to add to the penicillin vial so that we may withdraw 1 mL that contains 500,000 units of drug:

Set up the problem as follows:

$$\frac{\text{dose of drug ordered}}{\text{volume to add to the IV}} = \frac{\text{amount of drug in the vial}}{\text{amount of diluent added}}$$

This becomes:

$$\frac{500,000 \, \text{units}}{1 \, \text{mL}} = \frac{10,000,000 \, \text{units}}{X \, \text{mL}}$$

Cross-multiply:

$$\frac{500,000 \, \text{units}}{1 \, \text{mL}} \diagdown \frac{10,000,000 \, \text{units}}{X \, \text{mL}}$$

Divide:

$$\frac{\cancel{500,000\ \text{units}} \times X\,\text{mL}}{\cancel{500,000\ \text{units}}} = \frac{1\,\text{mL} \times \overset{20}{\cancel{10,000,000\ \text{units}}}}{\underset{1}{\cancel{500,000\ \text{units}}}} = 20\,\text{mL}$$

We add 20 mL to the vial and withdraw 1 mL for injection into the IV bag.

Problem: The label on a drug vial says to reconstitute with 8 mL of water to get 10 mL of a 500,000 units/mL solution. You add 10 mL to the vial by mistake. What would be the resulting concentration of drug?

Solution: If you had added the correct amount, the label says that you would have had 10 mL of a 500,000 units/mL solution. That being the case, the total amount of drug in the vial is:

$$\frac{10\ \cancel{\text{mL}} \times 500,000\ \text{units}}{\cancel{\text{mL}}} = 5,000,000\ \text{units using}$$

(concentration × volume = amount of drug)

Now, all we have to do is recalculate the dilution. We are now adding 10 mL instead of 8 mL, so the total volume is now 12 mL instead of 10 mL (the extra 2 mL is the volume taken up by the drug, which does not change). Now calculate the concentration:

5,000,000 units/12 mL = 416,667 units/mL

Occasionally, the technician may be asked to add an appropriate amount of drug to an IV bag that results in a particular concentration. In this case, use the ratio/proportion method to determine how much of a particular drug or drug solution is to be added.

Problem: The order is for 250 mL of a 0.2% calcium gluconate solution in $\frac{1}{2}$ NS to be delivered in 5 hours. You have a 20% solution of calcium gluconate on hand. How much do you add to the IV bag?

Solution: First, calculate the amount ordered in grams (250 mL of a 0.2% solution) and recall that 0.2% = 0.2 g/100 mL.

Set up the ratio/proportion:

$$\frac{0.2\,\text{g}}{100\,\text{mL}} = \frac{X\,\text{g}}{250\,\text{mL}}$$

Cross-multiply and divide:

$$0.2\ \text{g} \times 250\ \text{mL} = X\ \text{g} \times 100\ \text{mL},$$

so the amount of drug ordered (Xg) is then:

$$\frac{0.2\,g \times \cancel{250}^{5}\,\cancel{mL}}{_{2}\cancel{100}\,\cancel{mL}} = 0.5\,g \text{ of drug needed to fill the order}$$

Now, determine how much of the 20% solution should be added to the bag:

$$\frac{0.5\,g}{X\,mL} = \frac{2\cancel{0}\,g}{10\cancel{0}\,mL}$$

Cross-multiply:

$$\frac{0.5\,g}{X\,mL} \diagdown\!\!\diagup \frac{2\cancel{0}\,g}{10\cancel{0}\,mL}$$

Divide:

$$\frac{0.5\,g \times 100\,mL}{20\,g} = 2.5\,mL$$

The volume to be added is 0.5 × 5 mL or 2.5 mL

Problem: The order is for heparin 1,000 units/hr in 1 L D_5W, to be infused for 5 hours. Calculate the amount of heparin to add to the IV.

Solution: The order states that the dose is 1,000 units/hr for 5 hours. The amount to be added is therefore:

$$\frac{1,000\,units}{\cancel{hr}} \times 5\,\cancel{hr} = 5,000\,units$$

Chapter Review Questions

1. The order is for aminophylline 250 mg in 500 mL NS, to run for 8 hours. You have aminophylline 500 mg/5 mL on hand. How much do you put in the IV bag?

2. What is the final concentration of drug in the IV bag prepared in question 1?

3. You add 10 mL of 10% calcium gluconate to a 1 L bag of D_5W. What is the concentration of calcium gluconate in the bag?

4. How much dextrose is contained in 300 mL of D_5W?

5. How many milligrams of drug are in 10 mL of a 1:1,000 solution?

6. A drug label states that the addition of 8 mL of saline to the vial will result in a drug concentration of 250 mg/mL. Suddenly, you realize that you just added *13 mL* of saline to the vial. What is the actual concentration of drug in the vial?

7. You reconstitute a vial of drug with 2.5 mL of saline. The vial contains 2,500,000 units of drug. What is the final concentration of drug in the vial?

8. Your vial of potassium solution contains 20 mEq of potassium per 5 mL. You add 5 mL to a 1 L IV bag. What is the final concentration of potassium in the bag?

9. You reconstitute 1,000,000 units of penicillin with 20 mL of saline. What is the final concentration?

10. You add 5 mL of a 250 mg/mL solution of methotrexate to 250 mL IV bag. What is the final concentration of drug in the bag?

CHAPTER 17

Calculation of Dose per Time

Calculation of Drug Dose as a Function of Time

Calculation of the amount of drug infused per time, or dose per time, is simply a matter of using the following formula, which you should memorize:

Concentration × **F**low rate = **D**ose/times

$$\left(C \times F = \frac{D}{t} \right)$$

It is helpful to think of the process of intravenous medication and get a picture in your mind as to what is happening. A prescribed dose of drug is to be administered to the patient in a certain length of time, using a slow intravenous infusion.

Calculating the Concentration of Drug (C)

If you know how much fluid is in the IV bag and how much drug was put in, you can calculate the **concentration** of drug in the solution:

$$\frac{\text{the amount of drug in g or mg}}{\text{the volume of fluid in the IV bag}} = \text{the concentration of drug in the solution}$$

> **EXAMPLE**
>
> Aminophyllin 500 mg in NS 250 mL:
>
> $$\frac{500 \text{ mg aminophyllin}}{250 \text{ mL NS}} = 500 / 250 = 2 \text{ mg/mL}$$

Calculating the Flow Rate (F)

The flow rate is nothing more than the rate at which the IV fluid flows from the bag into the patient. This may be calculated in terms of drops per minute (gtt/min) or milliliters per minute (mL/min), or milliliters per hour (mL/hr). To determine the dose given per time, it is best to use mL/hr:

$$\frac{\text{the amount of fluid in the IV bag}}{\text{the time that it takes the bag to empty}} = \text{the flow rate}$$

> **EXAMPLE**
>
> A 1000 mL bag of NS runs in over 8 hours. What is the rate?
>
> $$\frac{1000 \text{ mL}}{8 \text{ hr}} = 125 \text{ mL/hr}$$

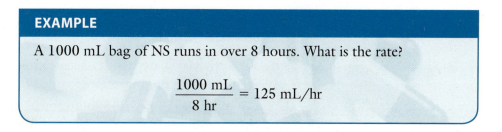

To convert the rate of an IV solution from mL/hr to mL/minute, you would simply divide the rate by 60 (60 minutes = 1 hour).

> **EXAMPLE**
>
> The rate is 125 mL/hr and you want to convert to mL/minute:
>
> 125 mL/hr = 125 mL/60 minutes = 2.08 mL/minute

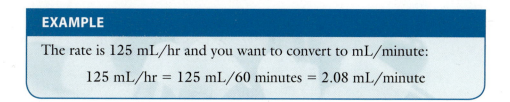

Calculating the Dose Administered per Time

To calculate the dose administered per time, we calculate the flow rate and concentration, and, using the formula plug in numbers:

EXAMPLE

You prepare a 500 mL bag of D$_5$W, containing 1,000 units of heparin. The solution is to be infused over 2 hours. The hourly dose of heparin administered to the patient would be calculated as follows:

$$F = \frac{500 \text{ mL}}{2 \text{ hr}} = \frac{250 \text{ mL}}{\text{hr}}$$

$$C = \frac{1,000 \text{ units}}{500 \text{ mL}} = \frac{2 \text{ units}}{\text{mL}}$$

$$\frac{D}{t} = \frac{2 \text{ units}}{\text{mL}} \times \frac{250 \text{ mL}}{\text{hr}} = \frac{500 \text{ units}}{\text{hr}}$$

The amount of drug per volume of fluid (*the concentration C*), multiplied by how fast the fluid flows into the patient, indicates the amount of drug flowing into the patient per time. When doing these calculations, remember that **dose** refers to the amount of **drug**, not the volume of fluid. Thus, your answer will always come out in a *weight* measurement (e.g., g/hr, mg/min, etc.). This formula is very versatile and can be used to calculate any of the parameters (*C*, *F*, or *D/t*), as shown below.

Problem: You have a 1 L bag of saline containing 1.5 g of antibiotic. The flow rate is 100 mL/hr. What is the hourly dose?

Solution: Step 1. Calculate the concentration (amount of drug per volume). The amount of drug added to the IV is 1.5 g. Convert: 1.5 g = 1,500 mg. The volume of the bag is 1 L (1,000 mL), so the concentration is 1,500 mg/1,000 mL = 1.5 mg/mL.

Step 2. Determine the flow rate. This is actually given in the problem: 100 mL/hr.

Step 3. Multiply:

$$\underset{\text{(concentration)}}{1.5 \text{ mg/mL}} \times \underset{\text{(flow rate)}}{100 \text{ mL/hr}} = \underset{\text{(dose per time)}}{150 \text{ mg/hr}}$$

Problem: You have 500 mL D$_5$W, containing 10,000 units of heparin. The order states that the patient is to receive 2,000 units of heparin per hour. Calculate the flow rate needed (in mL/hr).

Solution: Again, use the formula. The dose per time is given as 2,000 units/hr, and you can calculate the concentration (it is 10,000 units/500 mL, or 20 units/mL).

Using the formula, solve for the flow rate:

$$C \times F = \frac{D}{t}$$

$$\frac{20\,units}{mL} \times F = 2,000\,units/hr$$

$$F = \frac{\overset{100}{\cancel{2,000}}\,\cancel{units}/hr}{\underset{1}{\cancel{20}}\,\cancel{units}/mL} = 100\,mL/hr$$

If your flow rate is given in drops, rather than mL, an additional step is required. You would need to know the gtts/min rate and also the drop factor of the tubing used (gtts/mL) to calculate the mL/minute or mL/hr rate. By dividing the rate (gtts/min) by the drop factor (gtts/mL) you will get the mL/minute rate.

$$\frac{gtts/min}{gtts/mL} = mL/min$$

Problem: A 1 L bag of $\frac{1}{2}$ NS contains 1,000 mg of calcium gluconate. The flow rate is 25 gtt/min, and the drop factor is 15 gtt/mL. What is the hourly dose of calcium?

Solution: Use $C \times F = D/t$.

First, calculate the flow rate in mL/hour:

$$\frac{25\,\cancel{gtt}/min}{15\,\cancel{gtt}/mL} = 1.667\,mL/min$$

$$\frac{1.667\,mL}{\cancel{min}} \times \frac{60\,\cancel{min}}{hr} = 100\,mL/hr$$

Next, calculate the concentration:

$$\frac{1000\,mg}{1000\,mL} = 1\,mg/mL$$

Finally, use the formula:

$$\frac{1\,mg}{mL} \times \frac{100\,mL}{hr} = 100\,mg$$

Shortcuts

Those students who are very comfortable with this type of calculation may use a faster way of performing the calculation (the rest of us will stick to the main road).

The following illustrates an example of a shortcut through a calculation of dose per time.

Problem: A 0.5% solution of lidocaine is flowing at 50 mL per hour. What is the hourly dose?

Solution: We could use the formula, but there is an easy shortcut to this problem.

First, convert:

$$0.5\% = \frac{0.5\,g}{100\,mL}$$

as we need a dose in mg (or g)/time.

Next, use ratio/proportion (or just think and divide):

$$\frac{0.5\,g}{100\,mL} = \frac{X\,g}{50\,mL}$$

Since 50 mL goes into the patient per hour, the hourly dose is obtained by cross-multiplying the above equation and solving for X:

$$X = \left(\frac{0.5\,g}{100\,mL}\right) \times 50\,mL = 0.25\,g \text{ or } 250\,mg \text{ per hour}$$

Chapter Review Questions

1. You have an order for aminophylline 500 mg in 250 mL D_5W, which is to run for 5 hours. The drop factor is 60 gtt/mL.
   (a) What is the flow rate in gtt/min?
   (b) What is the dose per minute?

2. An IV solution of heparin contains 5,000 units in 500 mL and takes 2 hours to infuse. How much drug is infused in 30 minutes?

3. The IV solution in question 2 (5,000 units/500 mL) is to be infused so that the patient gets 1,000 units of heparin per hour. Calculate the flow rate in mL/hr.

4. You add 10 mL of a 10% solution of calcium gluconate to a 500 mL IV bag. The flow rate is 30 gtt/min with an infusion set labeled 15 gtt/mL. How much drug does the patient get per hour?

5. A 1000 mL IV bag contains 40 mEq of potassium and infuses at 50 mL/hr. In 2 hours, how many mEq of potassium are administered to the patient?

6. A solution of 10,000 units of heparin in 500 mL of D$_5$W infuses in 8 hours. What is the hourly dose?

7. You add 5 g of drug to 1 L of saline. The hourly dose is to be 250 mg. Calculate the flow rate. How long will the IV run?

8. You add 1 g of Aminophylline to 1 L of NS. The patient is to receive 50 mg/hr. What is the flow rate?

9. You have a solution of 0.5% calcium gluconate, which infuses at 100 mL/hr. Calculate the hourly dose.

10. An IV is running at 80 mL/hr. What is the gtts/min rate using a 20 gtt/mL tubing?

CHAPTER 18

Compounding

Quick Study

I. Compounding drugs—importance of written procedure

   A. Compounding of drugs according to a specific written procedure. This may legally be done by the technician.
   B. Bulk compounding—the compiling of drug product for general use, according to a specific written procedure. This may legally be performed by the technician.
   C. Extemporaneous compounding—the compiling of a drug product for a specific patient, where no written procedure exists. This may be done only by the pharmacist, unless a specific written procedure is generated.

II. Reducing and enlarging formulas

   A. Use of a conversion factor to change amounts of individual ingredients in a formula
   B. Calculating conversion factors: amount needed amount specified in the procedure

III. Procedures for compounding

   A. Compounding based on weight
   B. Compounding based on percentage

IV. Preparing solutions

Compounding Drugs by Procedure

On occasion, it may be necessary to make a drug formulation "from scratch." It is permissible for the technician to do this, *if a written procedure exists* for making the product. This is called **bulk compounding**.

If no written procedure exists for making the formulation, the drug product must then be made by the *pharmacist*. Perhaps a physician wants a drug that is normally given orally to be put into suppository form for a patient who is NPO (receives nothing by mouth). Or perhaps a drug for oral dosage is to be made into a cream. This type of compounding requires the professional judgment of the pharmacist and is called **extemporaneous compounding**, in which a special drug dosage form is made *for a particular patient*.

Reducing and Enlarging Formulas

Compounding may only be done by the technician if a written procedure exists. If no written procedure exists (extemporaneous compounding), compounding must be done by the *pharmacist*. Once a specific written procedure is generated by the pharmacist, the dosage form may be prepared by the technician.

When compounding a drug formulation, it is sometimes necessary to reduce or enlarge the formula, according to the amount of drug needed. Let's start with a problem that requires enlarging the formula.

EXAMPLE

A procedure for making 500 g of antibiotic ointment is as follows:

Neomycin	2.5 g
Bacitracin	4.0 g
Polymixin B	320 mg
Liquid petrolatum	150 g
White petrolatum	343.18 g

In our pharmacy, the antibiotic ointment is a big seller, and 500 g is not enough. We need to make 1,000 g. To find out how much of each component to add in order to make 1,000 g of ointment (instead of 500 g), we must multiply the amount of each ingredient listed in the procedure by a *conversion factor*—a number that will allow the ingredients, when mixed together, to equal 1,000 g of ointment.

We determine this conversion factor by *dividing the amount needed by the amount specified in the procedure*. In this case, combining the specified amounts of each ingredient in the procedure will give us *500 g* of ointment, and we need *1,000 g*:

$$\frac{1,000\,g}{500\,g} = 2.$$

So, we multiply the amounts of all of the ingredients by 2. The enlarged recipe for 1,000 g of ointment looks like this:

Neomycin	5 g
Bacitracin	8.0 g
Polymixin B	640 mg
Liquid petrolatum	300 g
White petrolatum	686.36 g

Now, suppose instead that the antibiotic cream *doesn't* sell well. We now want to make less than the procedure specifies. We only want to make 200 g from the procedure that makes 500 g. Calculate the conversion factor. The amount needed = 200 g. The amount specified in the procedure is 500 g, so, dividing:

$$200 \text{ g}/500 \text{ g} = 0.4$$

We now multiply all of the original amounts by 0.4, to obtain:

Neomycin	1 g
Bacitracin	1.6 g
Polymixin B	128 mg
Liquid petrolatum	60 g
White petrolatum	137.2 g
Total	200 g

Making Preparations by Percentage

A procedure for preparing a drug formulation may be expressed in percentages. If this is the case, you will have to convert the percentages to numerical form first, before measuring or calculating.

EXAMPLE

A procedure for preparing calamine lotion reads as follows:

Calamine	8%
Zinc oxide	8%
Glycerol	2%
Bentonite	25%

q.s. (fill to the proper volume) with 2% calcium hydroxide solution to 1 L.

Step 1. Convert the percentages to grams: 8% w/v = 8 g/100 mL

Step 2. Set up a ratio/proportion problem to determine how much of each component to add—1 L (1,000 mL) is being made, so:

$$\frac{8 \text{ g}}{100 \text{ mL}} = \frac{X \text{ g}}{1,000 \text{ mL}}$$

Cross-multiply and divide:

$$X = 80 \text{ g}$$

Step 3. Convert the other percentages the same way and tabulate them:

Calamine	80 g
Zinc oxide	80 g
Glycerol	20 g
Bentonite	250 g

q.s. with 2% calcium hydroxide solution to 1 L

Making Solutions by Percentage

On occasion, a technician might be required to make a simple salt or drug solution by percentage. This simply involves calculating the amount of salt and adding the water.

EXAMPLE

Prepare 2 L of saline (0.9% NaCl).

Step 1. Set up the ratio/proportion:

$$\frac{0.9\,g}{100\,mL} \diagdown\!\!\!\!\diagup \frac{X\,g}{2,000\,mL}$$

Cross-multiply and divide:

$$X = 18\ g$$

Step 2. Add 18 g of sodium chloride to 2 L of water.

Chapter Review Questions

Consider the following procedure for making 1,000 g of a bulk laxative:

psyllium	500 g
dextrose	487g
citric acid	5 g
sodium bicarbonate	5 g
lemon flavoring	3 g

1. What is the percentage of psyllium in the preparation?

2. We want to make 500 g of laxative. How much psyllium do we need?

3. What is the percentage of sodium bicarbonate in the preparation?

4. How much of each ingredient would be necessary to make 250 g of laxative?

Consider the following procedure for calamine lotion with antihistamine:
q.s. with 2% calcium hydroxide solution to 1 L

calamine	80 g
zinc oxide	80 g
glycerol	20 g
bentonite	245 g
diphenhydramine	5 g

5. What percentage of antihistamine (diphenhydramine) is added?

6. How much diphenhydramine is needed to make 5 L of lotion?

7. How much lotion can we make with 60 g of zinc oxide?

8. How much glycerol is needed to make 240 mL of lotion?

9. If the ingredients in the preparation take up a volume of 50 mL, the total amount of calcium hydroxide added to the preparation would be:
   a. 1 L
   b. 850 mL
   c. 950 mL
   d. 1,000 mL

10. We need 200 mL of a 2% solution of calcium hydroxide. How much calcium hydroxide do we need to make the solution?
    a. 5 g
    b. 2.5 g
    c. 4 g
    d. 8 g

CHAPTER 19

Commercial Calculations

Quick Study

I.   Cost and markup
- The cost of the drug or device to the pharmacy ("cost price")
- The markup: the percentage of the cost price that is added to the cost price

A.   Calculating the selling price
- Cost markup selling price
- Dispensing charges: additional fees added to the selling price (calculated by percentage or a flat fee)

Cost and Markup

Cost price—wholesale price or acquisition cost

Markup—a percentage of the cost price

Selling price—cost + markup

Profit—markup amount less expenses

In the pharmacy, prescription and over-the-counter drugs are normally ordered in large amounts (by the case or *gross*), in order to get a lower price for high-use items. The *price that the pharmacy pays for a drug* or supply item is called the **cost price**. The drug or item cannot then be sold at the same price that was paid for it—there would be no profit to the pharmacy, which, after all, is a business. So, a *percentage of the cost price* (the **markup**) is added. Thus, when the pharmacy sells the item it makes a profit. The amount of profit equals the markup amount minus the associated costs, such as charges for building electricity, salaries of personnel, etc.

Calculating the Selling Price

The selling price is based on what the pharmacy paid for the item, plus a reasonable profit.

> ### EXAMPLE
>
> Think of a man buying a pound of potatoes. He pays $1 for them. He then takes them to his neighbor and charges his neighbor $2, which is the cost price plus an extra $1 for buying the potatoes and driving them home. The cost price of the potatoes was $1 and the selling price was $2, so the markup on the potatoes was $1, or 100% of the cost price. The actual profit that the man made is less than the markup that he charged, as it cost him 50 cents in gas to drive to the store. The net profit on the sale would then be $1-$0.50, or 50 cents.

Problem: The pharmacy buys a case of cold remedy for $20 (the cost price). It marks the price up by 100% (the markup). Calculate the selling price.

$$\boxed{\$20} + \boxed{100\% \times \$20 = \$20} \longrightarrow \boxed{\$40}$$

$$\text{Cost} + \qquad \text{Markup} \qquad = \text{Selling price}$$

This is an important formula to remember. With slight variations, all of the commercial calculations use this formula. For example, we can make the problem we just did more complicated. Normally, we do not sell products from the pharmacy by the case. We sell them individually. So, let's take the same problem and compute the selling price of each individual bottle of cold remedy.

Problem: The pharmacy buys a case of cold remedy for $20. There are 10 bottles per case. The bottles of cold remedy are marked up by 100%. Calculate the selling price per bottle.

Solution: To calculate prices for individual items, we must know the price per case and the number of items per case. In this problem, the price per case is $20 and there are 10 bottles per case. Cost price per bottle is thus $20/10 = $2 per bottle.

Using the formula Cost + Markup = Selling price, we calculate:

$$\text{Cost} = \frac{\$20\,\text{per case}}{10\;\text{bottles per case}} = \$2$$

$$\text{Markup} = 100\% \text{ of } \$2 = \$2$$

$$\text{Selling price} = \$2 + \$2 = \mathbf{\$4}$$

Problem: The pharmacy pays $250 for a stock bottle of Tegretol, which contains 1,000 tablets. The markup is 200%. What is the selling price for 100 tablets?

> Remember: Cost + Markup = Selling Price

Solution: The cost price per tablet is $250/1,000 = $0.25 per tablet.

The markup would be $0.25 × 2, or $0.50. Using the formula:

Cost + Markup = Selling price

$0.25 + $0.50 = **$0.75** per tablet

The selling price for 100 tablets would be $0.75 × 100, or $75.

The Dispensing Fee

The pharmacy may add an additional amount to the price of a prescription drug: the **dispensing fee**. This amount may be a flat fee or a percentage of the selling price, depending on the rules of the institution or pharmacy chain. The dispensing fee is added *only* on drugs *actually* dispensed from the pharmacy, not those sold over the counter.

Chapter Review Questions

1. A pharmacy sells a tube of Ben-Gay for $6.90, with a 200% markup. What was the cost of the Ben-Gay to the pharmacy?

2. Referring to question 1, how much gross profit will the pharmacy make on a case of 50 if it sells the Ben-Gay for 50% off?

3. You have a vial of ampicillin sodium for injection, containing 5 g of drug. You dilute it to 500 mg/mL. The cost of the vial is $15, and the markup is 200%.
   (a) How much does the entire vial sell for?
   (b) How much gross profit will be made on the one vial?

4. You get an order for ampicillin sodium 1 g IV bid. Disregarding dispensing fees, how much would the patient be billed for one dose? For a daily dose? (Hint: Use the information from question 3.)

5. You have a 10% solution of calcium gluconate, priced at $2 per 10 mL. There is a 200% markup on the drug product. Your order is for 1 g of calcium gluconate in a saline drip.
   (a) What would the patient be charged for the drug?
   (b) How much gross profit would the pharmacy make on this dose?

CHAPTER 20

Math Test with Solutions

The following questions will test your ability to solve pharmacy-oriented questions in a multiple-choice format. Choose the *best* solution.

1. 50 mL =
   a. 0.5 L
   b. 50,000 mcl
   c. 0.05 L
   d. both b and c

2. 10% of 50 g =
   a. 500 mg
   b. 5,000 mg
   c. 5 g
   d. both b and c

3. On a written prescription, gr xii would mean:
   a. 5 g
   b. 22 g
   c. 8 grains
   d. 12 grains

4. The instructions "one gtt AU qod" would be transcribed on the label as:
   a. 1 gram by mouth twice a day
   b. place one drop in either eye every day
   c. place one drop in each ear every other day
   d. place one drop in both ears every other day

5. You receive a box of gold. You would prefer it to weigh:
   a. 5 grams
   b. 5 grains
   c. 1 scruple
   d. 1 milligram

6. Which of the following is the smallest amount?
   a. 1 dram
   b. 1 Liter
   c. 1 teaspoon
   d. 5 milliliters

7. You receive an order for 25 units of U-100 insulin. Which of the following should be dispensed?
   a. a low-dose insulin syringe, containing 0.25 mL insulin
   b. a low-dose insulin syringe, containing 25 units of U-100 insulin
   c. a U-100 syringe, containing 25 units of insulin
   d. a tuberculin syringe, containing 25 mcL of U-100 insulin

8. A prescription drug order reads "diazepam 2.5 mg IM bid." The available stock is in a sealed 1 mL vial containing 5 mg/mL. A daily dose would be:
   a. one vial
   b. two vials
   c. 5 mL
   d. 10 mL in a 10 mL syringe

9. You have an order for "codeine gr i tid prn." You have 30 mg tablets in stock. The label on the dispensing bottle should read:
   a. take one tablet twice a day, as needed
   b. take two tablets twice a day
   c. take two tablets three times a day, as needed
   d. none of the above—the prescription must be filled exactly as written

10. A patient is to take 15 mL of elixir twice a day. You would label the bottle with instructions to take _____ twice a day.
    a. 1 tablespoon
    b. 1 dram
    c. 32 teaspoons
    d. either a or c

11. gr ss = _____ mg
    a. 5
    b. 15
    c. 30
    d. 60

12. ℥ i =
    a. 20 mL
    b. 5 mL
    c. 15 mL
    d. 30 mL

13. 500 cc
    a. 0.5 L
    b. 500 mL
    c. the volume contained in a cube with dimensions of 1 cm per side
    d. a and b only

14. A patient has a temperature of 37°C. If normal temperature is 98.6°F, he:
    a. is cold
    b. has a fever
    c. is perfectly normal
    d. is sick

15. To reconstitute a drug, you would:
    a. add a second drug to it
    b. add water to it
    c. dilute with an appropriate solution
    d. none of the above

16. Your order is for cefoperazone 250 mg bid. Your stock is CefoBid suspension, 100 mg/mL. For a single dose, you would dispense:
    a. 5 mL
    b. 10 mL
    c. 2.5 mL
    d. 0.5 mL

17 For a daily dose of the prescription in question 16, you would dispense:
    a. 2.5 mL
    b. 5 mL
    c. 10 mL
    d. 8 mL

18. A 10% solution would be:
    a. 10 g/100 mL
    b. 100 g/L
    c. 100 mg/10 mL
    d. a and b

19. The order "Valium 20 mg IM stat" means to deliver:
    a. one tablet of Valium right now
    b. 10 mL of Valium as soon as possible
    c. an injection of 20 mg of Valium immediately
    d. 20 mL of Valium in a dosage cup right away

20. Your order is for codeine IM gr i. Available stock is 20 mg/mL. You dispense:
    a. 0.3 mL in a 1 mL syringe
    b. 3 mL in a 3 mL syringe
    c. 0.6 mL in a 1 mL syringe
    d. 1.5 mL in a 3 mL syringe

21. Your order is for furosemide 80 mg bid po. Your stock is Lasix 40 mg tablets. You dispense:
    a. two tablets per dose
    b. $\frac{1}{2}$ tablet per dose
    c. four tablets per dose
    d. both a and c are correct

22. A drug order is for nafcillin 0.25 g. In stock are 250 mg tablets. Dispense:
    a. four tablets
    b. two tablets
    c. one tablet
    d. ten tablets

23. 1 tab qid could be interpreted as:
    a. take one tablet twice a day
    b. take one tablet four times a day
    c. take one tablet every 6 hours
    d. both b and c

24. 3 mL could not be accurately measured in:
    a. an oral syringe
    b. a syringe for injection
    c. a calibrated spoon
    d. a dosage cup

25. An insulin syringe:
    a. holds 1 mL or less
    b. is calibrated in units
    c. is the same as a tuberculin syringe
    d. a and b

26. How much drug is contained in 20 mL of a 10% solution?
    a. 200 mg
    b. 20 mg
    c. 2 g
    d. 0.2 g

27. The instructions on a prescription include the notation "1gtt OD am hs." The drug would be placed into the:
    a. right eye twice a day
    b. left eye three times a day
    c. right eye in the morning and evening
    d. right eye in the morning and at bedtime

Match the following to the correct description:

    a. dosage strength
    b. dosage form
    c. supply dosage

28. a tablet

29. a capsule

30. 10 mg

31. 10 mg/tablet

32. parenteral solution

33. 10,000 units/10 mL

34. 20% solution

35. 10,000 units

36. tincture

37. syrup

38. Your order is for 2,000 mL of D_5W to run for 12 hours. The drop factor is 10 gtt/mL. The flow rate in gtt/min is:
    a. 12
    b. 14
    c. 28
    d. 17

39. Your order is 500 mL NS to run for 5 hours. The drop factor is 60 gtt/mL. The flow rate is ____ mL/min and ____ gtt/min.
    a. 0.8, 50
    b. 1.67, 100
    c. 1.8, 150
    d. 0.4, 24

40. You have an order for 75,000 units of heparin to be infused over 4 hours. The 1 L bag contains 150,000 units of heparin. The flow rate needed to deliver the dose is:
    a. 200 mL/hr
    b. 150 mL/hr
    c. 125 mL/hr
    d. 100 mL/hr

41. The recommended child dose of Keflex is 25 mg/kg/day in two divided doses. If a child weighs 66 lb, what is the correct dose?
    a. 375 mg bid
    b. 750 mg bid
    c. 700 mg qd
    d. 412 mg bid

42. The prescribed dose of drug for a child is 10 mg/m². His BSA is 0.8 m². The order would call for:
   a. 80 mg of drug
   b. 0.08 mg of drug
   c. 8 mg of drug
   d. 47 mg of drug

43. An IV bag containing a 2% solution of drug is running at 100 mL/hr. The hourly dose is:
   a. 20 mg
   b. 200 mg
   c. 2 g
   d. 2 mg

44. An order is for penicillin, to be infused at 100,000 units/hr. A 1 L IV bag containing 1,000,000 units of penicillin is used. The flow rate should be:
   a. 5 mL/min
   b. 50 mL/hr
   c. 100 mL/hr
   d. 2 mL/min

45. An adult dose of cefaclor is 500 mg. The dose for a 66 lb child would be:
   a. 50 mg
   b. 180 mg
   c. 220 mg
   d. 198 mg

46. The child in question 45 is eight years old. Using Young's Rule, the dose would be:
   a. 79 mg
   b. 174 mg
   c. 200 mg
   d. 80 mg

47. The adult dose of a drug is 40 mg/kg. A child weighs 62 pounds. The child's dose would be:
   a. 240 mg
   b. 663 mg
   c. 1,127 mg
   d. 100 mg bid

48. The adult dose of a drug is 100 mg. The dose for a child weighing 50 pounds would be:
   a. 75 mg
   b. 50 mg
   c. 150 mg
   d. 33 mg

49. A 10-year-old child receives the drug in question 48 The dose prescribed would be:
   a. 50 mg
   b. 75.2 mg
   c. 45.45 mg
   d. 30.6 mg

50. Your order is for 2,000 mL of D_5W to run for 12 hours. The flow rate in mL/min would be:
    a. 10 mL/min
    b. 12 mL/min
    c. 5 mL/min
    d. 2.8 mL/min

51. Your order is for 500 mL of NS to run for 4 hours. Your infusion set is labeled 10 gtt/mL. The flow rate in gtt/min would be:
    a. 2 gtt/min
    b. 20 gtt/min
    c. 21 gtt/min
    d. 60 gtt/min

52. Your order is for 75,000 units of heparin to be infused over 8 hours. Available is a 1 L bag containing 100,000 units of heparin. The flow rate should be:
    a. 50 mL/hr
    b. 100 mL/hr
    c. 94 mL/hr
    d. 45.2 mL/hr

53. 100,000 units of penicillin is infused in 5 hours. The hourly dose would be:
    a. 10,000 units
    b. 20,000 units
    c. 50,000 units
    d. Cannot be calculated from the information given

54. A patient receives D_5W at a rate of 100 mL/hr. The amount of dextrose administered per hour is:
    a. 50 mg
    b. 1 g
    c. 50 g
    d. 5 g

55. A patient receives 500 mL of a 1% calcium gluconate solution in 2 hours. The rate of infusion of calcium is:
    a. 50 mg/min
    b. 200 mg/hr
    c. 1.5 g/hr
    d. 41.7 mg/min

56. The recommended child dose of Keflex is 25 mg/kg/day, divided into two doses. If a child weighs 73 lb, how much drug would be prescribed for one dose?
    a. 825 mg
    b. 415 mg
    c. 375 mg
    d. 500 mg

57. A physician frequently orders rectal suppositories for hemorrhoids. The suppositories contain:

    0.5% epinephrine

    2% zinc oxide

    0.25% mrystic acid

    q.s. with white petrolatum

The stock of epinephrine on hand is a 1:100 solution. What volume of epinephrine will be required?

58. A 200 lb man is prescribed cephalexin 500 mg IV, for a 4-hour infusion. The drug is added to a 500 mL bag of saline. What is the flow rate?

59. A patient is to receive 1 L of D_5W/0.45 NS with 30 mEq of KCl IV on a 6-hour infusion. What is the hourly dose of potassium?

60. A physician writes instructions for the preparation of an antiemetic mixture:

Milk of magnesia	80 mL
Lidocaine viscous 1%	10 mL
Meclizine elixir 0.5%	10 mL

    Sig: ii or iii teaspoons ac. h.s.

    The proper size of the dispensing container to be used for the mixture would be:
    a. a 1 oz bottle
    b. a 4 oz bottle
    c. a 2 oz tube
    d. a container that holds 200 mL

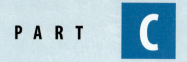

PART C

Pharmacology

CHAPTER 21

Introduction to Pharmacology

Quick Study

I.   Learning drug nomenclature—proprietary vs. generic names

II.   The therapy of illness—drugs of choice; first-, second-, and third-line drugs

    A.   Drug of choice—the most efficacious drug for the condition

    B.   First-line drugs—maximum efficacy with most acceptable adverse effect profile

    C.   Second-line drugs—somewhat decreased efficacy, as compared to first-line drugs, and/or with less acceptable adverse effect profile

    D.   Third- and fourth-line drugs—efficacious but unfavorable adverse effect profile. Often useful in specific forms or presentations of a disease (e.g., refractory patients, patients with concurrent behavioral abnormalities, etc.)

III. Drug mechanism of action, therapeutic uses, adverse effects, and contraindications

IV.   Frequently prescribed drugs of a class

    A.   Dosage forms and strengths available

    B.   Advantages, disadvantages, differential uses over other drugs of the class

    C.   Secondary uses

V.   Pharmacokinetics and pharmacodynamics

    A.   Absorption

    B.   Distribution

    C.   Metabolism

    D.   Drug clearance and elimination

VI. General mechanisms of drug interactions

A. Synergism: A potentiation of the effects of one drug by a second drug. This potentiation may relate to both therapeutic and toxic effects.

B. Additive effects: When a second drug contributes to the therapeutic effects of another drug.

C. Antagonism: A drug blocks the effects of another drug.

Introduction

The amount and depth of pharmacology, which the technician will be required to know, has expanded greatly since the first writing of the exam. Liability issues and a greater area of responsibility now require the technician to be knowledgeable in pharmacology. The PTCB exam now requires examinees to know not only drug names (generic and proprietary), but also their mechanisms of action, drug classifications, general uses, side effects, and interactions. Attention should be paid in this chapter and the following chapters to the general therapeutic action of a particular drug and the drug class (tricyclic antidepressant, benzodiazepine, opiate, etc.), in addition to:

- The mechanism of action of the drug
- The *physiological* actions of the drug. What are the effects of a drug on normal body function (e.g., effects on blood sugar, heart rate)?
- Possible adverse effects
- Possible drug interactions
- Food and lifestyle contraindications
- Contraindications to pregnancy or nursing
- Generic and proprietary (brand) names available

The availability and the specific uses of particular drug dosage forms, as well as the dosage and strengths (e.g., 10 mg tablet) should also be familiar to you.

Form vs. Use—Recognizing Various Forms of a Generic Drug

Note that many drugs have been treated with an acid or base and thus are salts of the original drug. This has been done to make the drug more easily utilized by the body when administered by a certain route (e.g., orally, intravenously, etc.). These drugs may have words such as "mesylate," "tartrate," "citrate," or "hydrochloride (HCl)" after their names, or the words "sodium" or "potassium." Penicillin G potassium (Penicillin G-K) is the potassium salt of penicillin, for example. Various chemical forms of a particular drug have different clinical uses. Take, for example, the antibiotic erythromycin, which is available in several chemical forms, each useful by a different route: Erythromycin gluceptate is used by parenteral route, erythromycin succinate is used orally, and erythromycin estolate is a highly absorbable form of erythromycin. Specification of the type of salt to the name of the drug may not always be seen in practice, especially if only one form of the drug exists. Drugs are normally referred to simply by name (e.g., trazodone, rather than trazodone hydrochloride). A particular drug salt is normally only specified on a medication order if the particular form is necessary for effective administration by a particular route, or is the best choice for a particular patient's condition.

Addition of letters to a drug name is also important, however. For example, penicillin G is the form of penicillin normally given by parenteral route, while penicillin V is given orally. In addition, letters appearing after the name of a drug may denote a certain type of formulation—for example, the addition of the letters "SR," "LA," or "XR" after a drug name denotes a sustained release formulation, and "NPH" (neutral protamine hagadorn) insulin is a complexed form of insulin that is longer acting than regular insulin.

Proprietary Drug Nomenclature

Drugs may be named according to a particular quality or property of the drug—for example, what they do, or their drug classification. Less frequently, names may reflect some other property that the drug has, such as fast onset (Allegra), long duration (Cardura), or established dosing interval (Cefo*bid*— as in "bid" or twice daily dosing). In many cases, the use and/or class of a drug can be determined from the name.

> ### EXAMPLE
>
> Take the trade name Tegopen. This drug is a penicillin derivative—the name ends in *pen*. The drug is actually cloxacillin.

Many drugs simply take part of the generic name as the trade name—for instance, **Amox**il is *amoxi*cillin, **Busp**ar is *buspir*one, **Platin**ol is cis*platin*, and **Pilocar** is *pilocar*pine. Most of the cephalosporin antibiotics have "*cef*" or "*kef*" in the name, such as **Cef**obid, **Kef**lex, Bio**cef**, and **Kef**tab. Most proprietary names reflect the class, properties, or use of the drug, and trade names by different manufacturers for the same drug are often similar (e.g., **Amox**il and Poly**mox** are both amoxicillin). A trade name may also reflect the *dosage form* (e.g., Cef**tabs**), or strength of the drug, as well.

You should keep these concepts in mind so if you are faced with a question on the exam and you are not familiar with the drug name, you can make an educated guess. (When working in the pharmacy it is, of course, better to use the "generic-to-brand" book. Unfortunately, you cannot bring it to the exam.)

Recognizing Proprietary Drug Names

When memorizing a proprietary name, you should look for the similarities between the proprietary name and the generic name, or find a part of the name that reflects the drug's function. This will help you recognize the name and associate it. Also, when memorizing names of drugs, it is very helpful to prepare flash cards. In addition, a pharmacology text or nurse's drug reference might be a source of drug names and classifications to memorize. If you come across an unfamiliar drug on the exam and can recognize the similarities between a generic name or therapeutic use, you may be able to recognize drug names that you have not memorized.

Understanding the Pharmacology of Chemotherapeutic Agents

The mechanism of action and adverse effects are similar for drugs within a class. Only differences in lipid solubility, duration, etc., may be seen.

The following chapters present the drugs that are most frequently used in the therapy of certain medical conditions. The drugs are presented by *class*, and in the order in which they would be chosen for therapy. The generic name and major proprietary names of each drug are listed, as well as the dosage forms that are commercially available.

Classification of Drugs by Mechanism of Action

The mechanism of action of a drug is a specific action on a biological or biochemical process. For example, a drug could stimulate or antagonize (block) receptors for a particular neurotransmitter, interfere with cellular metabolism, inhibit cellular replication, or disrupt bacterial cell wall synthesis.

NOTE

Drugs within a class tend to have similar mechanisms of action, adverse effects, and contraindications!

Drugs work by creating various biological and biochemical changes within the body. This is termed the **mechanism of action** of the drug. Drugs within a class tend to have similar mechanisms of action, adverse effects, and contraindications. Thus, for each classification of drug, the mechanism of action has been presented and a brief description of physiological effects and adverse (unwanted or detrimental) effects.

Choice of Drug Therapy

For any illness or condition, there are certain drugs that are prescribed more frequently, as they are more effective (efficacious) for the condition. A certain drug or drug class may be by far the most effective in treating a particular condition and so would be most frequently prescribed. This drug (or class of drugs) is called the "**drug of choice**" (DOC), and would be the first choice for therapy. Drugs that are very effective in treating a certain condition, and that have an acceptable adverse effect profile, are called **first line drugs**, because they are the first drugs to be prescribed. If a patient is *refractory* to the effects of the first-line drug (the drug doesn't work, for some reason specific to that patient), a second- or third-line drug, or even a fourth-line drug, is prescribed. These drugs are progressively either less efficacious in treatment, or have a lot of undesirable effects (a negative adverse effect profile), and are prescribed as second, third, or fourth choices, respectively.

Understanding Therapeutic Effects

> If you understand the mechanism of action of a drug, and its effects on physiology, then you have a good understanding of what the drug does in the body!

Understanding the therapeutic effects of a drug is normally nothing more than an understanding of its physiological effects. The actions of drugs are often quite complex, but in most instances can be distilled down to simpler concepts. For example, say that the drug in question works by stimulating an adrenergic alpha receptor (α_1). If you know what an α_1 receptor does, you have an idea of what the drug does. Of course, this may be a bit simplistic, as drugs that act primarily at one receptor will often stimulate others, but it is a good way to orient your thinking!

Pharmacokinetics and Pharmacodynamics—What Happens to the Drug After It Is Administered?

Pharmacokinetics is a study of the movement of and changes in the drug within the body. It consists of four parts:

- **Absorption**: how the drug gets into the bloodstream.
- **Distribution**: where the drug goes in the body (e.g., fat storage, storage in bloodstream formation of drug-protein complexes, etc.).
- **Metabolism**: how the drug is changed in the body. This change can result in the activation *or* the elimination of the drug.
- **Elimination**: how the body gets rid of the drug.

This is called the ADME process.

Absorption

Absorption refers to how a drug gets into the bloodstream from outside of the body (e.g., drugs administered orally, rectally, transdermally, sublingually, intranasally, etc.). *By definition, drugs administered by intravenous injection are not absorbed, as they are injected directly into the blood.*

What Determines the Amount of Drug Absorbed?

The amount of drug absorbed into the body from a specific body compartment (e.g., the stomach or small intestine) is determined by several factors:

- *The pH of the compartment*: When a drug enters a particular body compartment (e.g., the stomach), it reacts with the environment of that compartment. Depending on the nature of the drug (i.e., whether it is a weak acid or base) and the difference in acidity between the drug and its environment, the drug may either remain intact (as would happen when the environment and drug are similar), or ionize (when they are dissimilar). Drugs are absorbed *better* as intact molecules, not as dissolved salts or charged (ionized) particles. Ionization of a drug is determined by the pH of the compartment where it is administered (e.g., the stomach) and the ionization constant of the drug. Most drugs are either weak acids or weak bases. A weak acid will ionize in a basic environment (e.g., the duodenum), but not in an acid environment (e.g., the stomach). Therefore, it is better absorbed from the acid environment, as less of the molecule is ionized (charged). Examples of drugs that are weak acids include aspirin and acetaminophen. Drugs that are weak bases include diazepam (Valium) and chlordiazepoxide (Librium).

- *Lipid solubility*: Cell membranes are made of fats. Therefore, a drug that is lipid soluble will pass more easily through the cell membrane. It will not, however, tend to remain in the plasma, as plasma is primarily composed of water. Drugs that are highly lipid soluble include most CNS drugs and anesthetics.

- *Vascularity of the administration site*: Since the drug is being absorbed into the blood, the more blood vessels at the absorption site, the more rapidly the drug will be absorbed.

> ### EXAMPLE
> Sublingual administration provides rapid absorption, as the area underneath the tongue contains a large number of blood vessels.

> ### NOTE
> If the pH of a body compartment is altered, drug absorption will be altered as well.

> ### EXAMPLE
> Aspirin is absorbed well in the acid environment of the stomach. If an antacid is taken concurrently, the acidity of the stomach fluids will be reduced, and less of the aspirin will be absorbed!

The Distribution of the Drug in the Body

Distribution refers to where the drug goes once it is absorbed, and how it is stored. Once the drug is in the bloodstream, it disseminates throughout the body, or is **distributed**. Part of the drug will be free in the plasma (this is the drug that will actually be working in the body). The rest may be stored in some way, such as bound to plasma proteins, or stored in fat.

How Drug is Stored in the Body

> Drugs exist either free in the plasma, or stored.

Storage sites for drugs may be fatty tissue (e.g., the liver, spleen, CNS, or stored fat) if the drug is highly lipid soluble, or protein-drug complexes. These complexes may exist as drugs that are stored bound to either plasma proteins (e.g., albumin) or tissue proteins. Binding of the drug to plasma proteins stabilizes the drug and also keeps it from being broken down by the liver or filtered out and excreted by the kidneys (the proteins are too big to be filtered).

> In order for a drug to work, it must be free in the plasma.

Drugs bound to proteins exist in an equilibrium between bound drug and drug that is free in the plasma. Only the free drug is available to have a therapeutic effect or to be cleared (**eliminated**) from the body (free drug may produce toxic effects, as well, if the levels are too high). As free drug is cleared from the plasma, it is replaced by drug that is released from the drug-protein complexes. Thus, an equilibrium exists between the drug that is complexed to protein (bound drug) and that which is free in the plasma. Similarly, if more drug is absorbed (i.e., when the patient takes another dose), causing plasma levels of free drug to increase, more of the free drug will now begin to bind to proteins, so that the equilibrium between bound and free drug is maintained. Note that this is not necessarily a 1:1 ratio—the amount of drug complexed to proteins does not necessarily equal the amount that is free in the plasma.

Maintaining Plasma Concentrations of Drug—The Equilibrium

A state of equilibrium will occur, regardless of how the drug is stored—if it is stored in the fat, for example, rather than in a drug-protein complex, drug will leave the fatty tissue storage site as blood levels decrease, and enter fatty tissue as blood levels increase, in order to maintain the equilibrium between stored drug and drug that is free in the plasma.

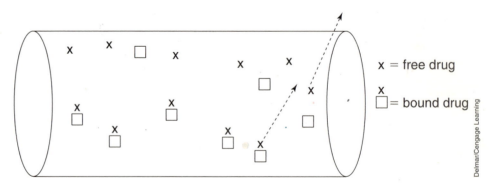

x = free drug

x
☐ = bound drug

Delmar/Cengage Learning

The Volume of Distribution and Loading Dose

The volume of space that the drug occupies in the body is called the **volume of distribution**. The volume of distribution (V_d) is important, as it gives an idea of how much drug must be taken before a state of equilibrium is reached.

A large volume of distribution means that the drug is distributed within many body compartments (e.g., plasma, tissues, the central nervous system), and a small volume of distribution means that the drug is concentrated primarily in one place (e.g., blood plasma). The more places that a drug can distribute to, the smaller the plasma concentration, with a given dose of drug. Since it is the free drug in the plasma that determines the therapeutic effect, a relatively large amount of drug may have to be taken before the distribution sites fill up, allowing plasma levels to increase to the point where consistent therapeutic actions are seen. Often, patients beginning a new regimen with this kind of drug are prescribed a rather large dose at the beginning of the regimen (a "loading" dose) in order to more quickly reach therapeutic levels in the blood.

Metabolism

> Drug metabolism is normally accomplished using a group of liver enzymes or group of enzymes called the cytochrome mixed function oxidase system, or cytochrome P_{450}.

Many drugs undergo chemical changes in the body. This is called metabolism. Metabolism of a drug may happen in almost any organ, but the majority of drugs are metabolized in the liver. The liver contains a large number of enzymes, which are metabolic enzymes. The most important of these, pharmacologically, is actually a system or group of enzymes called the **cytochrome mixed function oxidase system**, or **cytochrome P_{450}**. Cytochrome P_{450} is involved in the metabolism of most drugs. Some drugs (e.g., cimetidine, barbiturates) will alter the activity or levels of this enzyme, which may result in changes in the rate of metabolism of other drugs that the patient may be taking. It should also be noted that other enzymes may be involved in drug metabolism, as well, and that the levels of these enzymes may be influenced by age or gender—for example, neonates and geriatric patients may not have the necessary enzymes for metabolism of a certain drug.

> ### EXAMPLE
>
> The antibiotic chloramphenicol causes a syndrome in neonates called grey baby syndrome. This occurs because the infants do not have the enzyme (*glucuronidase*) necessary to metabolize the drug.

Drug Clearance and Drug Elimination

Elimination of a drug is the removal of the drug *from the body*, while **clearance** of a drug is removal of the drug *from the bloodstream*. Drug clearance is normally accomplished by the kidney or liver (sometimes by the lung). Drug is filtered out in the kidney (provided that it is not lipid soluble or protein bound) or secreted from the liver into the bile and then into the feces. If a drug is lipid soluble, it will not be directly eliminated by the kidney. It must be eliminated (or at least processed) by the liver. *Care must be paid to the route of elimination of the drug and the state of health of the patient!* If a drug is eliminated primarily by the kidney, for example, it should be given with caution to a renally compromised patient, and dosage should be reduced in the elderly and neonates.

Drug Half-Life

> Mathematically, the half-life of a drug is the amount of time that it takes one half of a drug dose to be cleared from the body.

Every drug has a limited amount of time in which it will remain active in the body. This amount of time is measured by the drug half-life ($T_{1/2}$). Mathematically, the half-life of a drug is the amount of time that it takes one half of a drug dose to be cleared from the body (see Chapter 2). The half-life is determined by the clearance rate—which is influenced by:

1. The rate of elimination of the drug.
2. How quickly the drug might be inactivated in the body (e.g., by enzymes, etc.).

EXAMPLE

Acetylcholine is not used therapeutically as a drug because it is rapidly inactivated by plasma enzymes called *cholinesterases*. Since it is cleared (inactivated) so rapidly, its half-life is only a few seconds.

EXAMPLE

Some lipid-soluble drugs have very long half-lives because they pass through the liver and are excreted into the bile. However, instead of being *eliminated* from the body, when the bile (containing the drug) is released into the intestine from the liver and gallbladder, the drug is reabsorbed through the intestinal wall. This phenomenon is called **enterohepatic recycling**. The drug, instead of being eliminated from the body, is instead reabsorbed. Thus, it is cleared from the body very slowly, as it keeps being reabsorbed from the intestine. This results in a long half-life (the half-lives of these drugs can be as long as several days).

Alteration of Drug Half-Life

It should be noted that the half-life of a drug may also be altered by altering the clearance of the drug. Drugs excreted through the kidney, for example, will ionize in urine that is of a different pH, or remain intact when the urine pH is favorable. Just as in the stomach and intestine, intact drug will be *reabsorbed* into the body, while ionized drug will be excreted. Depending on the drug, changes in the rate of drug elimination may happen when body pH becomes altered (e.g., ingesting very acidic drinks, decreasing respiration rate or taking bicarbonate for an upset stomach). An increased rate of elimination may also be seen with severe illness, which changes the balance of proteins in the blood, causing changes in the amount of free drug in the plasma and thus influencing the rate of elimination.

The half-life of a drug also depends on the ability of the patient to clear the drug. A person with poor renal function, or decreased liver function, for example, may clear a drug very slowly (depending on the nature of the drug), effectively increasing the half-life.

The Adverse Effect Profile

> A drug with a negative adverse effect profile produces serious adverse effects that occur in a large number of patients.

> The number and frequency of occurrence of adverse effects makes up the adverse effect profile of a drug.

Every drug produces a spectrum of unwanted effects, which we call **adverse effects**. These can range from uncomfortable effects, such as nausea and edema, to potentially life-threatening effects, such as cardiac dysrhythmias and liver or kidney failure. These effects are erroneously (and inaccurately) referred to as "side effects."

Any effect that produces end organ toxicity is a **toxic effect**. These would include ototoxicity (damage to the ear and loss of hearing), such as that produced by loop diuretics and aminoglycoside antibiotics; nephrotoxicity (damage to the kidney), such as that produced by platinum-containing antineoplastic drugs; cardiotoxicity (produced by many agents, for example, the antibiotic antineoplastic agent doxorubicin); and hepatotoxicity (produced, for example, by acetaminophen). The more serious and frequent the adverse effects, the more "negative" the adverse effect profile.

Anticipating an Adverse Drug Effect

It is always best if you do not memorize all of the adverse effects of a drug or drug class. Instead, understand the *mechanism* of the drug's action, and, using your knowledge of physiology, anticipate its physiological effects.

EXAMPLE

Monoamine oxidase inhibitors, used in the therapy of depression, inhibit the enzyme monoamine oxidase, which breaks down catecholamines, such as epinephrine and norepinephrine. This results in elevated levels of these substances and improved mood.

Think! What would you expect the adverse effects of the drug to be?

To predict the adverse effects of this drug, first think of what effects norepinephrine normally produces. Elevated levels would just produce a magnified effect. A few things that come to mind might be that norepinephrine:

- Increases heart rate and blood pressure
- Increases blood sugar
- Decreases appetite

Therefore, for adverse effects, we might expect hypertension, cardiovascular abnormalities, negative interactions with diabetic patients, and anorexia. Norepinephrine also produces central nervous system effects, such as insomnia, restlessness, and nightmares, so you might expect nervousness and sleep disturbances in the patient, as well.

Hint: The adverse effect profiles of drugs within a class will be somewhat similar!

If you understand the physiology behind how the drugs work, and their mechanism of action, you need only think for a minute to predict both therapeutic and possible adverse effects.

Drug-Drug Interactions

There are many ways in which drugs can interact with each other within the body to cause problems. Many adverse interactions happen because the drugs do different things that interfere with their mechanism of action, or the way that they work. Many others occur because of the way that the drugs are stored or distributed within the body or the way in which they are eliminated from the body. Drug interactions at the following levels are described: absorption, distribution (protein binding), and clearance.

Drug-Drug Interactions at the Level of Absorption

In order for a drug to work, it must be *free in the plasma*. Thus, if it is taken orally, the drug must be *absorbed* from the gastrointestinal (GI) tract into the bloodstream. Drugs taken concurrently may interfere with absorption in various ways, such as competition for transport across the intestinal wall. Sometimes two drugs are absorbed into the body in the same way and so interfere with each other's absorption by competing for transport sites into the body. The higher the concentration of a drug, the more likely it is to gain access to the transport system.

- *Binding interactions*: Some drugs decrease the absorption of other drugs by binding to them in the stomach or intestine and preventing their absorption into the body.

> **EXAMPLE**
>
> Sucralfate, a drug used to promote healing of the stomach lining, binds to many drugs in the digestive tract and prevents or decreases their absorption; the tetracycline drugs (tetracycline, doxycycline, minocycline, etc.), if taken with meals or with mineral supplements (which contain iron, calcium, and magnesium), bind to these minerals in the intestine and cannot be absorbed into the body.

- *Changing the pH of the environment*: Drugs that influence the pH of a particular compartment may result in increased or decreased absorption of a second drug.

> Antacids decrease the acidity of the stomach and thus may alter the absorption of other drugs.

EXAMPLE

Antacids or other drugs that decrease stomach acidity (e.g., cimetidine, ranitidine) will decrease the absorption of aspirin or other acidic drugs into the body, thus decreasing the drug's effectiveness. In contrast, the decrease in acidity might increase the absorption of a drug that is more basic in nature (e.g., diazepam).

Changes in body pH due to the ingestion of an acidic or alkaline drug or substance can influence the rate of clearance of the drug, as well.

- *Changes in local blood flow*: Drugs that alter local blood flow may influence the rate of absorption of a second drug.

EXAMPLE

Drugs are injected intramuscularly because they are absorbed more slowly than with intravenous injection. Including a vasoconstrictor, such as norepinephrine, or local anesthetic (e.g., procaine) will decrease local blood flow and reduce the rate of absorption even further. This allows more drug to be injected, which is then absorbed over a long period of time.

Drug Distribution—Protein-Binding Interactions

Many drug interactions occur because two or more drugs bind to the same plasma proteins. The one that binds the tightest and the fastest "wins," leaving the "loser" floating in the plasma. This results in too much of the "loser" drug as free drug in the plasma. Remember that a drug, in order to work, must be free in the plasma—a stored drug is not available to work. The more free drug in the plasma, the greater is the effect and the greater the potential for toxicity. Since increased amounts of the free drug are available to work in the body, this drug may cause toxic effects. Also, remember that the free drug is more quickly metabolized or filtered out by the kidney, so it will be eliminated from the body faster as well. When two drugs that both bind extensively to plasma proteins are taken concurrently, the doses must be adjusted to reflect the change in plasma free drug concentrations, due to protein-binding interactions.

A good example of a drug that is highly plasma protein bound is warfarin (Coumadin). This drug has protein-binding interactions with many drugs.

The majority of protein-binding interactions occur with drugs bound to the plasma protein albumin. These drugs are many, and include carbamazepine, warfarin, propylthiouracil, oral hypoglycemic drugs (e.g., tolazamide, chlorpropamide), and erythromycin.

Drug-Drug Interactions at the Level of Drug Clearance

Whenever a patient takes a drug, that drug is designed to do its job and leave. The body *eliminates* the drug after a period of time, by expelling the drug through the lungs, urine, or bile. The drug may be broken down with enzymes (*metabolism*) in the liver and/or be filtered out of the blood by the kidneys and dumped in the urine.

The lungs may be involved in breaking down a drug, or may simply expel the drug into the air, eliminating it from the body. Drugs that are metabolized may go into the bile and out through the intestine, or, if the actions of the enzymes in the liver make them water soluble (so that they can be dissolved easily in water), they may go out through the urine. Some drugs are not metabolized and (if they are soluble in water) may go directly out in the urine; other drugs that are lipid soluble and not metabolized are excreted through bile, not urine.

Drug-Drug Interactions—Competition for Drug Clearance

A very important drug interaction occurs when more than one drug is being metabolized at the same time (this includes drugs such as alcohol). Some drugs interact by competing with each other for the same enzyme or altering the activity of a liver enzyme.

Enzymes are proteins that break down drugs. Many drugs are metabolized by a particular group of enzymes called cytochrome P_{450}. Drugs, such as cimetidine (Tagamet) and alcohol, alter the activity and amount of these enzymes, which changes the metabolism of other drugs that are cleared by the same enzymes. This means that the drug levels in the blood will continue to increase as the patient keeps taking the prescribed doses.

Effects of Age, Organ Damage, and Drug Use

An important thing to consider is a *patient's age*. Because drugs are cleared out of the body by the liver and kidney and the functions of these organs decrease with age, the dosage of the drug must be adjusted to compensate. Another important factor, especially when assessing drugs eliminated by the liver, is *whether the patient is an abuser of alcohol* or has *preexisting liver damage* (e.g., from hepatitis). Any existing damage to the liver could decrease the rate of clearance of the drug, causing the blood levels of drug to build up to toxic levels over time.

Drug Toxicity and Interactions

All drugs are, to some extent, poisons and have harmful effects. The dosages established for the patient are designed to minimize the harmful effects while maximizing the beneficial effects. However, taking more than one drug concurrently may cause a problem; sometimes one drug can set the stage for the harmful effects (toxic effects) of another.

EXAMPLE

Isoproterenol (a sympathetic agonist at beta receptors) acts on the heart to increase heart rate and increase electrical conduction through the heart tissue. Too high of a dose can cause tachycardia and arrhythmias. Thyroid drugs sensitize the heart to the effects of norepinephrine and epinephrine, which are produced under stress (and have effects on the heart similar to isoproterenol). Taking both drugs together could increase the probability of a fatal arrhythmia.

EXAMPLE

Drugs, such as furosemide and thiazide diuretics, cause a large amount of potassium loss. The heart is very sensitive to potassium levels and when other drugs that alter potassium are taken concurrently (e.g., sotalol), severe arrhythmias may result.

Drug Agonism and Antagonism

Many drugs are designed to mimic or interfere with the actions of a substance in the body (an *endogenous* substance). A drug that mimics the actions of an endogenous substance is called an **agonist**. An agonist may work in a variety of ways—through stimulating a cellular or biochemical pathway, for example, or inhibiting the breakdown of the endogenous substance (this is called *indirect* agonism). A common way for an agonist to work is by stimulating a receptor for an endogenous substance.

EXAMPLE

The lining of the blood vessel (the vascular *endothelium*) normally produces a vasodilating substance, nitric oxide (NO—also called "endothelin"). The nitrous oxide is used to activate an enzyme, which makes cyclic GMP, a potent vasodilating agent. The antianginal drug nitroglycerin is a glycerol molecule with three nitro groups attached to the molecule (NO_2). These nitro groups are removed from the molecule and converted to nitrous oxide. The nitrous oxide then inserts itself into the metabolic pathway and cyclic GMP is formed, just as with the endogenous substance.

EXAMPLE

The drug edrophonium binds to an enzyme, acetylcholinesterase, and inhibits it. Acetylcholinesterase is used by the body to break down acetylcholine, a neurotransmitter. Edrophonium, by inhibiting the enzyme, increases the amount of acetylcholine available, and thus magnifies its effects. This drug does not increase the actions of acetylcholine directly, but it is an *indirect* agonist.

Physiology Review

Receptors are proteins that communicate within the cell. A membrane-bound receptor, when stimulated by a hormone or neurotransmitter, communicates this stimulus to a *secondary messenger* within the cell. This messenger activates a cascade of events, resulting in changes within that cell. A receptor is only stimulated at the instant of contact with the transmitter—the transmitter molecule must detach and reattach in order to cause further stimulation of the receptor. Thus, if a substance is administered that binds to the receptor and either does not stimulate it or stimulates it once and then does not leave, that substance blocks that receptor to agents that may be available to stimulate it. Thus, this substance is termed an **antagonist** to the receptor and prevents the function of the receptor. Conversely, if the substance activates the receptor, it is termed an **agonist** to the receptor, and increases the receptor's function.

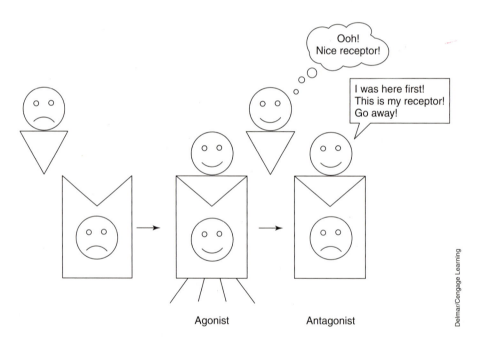

Agonist   Antagonist

Delmar/Cengage Learning

EXAMPLE

The α_1 receptor for norepinephrine causes vasoconstriction when stimulated. The drug prazosin binds to the same receptor and blocks the binding of norepinephrine in a competitive manner (both the drug and NE bind and detach, then repeatedly bind and detach, so there is competition for the receptor). Thus, the effects of norepinephrine are *antagonized* by the prazosin, as the NE cannot always bind to the receptor and exert its effects.

EXAMPLE

A patient produces high levels of norepinephrine when sleeping. This keeps him awake. When he is doing a stressful activity, the levels are too low.

DISCUSSION

We need to increase the actions of norepinephrine during periods of activity and decrease them during sleep. A partial agonist drug has weak activity. When levels of norepinephrine are low (e.g., when he is engaged in stressful activity) and there is not much of the strong agonist to stimulate receptors, it acts as an agonist at the receptors. When norepinephrine levels are too high (e.g., when he is sleeping), the drug, which has comparatively little activity, will occupy the receptor and block the strong agonist from binding. It is acting as an *antagonist*. So, when norepinephrine levels are low, the drug increases activity and when it is high, activity is inhibited.

Partial Agonists

These drugs are weak agonists. They act as agonists at the opiate receptors if no stronger agonists are present. If a stronger agonist is present, these drugs will block the receptor and act as antagonists, as they don't have much activity:

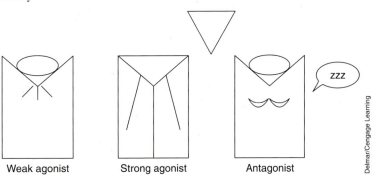

Weak agonist   Strong agonist   Antagonist

Delmar/Cengage Learning

Use of a Partial Agonist

Partial agonists normalize activity—they are useful when there are erratic levels of the strong agonist.

EXAMPLE

A patient is addicted to morphine. Normally, his level of opiates produced is low. When he gets some morphine, it is high. We want to prevent him from getting "high."

> **DISCUSSION**
>
> To do this, we give a partial agonist. This drug keeps activity constant, as it acts as an agonist when levels are low and antagonizes the morphine that comes in from outside. Thus, the "high" is cut off at the knees, but the body's normal opiate activity is not decreased (which would make the patient uncomfortable).

Additive, Synergistic, and Antagonistic Effects

Therapeutic Effects

Drugs that produce the same physiological effects may behave differently when taken together.

> **EXAMPLE**
>
> If two drugs both lower blood pressure by the same mechanism (e.g., blocking calcium channels) and both are seen to lower systolic pressure by 5%, then, by taking both drugs concurrently, we would expect a 10% decrease in systolic pressure. This is called an *additive* effect—the amount of effect of one drug is adding to that of another.

> **EXAMPLE**
>
> Two drugs have the same therapeutic effect but do not work by the same mechanism—say, one drug blocks calcium channels, reducing systolic pressure by 5%, and the other blocks norepinephrine receptors (also reducing systolic pressure by 5%)—this time, taking both drugs concurrently produces a decrease in systolic pressure of 15%. This is called *synergism*—two drugs taken together producing a physiological effect that is much greater than the effects of each drug added together (5% + 5% = 10%, not 15%). A drug may also *interfere* with the actions of another drug, reducing the physiological effect. This is called *antagonism*.

Additive and Synergistic Drug Toxicity

Many drugs have adverse effects that will be additive or synergistic with those of another drug. This may produce toxicity to an organ or system.

> **EXAMPLE**
>
> Furosemide and streptomycin both produce ototoxicity—furosemide lowers the fluid volume in the inner ear, reducing stimulation of the auditory nerve, and aminoglycoside antibiotics (e.g., streptomycin) are directly toxic to the auditory nerve. When these drugs are taken alone, the effects are manageable; however, when taken concurrently, the effect on the auditory system more than doubles. These drugs synergize and can produce significant damage to the ear, with much more ototoxicity than would be expected from either drug alone.

> **EXAMPLE**
>
> The interaction between a central nervous system (CNS) depressant and an antihistamine. Antihistamines produce a small amount of CNS depression, some more than others. However, when antihistamines are taken with another drug that produces a large amount of CNS depression, such as anticonvulsants, antipsychotics, or even alcohol, the effect can be lethal. The same is true with ethyl alcohol, which is an extremely potent CNS depressant.

Effects of Alcohol with CNS Depressants

If alcoholic beverages are taken with sedating drugs, such as antiseizure medications, antipsychotics, antidepressants, or barbiturates, the central and autonomic nervous systems can be depressed to an extent that they are unable to function, and death could result. Since the depressant effect is so much greater when both drugs (e.g., alcohol and CNS depressants or certain antihistamines) are taken concurrently, this is a *synergistic* effect.

Synergistic Therapeutic Effects—Too Much of a Good Thing

Some drugs may **synergize** to produce too much of a beneficial effect, as well.

> **EXAMPLE**
>
> The effects of aspirin and warfarin. Aspirin is an **antithrombotic** drug; it affects platelets in the blood, to make them less "sticky," reducing the formation of small **thrombi** (clots). The reduction in the "stickiness" of the platelets may decrease the activity of clotting factors on the platelets as well, and thus reduce clotting.

Warfarin is an **anticoagulant** that works by interfering with the recycling of vitamin K, which is required for many of these clotting factors to work properly. When aspirin and warfarin are taken together, the effects of the two drugs synergize and blood clotting is decreased to the extent that internal bleeding may occur.

Additive Therapeutic Effects

EXAMPLE

The antithrombotic drugs aspirin and dipyridamole are drugs that have **additive** therapeutic effects. Since both drugs have the same physiological effect (inhibition of platelet function), the overall therapeutic effect of combination therapy will be predictable—approximately the sum of the effects from each drug. Concurrent therapy may be beneficial, as lower doses of each drug may be given, reducing the level of side effects from each drug, while the therapeutic effect is maintained.

Antagonism of Therapeutic Effects

Some drugs may **antagonize** (block) the effects of others. This antagonism might be a direct antagonism, where one drug physically blocks the binding or actions of another, or it might be more indirect in nature (e.g., blocking the activation of the second drug or creating an environment in which it is unfavorable for the other drug to work.

EXAMPLE

Probenecid, a drug used for gout, must be transported into the kidney tubules in order to be effective. Aspirin uses the same transport system to enter the kidney tubules and be excreted. Concurrent therapy with aspirin would thus antagonize the effects of probenecid, as it would inhibit transport of the drug to its site of action.

EXAMPLE

A patient with Parkinson's disease might be taking Sinemet, which is a combination of L-dopa and the enzyme inhibitor carbidopa. The carbidopa inhibits the actions of the enzyme dopa decarboxylase, which normally converts L-dopa into dopamine. The same patient might also be prescribed amethyldopa, for hypertension. In order to be effective, this drug must first be converted to a-methyl dopamine in the sympathetic neuron, using the same enzyme pathway as the L-dopa. By inhibiting the actions of dopa decarboxylase, the Sinemet would also inhibit the actions of the amethyldopa, by inhibiting its activation.

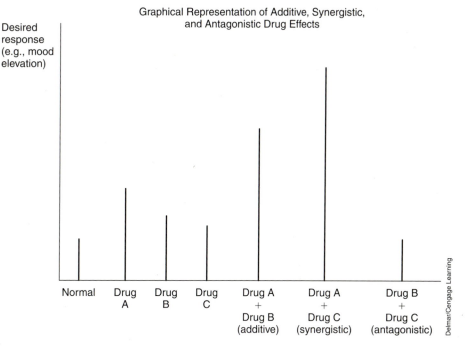

Graphical Representation of Additive, Synergistic, and Antagonistic Drug Effects

Drug-Food Interactions

In addition to interactions between *drugs* in the body, there are also many drugs that interact with chemicals found in certain foods that should be avoided during therapy. It is the responsibility of the pharmacy, as well as the prescriber, to be sure that the patient knows to avoid these types of foods.

> **EXAMPLE**
>
> The anticoagulant warfarin works by decreasing vitamin K, which decreases the activity of the vitamin K-dependent clotting factors. Vitamin K is present in foods such as green leafy vegetables. Vitamin K absorbed from the green vegetables replaces the vitamin K lost through the action of the drug, and reduces the efficacy of the drug (a *drug-food antagonism*).

> **EXAMPLE**
>
> Monoamine oxidase (MAO) inhibitors inhibit the breakdown of norepinephrine and elevate mood. A chemical called tyramine (present in foods such as cheese, chocolate, wine, and other types of food and drink) is normally metabolized by MAO. Tyramine can cause norepinephrine to be released in large quantities. If these foods are eaten during therapy with a MAO inhibitor, large amounts of norepinephrine will be produced that now cannot be broken down, as breakdown of norepinephrine has been substantially inhibited by the drug. This rapid and large increase in norepinephrine levels can cause a hypertensive crisis, which could be fatal (a *drug-food synergism*).

Blood Laboratory Values

You may be required to be familiar with basic laboratory tests, what they refer to, and general normal values. You might especially be aware of common laboratory tests for renal clearance, respiratory function, and liver function. Some commonly used blood tests include:

- *Tests for renal function*: These include the blood urea nitrogen (BUN) and creatinine levels. The rate at which the kidney clears creatinine (a product of muscle breakdown) is an indicator of kidney function. A high rate of creatinine clearance indicates proper kidney function, while a low rate indicates that the patient may have renal impairment. A high level of urea (BUN) may also be an indicator of poor renal function. Too high of a level of urea may also be indicative of gout. The ratio of blood urea nitrogen to creatinine is also an indicator of renal function.

- *Liver function*: Liver function is measured by means of the activity and levels of serum enzymes. In general, the lower the levels of liver enzymes, the better. Tests for liver function include the serum glutamic oxaloacetic transaminase (SGOT), serum glutamic pyruvate transaminase (SGPT), lactate dehydrogenase (LDH), alanine aminotransferase (ALT), and aspartate aminotransferase (AST). Elevated levels of SGOT may be seen in various conditions, such as rheumatoid arthritis, pancreatitis, muscular dystrophy, and asthma. Falsely elevated SGOT levels may be seen in certain conditions (e.g., inhalation of calcium dust or therapy with opiates and certain antibiotics). An elevated AST/ALT ratio may indicate liver damage due to alcohol (cirrhosis), or hepatitis.

- *Blood glucose levels*: Blood glucose is normally measured in either the fasting state (the patient has had no food in 12 hours) or the postprandial state (the patient has eaten recently). A high level of blood glucose may indicate that the patient is an uncontrolled diabetic, while low levels may indicate hypoglycemia. A diagnosis of either condition is not made on the basis of one serum glucose determination, but requires a long and involved test called the *glucose tolerance test*, where serum levels of glucose are measured at intervals after the patient drinks a concentrated solution of glucose ("Glucola"). Another common test is the measure of HbA1c levels.

- *Serum blood gasses*: A determination of respiratory function may be made by analyzing the "partial pressures" of oxygen and carbon dioxide in the blood (partial pressures are noted as Po_2 for oxygen and Pco_2 for carbon dioxide). A low oxygen level or high level of carbon dioxide may indicate depressed respiratory function.

- *Electrolyte levels*: These are often assessed in a hospital setting, to be sure that the serum levels of sodium, potassium, and calcium are within normal levels. The most important of these is the potassium level, which *may* need to be supplemented to protect heart function, particularly before a surgical procedure, those receiving excessive fluids, or patients taking a diuretic.

Normal Values of Some Common Blood Tests

BUN	5–20 mg/ dL
BUN/Creatinine ratio	10:1 to 20:1
Creatinine	0.6–1.2 mg/ dL
Creatinine clearance	75–125 mL/min
Serum glucose	70–110 mg/dL (fasting)
Po_2	75–105 mm Hg
Pco_2	35–45 mm Hg
Electrolytes:	
Sodium	145–147 mEq/L
Potassium	3.5–5 mEq/L
Calcium	8.8–10.4 m/ dL
Chloride	95–105 mEq/ dL

Normal Levels of Common Liver Enzymes

Enzyme	Normal Range (Males)	Normal Range (Females)
SGOT	5–40 IU/L	5–33 IU/L
AST	5–40 IU/L	5–33 IU/L
SGPT	7–46 IU/L	4–35 IU/L
ALT	7–46 IU/L	4–35 IU/L
GGT	4–23 IU/L	3–13 IU/L

Chapter Review Questions

1. An example of a drug's mechanism of action would be:
   a. blockade of serotonin receptors
   b. inhibition of muramic acid crosslinking in a bacterial cell wall
   c. decreased inflammation
   d. a and b only

2. An adverse effect is:
   a. an unwanted effect
   b. a potentially toxic effect
   c. an effect that only occurs at high doses
   d. a and b

3. An example of a drug-induced toxic effect would be:
   a. hearing loss produced by gentamicin
   b. nephrotoxicity produced by cisplatin
   c. congestive heart failure produced by doxorubicin (Adriamycin)
   d. all of the above

4. The monoamine oxidase inhibitor tranylcypromine inhibits the metabolism of norepinephrine. It may produce a hypertensive crisis if certain foods are eaten during therapy. Phenelzine, another monoamine oxidase inhibitor, would most likely:
   a. have similar effects
   b. have the same mechanism of action as tranylcypromine, but not have food interactions
   c. have a different adverse effect profile
   d. act completely differently

5. Tetracyclines are drugs of choice for rickettsial infections, such as Rocky Mountain Spotted Fever. This means that they:
   a. are the only drugs effective against the condition
   b. are the most effective drugs for the condition
   c. are the first drugs to be prescribed
   d. are the only drugs prescribed

6. Which of the following drugs would require a dosage adjustment in a 70-year-old patient?
   a. Cefaclor (eliminated in the urine)
   b. Oxazepam (eliminated through the bile)
   c. both a and b
   d. neither drug would require dosage adjustment

7. A patient is taking phenelzine. With each dose of drug:
   a. plasma levels of drug rise
   b. plasma levels of drug remain the same, as the drug is stored
   c. plasma levels of drug rise and then fall as the drug is distributed
   d. more and more drug binds to proteins in the liver

8. A patient with cirrhosis of the liver is prescribed a fat-soluble drug (e.g., Valium). Which of the following could occur?
   a. plasma levels will reach toxic levels, as the drug cannot be cleared properly
   b. renal failure will occur
   c. a loss of activity may occur, as the drug could not be transformed into its active form
   d. either a or c could occur

9. Which of the following is not absorbed?
   a. a 40 mg Lasix tablet
   b. Nicotine from a transdermal patch
   c. Compazine from a rectal suppository
   d. 100,000 units penicillin G potassium in an intravenous drip

10. A patient is taking Valium (a weak base) orally. It will most likely be absorbed:
   a. in the stomach (pH 2)
   b. in the liver (pH 7.4)
   c. in the small intestine (pH 8)
   d. directly into the blood

11. A lipid-soluble drug, such as a general anesthetic, would most likely be concentrated in:
   a. the plasma
   b. fatty tissues
   c. the liver
   d. the kidney

12. The addition of a vasoconstrictor, such as norepinephrine, to an IM injection is done for the following reason(s):
   a. the addition of norepinephrine allows the dosage to be small
   b. to slow the absorption of the drug
   c. to allow maximum drug effect
   d. to allow the drug to diffuse into the tissues more rapidly

13. A drug that is active in the body must be:
   a. bound to plasma proteins
   b. changed by the liver
   c. free in the plasma
   d. given orally

14. A patient comes in with a prescription for phenytoin in 30 mg capsules. The instructions state ii bid q2d, then i bid. This drug:
   a. is prescribed in overdose
   b. requires a loading dose
   c. is not appropriate for the patient
   d. is prescribed for a small child

15. The trade name of a drug is Cefobid. Which of the following is probably true?
   a. the drug is an antiseizure medication
   b. the drug is an antibiotic
   c. the drug is taken twice a day
   d. both b and c are correct

CHAPTER 22

Central Nervous System Agents

Antidepressants

Depression is thought to be caused by an imbalance of neurotransmitters in the brain. Older therapies focused on elevating levels of norepinephrine in the central nervous system, which appears to have a clinical benefit; however, it is now accepted that the main neurotransmitter involved in the etiology of depression is serotonin.

Drugs of Choice in the Therapy of Depression

Drugs of choice for depression are now the serotonin reuptake inhibitors (SSRIs), which block the reuptake of serotonin at the neuronal ending, resulting in increased levels of serotonin in the synapse and increased receptor stimulation. These drugs are also very specific in their effects, unlike the older antidepressants, and have fewer adverse effects. Serotonin is a potent vasodilator so SSRI's are thus used in the *therapy of migraine headache*, as well although the mechanism of action is unknown.

Second-Line Drugs in the Therapy of Depression

Tricyclic antidepressants are often prescribed for depression. They inhibit the reuptake of norepinephrine, dopamine, and serotonin (depending on the particular drug of the class) into the neuronal ending, resulting in increased synaptic concentrations.

Third- and Fourth-Line Drugs in the Therapy of Depression

Third- and fourth-line drugs include *bupropion* (the mechanism of action of bupropion is still unclear), and a new class of drugs, the *heterocyclic antidepressants,* which are thought to increase the production and release of serotonin by inhibiting negative feedback at the neuronal ending.

If SSRIs are the most effective drugs in the therapy of depression, why prescribe other drugs? When choosing a drug therapy, we must keep in mind that we are treating living people. People are different and respond differently. (Different responses to drugs by different patients are called *idiosyncratic* reactions). A drug that is effective in one patient may not be effective in another. SSRIs also tend to have less adverse effects than other agents, and,

Physiology Review

Recall that neurotransmitters are packaged into small compartments, called *secretory vesicles* or *secretory granules*. These granules are stored in the neuronal ending, and, when the neuron is stimulated, release their contents into the *synapse*. Once released, the neurotransmitter stimulates *receptors* on the cell membrane of the next neuron in the pathway ("postsynaptic" receptors). If the neurotransmitter is stimulatory, it will cause this neuron to be stimulated, starting the process all over again. Some neurotransmitters, like GABA, are inhibitory, and inhibit neuronal stimulation—these will be discussed later.

Neurotransmitter molecules, in addition to stimulating receptors on the membrane of the next neuron in the pathway, may also bind to specialized receptors on the surface of the neuron that released them. These are called α_2 [alpha-2] receptors, and stimulation of these receptors alters the release of neurotransmitters. In this way, once a sufficient neurotransmitter has been made and released, it "shuts itself off" by way of a regulatory receptor at the neuronal ending. Once the neurotransmitter does its job, it is pumped back into the neuronal ending by a membrane protein "pump" for recycling.

> Drugs are "people specific." One drug might work very well for one person and not help another person.

depending on the person, the adverse effect profile also may be a factor in which drug to use.

Drugs rarely used now for depression include **monoamine oxidase inhibitors**, which inhibit the metabolism of norepinephrine and thus increase norepinephrine release. The side effects profile and interactions with other medications make them the last choice for treating depression.

Serotonin Reuptake Inhibitors (SSRIs)

Mechanism of action: These drugs inhibit the membrane protein pumps that transport released serotonin (*5HT*) into the neuronal ending for recycling. This results in more serotonin available in the synaptic cleft and an increased stimulation of postsynaptic receptors.

> **NOTE**
>
> The number of reuptake pumps blocked, and thus the amount of serotonin available in the cleft, is a function of drug dose.

Administration: SSRIs are administered orally.

Adverse Effects

Rash and skin abnormalities are not uncommon. In addition, these drugs bind to receptors for neurotransmitter substances, such as norepinephrine, acetylcholine, and histamine. Thus, common adverse effects include headache, dizziness, sedation, insomnia, restlessness, tremor, and gastrointestinal dysfunction and decreased libido, weight loss. Cardiovascular effects, such as palpitations, chest pain, and hypotension, may also be seen. These drugs can also cause *Serotonin Syndrome*, due to an increased level of serotonin in the CNS. This syndrome is characterized by fever, agitation, confusion, tremors, and cardiovascular abnormalities, which may progress to coma and death.

Interactions

SSRIs are highly plasma protein bound (the amount of binding differs with each individual drug) and so have the potential for drug interactions. They are also metabolized by the cytochrome mixed function oxidase system (cytochrome P_{450})—another potential for drug interactions.

Contraindications

SSRIs should not be used in combination with MAO inhibitors or within two weeks of terminating treatment with MAO inhibitors. Treatment after this time should then be initiated cautiously and dosage increased gradually until optimal response is reached. Conversely, MAO inhibitors should not be introduced within two weeks of cessation of therapy with an SSRI.

Treatment of psychiatric patients: SSRIs can cause a manic episode or exacerbate existing mania. They should therefore be used with caution, or not at all, in bipolar or manic patients. Additional medications are often prescribed to stabilize mood.

Drugs Available

Fluoxetine

Brand names: Prozac, Sarafem

Available as: 10 mg, 20 mg, and 40 mg capsules; 10 mg and 20 mg tablets; 90 mg, delayed-release capsules; 20 mg/5 mL syrup

Dosage: 20 mg/day, administered in the morning.

Dispensing: Dispense in a tightly closed, light-proof container.

Special notes:

- *Fluoxetine has a very long half-life,* due to hepatic metabolism, and the production of an active metabolite (norfluoxetine). The initial half-life is approximately two days after a single dose. With consistent (daily) dosing, the half-life increases to four days. After the drug is withdrawn completely, active drug remains in the plasma for as much as two months.

- *Fluoxetine has a lower incidence of adverse effects than other drugs of the class,* as it is more selective and does not bind to receptors for histamine and acetylcholine.

- *Fluoxetine is stored bound to plasma proteins*—94% of the drug is plasma protein bound. This may result in interactions with other drugs that are bound to plasma proteins.

- *Fluoxetine may have a longer duration in the elderly* because the drug is metabolized by the liver and eliminated by the kidney (both hepatic and renal function are decreased in elderly patients). Dosage adjustment in geriatric patients is required.

Fluvoxamine (fluvoxamine maleate)

Brand name: Generics only (Luvox brand no longer commercially available)

Available as: 25 mg, 50 mg, and 100 mg tablets

Dosage: 50 mg qd hs, increasing to 100–300 mg. Pediatric dose: 25 mg, administered as a single dose at bedtime. Maximum pediatric dose: 200 mg/day.

Dispensing: Dispense in a tightly closed container, as the drug is sensitive to humidity.

Special notes:

- Fluvoxamine has the shortest half-life of all the SSRIs—no active metabolites are formed.

- Fluvoxamine is less plasma protein bound (77%) than other drugs of the class.

- Sedation is more common with fluvoxamine than with other SSRIs.

- Anorexia and weight loss are less of a concern with fluvoxamine than with fluoxetine.

Paroxetine hydrochloride

Brand name: Paxil

Available as: 10 mg, 20 mg, 30 mg, and 40 mg tablets; controlled-release tablets: 12.5 mg, 25 mg, and 37.5 mg; oral suspension: 2 mg/mL

Dosage: Immediate release tablets or oral suspension: 20 mg/day, increasing in 10 mg/day increments to a maximum dose of 50 mg/day. Controlled release tablets: 25 mg/day as a single dose in the morning.

Dispensing: Dispense in a tightly closed, light-resistant container.

Special notes:

- Therapeutic uses of paroxetine are in the therapy of OCD, panic disorder, and depression.

- The mesylate form of paroxetine is more completely absorbed, as compared with the hydrochloride form, making the effects more predictable.

- Paroxetine is subject to a biphasic process of metabolic elimination—a significant first-pass effect is seen in the first phase. Increased bioavailability is observed with multiple dosing.

- A wide range of variation between patients is seen—dosage intervals may vary from patient to patient.

- Elimination half-life is prolonged in geriatric patients, so dosage adjustment is necessary.

Sertraline hydrochloride

Brand name: Zoloft

Available as: 25 mg, 50 mg, and 100 mg tablets; oral concentrate 20 mg/mL

Dosage: Initial therapy at 25 mg/day, increasing to 50 mg/day after one week. Maximum therapeutic dose: 200 mg/day.

Special notes:
- Sertraline has very little sedation and does not interfere with motor skills.
- Food increases the bioavailability of the drug. The drug should therefore be taken with meals, although not required.

Duloxetine hydrochloride
Brand name: Cymbalta

Available as: 20 mg, 30 mg, and 60 mg delayed-release capsules

Dosage: 40–60 mg daily in two doses

Special notes:
- Inhibits serotonin and norepinephrine and is a weak inhibitor of dopamine reuptake.
- Therapeutic use in major depressive disorder (MDD).
- Management of neuropathic pain.
- Fibromyalgia.
- Renal and hepatic precautions in patients with kidney or liver insufficiency.

Venlafaxine hydrochloride
Brand name: Effexor, Effexor XR

Available as: 25 mg, 37.5 mg, 50 mg, 75 mg, and 100 mg tablets. Effexor XR: 37.5 mg, 75 mg, and 150 mg extended-release capsules

Special notes:
- Effective in treating patients with melancholia.
- This drug is not a pure SSRI—it is heterocyclic as it also inhibits the reuptake of norepinephrine.
- An increase in blood pressure is possible.
- No contraindications for use in geriatric patients.
- The drug is less than 35% plasma protein bound. Therefore, protein-binding–induced drug interactions with venlafaxine are not expected.
- Half-life is prolonged in patients with liver disease.

Citalopram
Brand name: Celexa

Available as: 10 mg, 20 mg, and 40 mg scored tablets; 10 mg/5 mL oral solution.

Dosage: 20 mg daily dose initially, increasing to 40 mg. Maximum dose: 80 mg/day.

Special notes:

- Highly selective serotonin reuptake inhibitor (SSRI) with minimal effects on norepinephrine and dopamine neuronal reuptake.
- Very low receptor binding—decreased anticholinergic, antihistaminic, antiadrenergic effects.
- Decreased adverse effects, such as dry mouth, sedation, and cardiovascular effects.
- Dosage should be reduced in the elderly and patients with reduced hepatic function.
- Antifungal agents (e.g., ketoconazole, iatraconozole), macrolide antibiotics (e.g., erythromycin), and omeprazole may decrease citalopram clearance.
- Citalopram has been associated with symptoms resembling syndrome of inappropriate ADH secretion (SIADH), and produces hyponatremia.
- Citalopram has anticonvulsant effects and should be used with caution in patients with a history of epilepsy.

Escitalopram

Brand name: Lexapro

Available as: 5 mg tablets; scored 10 mg and 20 mg tablets; 5 mg/5 mL oral solution.

Dosage: 10 mg once daily

Special notes:

- Highly selective SSRI with minimal effects on norepinephrine and dopamine neuronal reuptake.
- 100-fold more potent than citalopram.
- Very low receptor binding—decreased anticholinergic, antihistaminic, antiadrenergic effects.
- Decreased adverse effects, such as dry mouth, sedation, and cardiovascular effects.
- 56% protein bound.
- Does not block ion channels significantly, resulting in less adverse cardiac effects.
- Half-life is doubled in patients with reduced liver function.

Drugs Used in the Therapy of Migraine Headaches

Serotonin Receptor Agonists (SRAs)

Mechanism of action: SRAs act as direct agonists at the serotonin ($5HT_1$) receptor. They mimic the effects of serotonin, causing an cerebral vasodilation. Drugs available include sumitriptan (the prototypical drug), and the newer SRAs, which include almotriptan, electripan, frovatriptan, naratriptan, rizatriptan, sumatriptan, and zolmitriptan.

Drugs Available

Sumatriptan succinate
Brand name: Imitrex

Classification: Serotonin receptor ($5HT_1$) agonist

Available as: 25 mg, 50 mg, and 100 mg tablets; 6 mg/0.5 mL injection; nasal spray, 5 mg and 20 mg.

Dosage: 50–100 mg per dose. Maximum daily dose: 200 mg.

Storage: Store between 2 and 30°C

Zolmitriptan
Brand name: Zomig

Classification: Serotonin receptor ($5HT_1$) agonist

Available as: 2.5 mg and 5 mg tablets; nasal spray, 5 mg.

Rizatriptan
Brand name: Maxalt, Maxalt MLT

Classification: Serotonin receptor ($5HT_1$) agonist

Available as: 5 mg and 10 mg tablets; 5 mg and 10 mg disintegrating tablets (MLT).

Tricyclic Antidepressants

The clinical benefits of the tricyclics and heterocyclic antidepressants are not seen for four to five weeks, while adverse effects are seen immediately. This leads to low patient compliance.

Mechanism of action: Tricyclic antidepressants inhibit reuptake of neurotransmitter into the neuronal ending. The primary neurotransmitters affected are norepinephrine and serotonin. The degree to which reuptake of a particular transmitter is affected depends on the drug.

Inhibition of reuptake occurs immediately, although the clinical benefits of the drug are not seen for four to five weeks. It is now thought that the major clinical action of these drugs is due to a decrease in beta receptors in an area of the brain called the limbic system (i.e., the increased concentration of norepinephrine causes an overstimulation of beta receptors, and leads to a decrease in receptor number or function).

Adverse Effects

> Mood elevation occurs only in depressed individuals! These drugs are not abusable drugs!

These drugs have very low patient compliance, due to the delayed onset of clinical effects and the prompt onset of adverse effects. Tricyclics are very nonspecific drugs and therefore have effects at various receptors—in particular, they have an affinity for muscarinic and histamine receptors. This results in major antimuscarinic effects, such as *tachycardia, sedation, dry mouth,* and *constipation,* as well as less frequently seen effects, such as palpitations and arrhythmias. Effects on histamine receptors cause increased sedation.

Interactions: Tricyclics are highly plasma protein bound, so drug interactions with other drugs that bind to plasma proteins may cause fluctuations in plasma concentration of the drug and potential toxicity.

Contraindications

- These drugs are contraindicated with any drug or substance that causes an increase in the levels of catecholamines (e.g., norepinephrine) or serotonin levels.

> **NOTE**
>
> Tricyclics should not be administered within 14 days of treatment with an MAO inhibitor. Doing so could result in a hypertensive crisis, due to radically increased levels of norepinephrine.

- Tricyclics should not be administered during the acute phase of recovery from a **myocardial infarction**, or to a patient with **glaucoma,** because of the drug's antimuscarinic effects.
- Tricyclics are contraindicated in **hyperthyroid** patients, or those on exogenous thyroid medication, because of the increased sensitivity to catecholamines in these patients.
- Because of the high degree of sedation, operating machinery and driving, etc., should be done with caution.

Tricyclic Antidepressants Available

Imipramine
Brand name: Tofranil
Administration: Oral

Available as: 10 mg, 25 mg, and 50 mg tablets (HCl); 75 mg, 100 mg, 125 mg, and 150 mg capsules (pamoate).

Dosage: 100 mg/day in divided doses, increasing to 300 mg/day for hospital patients. 75 mg/day increasing to 150 mg/day for outpatients. Maximum dose: 200 mg/day. Geriatric and adolescent doses: 30 mg to 40 mg/day. Maximum dose: 100 mg/day.

Special notes:

- Imipramine affects primarily serotonergic neurons; however, its metabolite, desipramine, affects primarily noradrenergic neurons. The drug, therefore, ultimately has approximately equal effects on both neuronal types.
- Imipramine is metabolized to an active metabolite, desipramine (which is also marketed separately). Thus, it has a long half-life. The half-life is shortened in hepatically compromised patients.
- Useful in the therapy of childhood nocturnal enuresis.

Desipramine

Brand name: Norpramin

Available as: 10 mg, 25 mg, 50 mg, 75 mg, 100 mg, and 150 mg tablets.

Special notes:

- Desipramine is the active metabolite of imipramine, thus the pharmacologic profile is similar. However, desipramine has potent effects on noradrenergic neurons, in contrast to imipramine's major effects on serotonergic neurons.

Amitriptyline

Brand name: Elavil

Classification: Tricyclic antidepressant

Available as: 10 mg, 25 mg, 50 mg, 75 mg, 100 mg, 150 mg tablets; and 10 mg/mL injection.

Special notes:

- Amitriptyline has its major effect on noradrenergic neurons, with a lesser effect on serotonergic neurons.
- Amitriptyline is structurally related to the thioxanthene antipsychotics, such as thiothixene, and therefore has effects on dopamine release. This property may make the drug more useful in the treatment of depression in the psychotic patient. Amitriptyline is also related to the skeletal muscle relaxant cyclobenzaprine, although amitriptyline is not believed to possess muscle-relaxant properties.

- Amitriptyline is useful in behavioral disorders, such as ADD and phobic disorder.
- Amitriptyline is metabolized to nortriptyline, which is also marketed separately.

Nortriptyline

Brand names: Aventyl, Pamelor

Classification: Tricyclic antidepressant

Available as: 10 mg, 25 mg, 50 mg, and 75 mg capsules; 10 mg/5 mL injection.

Dosage: 25 mg three to four times a day. Maximum daily dose: 150 mg geriatric/adolescent dosage: 35–50 mg/day in divided doses.

Dispensing: Dispense in a tightly closed container.

Special notes:

- Nortriptyline is the major metabolite of amitriptyline, and thus has similar pharmacologic properties. It is most selective for actions on noradrenergic neurons.

Doxepin

Brand names: Adapin, Sinequan

Available as: 10 mg, 25 mg, 50 mg, 75 mg, 100 mg, and 150 mg capsules; 10 mg/mL concentrated oral liquid.

Primary Uses: Psychoneurotic patients with anxiety and/or depressive reactions. Anxiety neurosis associated with somatic disorders. Psychotic depression, including manic-depressive illness.

Dosage: 75 mg/day (h.s.) initially, increasing to 150 mg/day. Maximum daily dose: 300 mg.

Adverse effects: Due to strong anticholinergic actions, the drug can cause changes in heart rate and conduction (producing a "quinidine-like" effect), possibly leading to heart block and/or arrhythmias. CNS effects such as headache, drowsiness, autonomic effects, and insomnia may also be seen, as well as seizures. GI disturbances and various other effects may be seen as well.

Special notes:

- Doxepin is a psychotropic agent with antidepressant and anxiolytic properties.
- Doxepin has pronounced sedative and anticholinergic effects. In the higher dosage range, it produces peripheral adrenergic blocking effects.

Amoxapine

Brand name: Ascendin

Classification: Tricyclic antidepressant, also considered to be a heterocyclic drug.

Available as: 25 mg, 50 mg, 100 mg, and 150 mg tablets.

Dosage: 200 mg to 300 mg/day. Dosage should start around 50–100 mg/day and gradually increase, to decrease sedation caused by the drug. Dosage may be increased to 400 mg after two weeks of therapy. Geriatric dosage: 25 mg two to three times daily, increasing to 50 mg. Maximum dose: 600 mg/day in two divided doses.

Dispensing: Dispense in a light-proof container.

Special note:

- Amoxapine has characteristics of both tricyclic and heterocyclic drugs. It has less anticholinergic activity than other drugs of the tricyclic class. It produces orthostatic hypotension in doses of greater than 400 mg/day. The drug lowers seizure threshold and produces low to moderate sedation.

Tetracyclic Antidepressants

Mechanism of action: These drugs are potent antagonists at central α_2 receptors, resulting in increased central levels of norepinephrine, which leads to mood elevation. Peripheral effects (e.g., cardiovascular effects) are minimized, as the drug has a predominantly central action. These drugs also affect certain subtypes of the serotonin receptor, resulting in less adverse effects, such as anxiety, insomnia, and nausea that occur with other agents, like the selective serotonin reuptake inhibitors (SSRIs).

Prototype Drug of the Class

Mirtazapine

Brand name: Remeron

Available as: 7.5 mg, 15 mg, 30 mg, and 45 mg tablets; 15 mg, 30 mg, and 45 mg disintegrating tablets.

Special notes:

- Antagonizes $5HT_2$, $5HT_3$, and adrenergic α_2 receptors.
- Has some antipsychotic activity.
- Is useful in the relief of nausea.

- May cause weight gain.
- Does not cause orthostatic hypotension or sexual dysfunction.
- Also used to treat insomnia associated with SSRI usage.

Maprotiline

Brand name: Ludiomil

Available as: 25 mg, 50 mg, and 75 mg tablets.

Special notes:
- May lower seizure threshold.
- Has been shown to induce seizures in previously seizure-free individuals.
- Contraindicated in patients with cardiovascular disease or hypothyroidism.

Heterocyclic Antidepressants

Mechanism of action: Serotonergic neurons also contain α_2 receptors, called heteroreceptors, which decrease serotonin release. These drugs block hetero-receptors, which results in increased release of 5HT.

> **NOTE**
>
> Mood elevation occurs *only* in clinically depressed persons. These are not abusable drugs!

Special notes:
- Therapeutic effects are delayed—effects take two to three weeks to manifest.
- Adverse effect profile is similar to that of SSRIs. (SSRIs are actually considered to be a subgroup of the heterocyclic antidepressants.)

Prototype Drugs

Nefazadone

Brand name: Generics only (Serzone brand no longer commercially available)

Available as: 50 mg, 100 mg, 150 mg, and 200 mg scored tablets; 250 mg unscored tablets.

Special notes:

- Hepatic metabolism results in the formation of an active metabolite—trazodone.

- Both a serotonin reuptake inhibitor (SRI) and a $5HT_2$ antagonist.

- Useful in the therapy of chronic pain.

- May cause orthostatic hypotension (drop in blood pressure upon standing).

- *Cases of life-threatening hepatic failure have been reported in patients treated with nefazadone.* Therapy should not be initiated in individuals with active liver disease or with elevated baseline serum transaminases. Patients should be advised to be alert for signs and symptoms of liver dysfunction (e.g., jaundice, anorexia, gastrointestinal complaints, malaise, etc.) and to report them to the doctor immediately if they occur.

Trazodone

Brand name: Desyrel

Available as: 50 mg, 100 mg, 150 mg, and 300 mg tablets.

Dosage: 150 mg/day in divided doses, which may be increased by 50 mg/day every three to four days. Maximum dose: 400 mg/day.

Dispensing: Dispense in a tightly closed, light-resistant container.

Special notes:

- It is highly plasma protein bound.

- It has been shown to cause priapism in young males.

- May cause cardiac arrhythmias.

- Causes sedation and often used for insomnia.

- Synergism with alcohol and/or barbiturates can produce CNS depression.

Monoamine Oxidase Inhibitors

> Abrupt discontinuation of MAOIs may cause withdrawal symptoms, such as restlessness, anxiety, depression, confusion, hallucinations, headache, weakness, and diarrhea.

Monoamine oxidase (MAO) is an enzyme that is attached to mitochondrial membranes within the neuronal ending. It breaks down catecholamines, such as norepinephrine and dopamine. There are two types of MAO: MAO_A, which breaks down norepinephrine and epinephrine, and MAO_B, which breaks down dopamine.

Monoamine oxidase inhibitors work by inhibiting MAO in a dose-dependent manner, which results in a decrease in the rate of metabolism of norepinephrine. This results in more norepinephrine available to be released from the neuron.

> Following discontinuation of any MAOI, dietary restrictions should continue for at least two weeks.

> MAOIs should be used with caution in patients with hyperthyroidism, as thyroid hormones sensitize the heart to the effects of catecholamines.

> MAOIs should not be taken with SSRIs, and are contraindicated with the use of sympathomimetics, such as phenylephrine or other direct-acting nasal decongestants. They are contraindicated with herbal agents, such as kava kava, valerian, and St. John's Wort, as well.

> MAOIs taken in conjunction with tryptophan may cause an overproduction of serotonin, and serotonin syndrome.

There are many problems with these drugs:

- First, *the effects of any drug that raises levels of norepinephrine will be potentiated,* as the increased levels of norepinephrine cannot be broken down. This can result in a *hypertensive crisis,* which can be life-threatening.

- Second, there are *food interactions:* "feel good" foods, such as wine, cheese, chocolate (and yes, even beans) contain a substance called tyramine, which is normally broken down by MAO shortly after ingestion. Without MAO present, the tyramine is absorbed and can enter the noradrenergic neuron and be converted to a false transmitter, octopamine, by enzymes that normally make norepinephrine. Octopamine is packaged with norepinephrine in the secretory vesicles and pushes out the norepinephrine, causing a huge release of norepinephrine. If MAO were active in the cell, the norepinephrine would be broken down in the neuron, but it is not, so huge amounts of norepinephrine are released again, leading to hypertensive crisis.

Adverse Effects

A serious adverse effect of MAOIs is the development of a hypertensive crisis. Symptoms of this disorder include: a change in heart rate (sinus tachycardia or sinus bradycardia), angina, palpitations, severe headache, light sensitivity, mydriasis, fever, profuse sweating, nausea/vomiting, and stiff or sore neck. Other adverse effects include:

- Orthostatic hypotension
- Peripheral edema and swelling of the legs
- Anticholinergic effects, such as sedation, miosis, confusion, blurred vision, and urinary retention
- Sexual dysfunction
- Tremors, insomnia, and fatigue
- Hematological reactions (e.g., anemia, pancytopenia)
- Liver toxicity (rare)

Phenelzine
Brand name: Nardil
Available as: 15 mg tablet
Dosage: 15 mg tid up to 90 mg qd

- No clinical response is seen until four weeks of therapy at 60 mg/day.
- Increases in dose should not exceed 100 mg/d after three days of therapy.

Storage: The sustained-release form may be refrigerated.

- Reversible MAO inhibitor
- Nonselective MAOI
- Also desensitizes receptors for serotonin, as well as adrenergic receptors

Unclassified Antidepressants

This group actually contains several agents, as many of the newer agents have properties of more than one class. The drug to be discussed here is bupropion, as the mechanism of action is still unclear for this drug.

Bupropion

Brand names: Wellbutrin, Wellbutrin SR, Wellbutrin XL, Zyban

Classification: Heterocyclic antidepressant

Available as: 75 mg and 100 mg tablets; sustained release: 100 mg and 150 mg tablets; Zyban: 150 mg tablets (for smoking cessation); XL: 150 mg and 300 mg tablets.

Dosage: 300 mg/day in two divided doses (SR) 100 mg tid (immediate release), q 6 h intervals. Increases in dose should not exceed 100 mg/day after three days of therapy.

Special notes:
- Four weeks of therapy may be necessary before clinical effects are seen.
- The mechanism of action of bupropion is not fully understood, but it has been shown that bupropion inhibits the neuronal uptake of dopamine.
- Clinical antidepressant effects are delayed—effects may be seen after two to three weeks of therapy, but full effects are not seen until four or more weeks of therapy.
- Bupropion has a high potential for causing drug-induced seizures if taken with alcohol.
- Bupropion is also indicated for use as an aid to smoking cessation—a sustained-release form is marketed under the proprietary name *Zyban* for this purpose (available in tablet form).
- Useful in treatment of psychiatric disorders, such as ADHD.

Sedative Hypnotics

Used in the therapy of anxiety and insomnia, sedative hypnotics are a group of drugs that decrease the frequency of neuronal conduction. They include two major drug classes—the *barbiturates* and the *benzodiazepines*, as well as lesser used drugs, like chloral hydrate.

> Due to the unique properties of benzodiazepines, it would be extremely difficult for a patient to overdose and die by accident — the patient never reaches beyond the stage of surgical anesthesia.

- Barbiturates and benzodiazepines have varied clinical uses—they may be used to reduce anxiety (**anxiolytics**), decrease the frequency of seizures (**anticonvulsants**), or induce sleep (**hypnotic agents**).

- Their effects are dose-related, progressing from sedation (a calming effect, such as that desired for control of anxiety) to hypnosis (sleep) to analgesia, surgical anesthesia (lack of sensation), and finally, with abnormally high doses, to coma and death.

- Barbiturates (pronounced bar-bih-TUR-ayts) follow a linear progression through these stages; benzodiazepines do not. The graph shows the relationship between dose and physiological effect of a barbiturate (e.g., secobarbital), shown as a solid line, and a benzodiazepine (e.g., alprazolam, diazepam), shown as a dotted line.

Barbiturates and Benzodiazepines

Mechanism of action: These sedative-hypnotic drugs work by augmenting the actions of the inhibitory neurotransmitter GABA. They thus decrease the frequency and amplitude (strength) of neuronal transmission. This results in

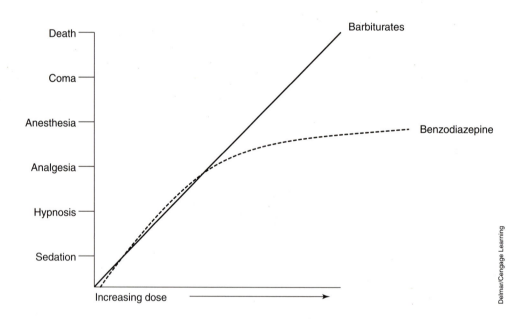

Delmar/Cengage Learning

Physiology Review

Excitatory neurotransmitters bind to receptors on the surface of a postsynaptic neuron and cause stimulation of that neuron, which results in synaptic transmission from the neuron and release of neurotransmitter. *Inhibitory* neurotransmitters bind to receptors and prevent neurotransmission. The inhibitory neurotransmitter GABA binds to a receptor, which permits chloride ions to flow through a membrane channel. This flow of negatively charged ions into the cell decreases excitation of the cell membrane.

decreased rate of firing of neurons, decreased mental acuity, relaxation, and eventually sleep.

In low doses, these drugs may be used for control of seizures, as they decrease the excitability of the neuron and thus decrease the potential for seizure activity. *Because their action is very generalized, however, they are not drugs of first choice as anticonvulsants.* Certain barbiturates, however, may be used in the therapy of status epilepticus, a life-threatening type of seizure.

In moderate doses, these drugs are used as hypnotics or sedatives—modern medicine chooses benzodiazepines for therapy rather than barbiturates, as a general rule, because there is less possibility of lethal overdose.

With very large doses of barbiturates, CNS function is depressed to the point where coma and, finally, death are seen.

> **NOTE**
>
> Benzodiazepines are effective skeletal muscle relaxants. They also produce an *anterograde amnesia*, which is useful in painful diagnostic procedures. (With anterograde amnesia, the patient does not remember anything in the hours that follow the administration of the drug. Thus, the procedure, while painful at the time, is not remembered. This same property has caused certain benzodiazepines to be used as "date rape" drugs.)

Adverse Effects

Benzodiazepines

These drugs have few serious adverse effects. The most commonly reported adverse effects are CNS related, and include:

- Sedation (drowsiness)
- Hangover effect
- Difficulty in movement (ataxia)
- Visual disturbances

Other adverse effects are:

- Changes in bowel and bladder function, skin rashes, and changes in libido.
- Sleep changes—benzodiazepines reduce the length of REM sleep. In addition, when used as hypnotic agents, they may produce a "rebound" effect (rebound insomnia) when the drug is withdrawn.

> Because of the possibility of paradoxical reactions, benzodiazepines should not be used in patients suffering from psychotic disorders. These drugs are also not effective in patients with obsessive compulsive disorders.

> Barbiturates, because of their respiratory depressant effect, should be used with caution or avoided altogether in patients with compromised lung function.

> Barbiturates tend to have very long half-lives, as they undergo extensive metabolism. For example, the half-life of phenobarbital is three days.

Serious adverse effects: These occur rarely, and include leukopenia, jaundice, hypersensitivity, and paradoxical reactions.

Paradoxical reactions: Benzodiazepines are unique in that patients taking these drugs may experience conditions opposite to the effects of the drug, particularly upon withdrawal of the drug. Paradoxical effects include hyper-excitability, anxiety, excitement, hallucinations, increased muscle spasticity, insomnia, rage, and sleep disturbances. If the patient experiences these symptoms during therapy, the drug should be withdrawn.

Pregnancy: Benzodiazepines have been associated with an *increased incidence of fetal malformations*. They are, therefore, contraindicated in the first trimester of pregnancy.

Withdrawal of benzodiazepines should be gradual. Abrupt discontinuation of benzodiazepines may produce withdrawal symptoms that may mimic or even magnify symptoms seen before treatment. These include irritability, nervousness, insomnia, agitation, and tremors. Convulsions, diarrhea, abdominal cramps, vomiting, and mental impairment may also be seen.

Adverse Effects Seen with Barbiturates

> It should be noted that the effects of barbiturates and benzodiazepines are synergistic. Indeed, the binding of barbiturate molecules to their receptors on the chloride channel increases the binding of benzodiazepine. It should also be noted that the effects of both drug classes are markedly potentiated by alcohol, and the consumption of alcoholic beverages with these drugs may result in death.

- *Respiratory depression*: Barbiturates cause respiratory depression, so should be avoided, or used with caution, in patients with compromised respiratory function (e.g., COPD, emphysema). The effects on respiration are dose-related, so little respiratory depression is seen with sedative doses, and more severe depression with hypnotic doses and doses that produce surgical anesthesia.

- *Changes in bowel function*: Barbiturates reduce motility and tone in the GI tract because of a central depressant effect.

- *Sleep changes*: Barbiturates have been shown to reduce the REM period of sleep, resulting in less restful sleep.

Interactions

- *Alcohol*: Both barbiturates and benzodiazepines are contraindicated with alcohol or other CNS depressants, as the effects are synergistic.

- *Opiates*: The administration of opiates is contraindicated with barbiturates, as the respiratory effects are additive.

- *Other CNS drugs*: Both barbiturates and benzodiazepines may potentiate the effects of or interact with other CNS-acting drugs, such as nonbarbiturate hypnotics, antihistamines, antipsychotic drugs, MAO inhibitors, tricyclic antidepressants, and anticonvulsants.

Addiction

- *Benzodiazepines are not considered to be physically addictive*—the addiction is considered to be a psychological addiction. They are thus classified under the Controlled Substance Act as C-III and C-IV. When discontinuing benzodiazepines, tapering the dose is suggested to prevent the possibility of seizures.
- *Barbiturates are considered to be both physically and psychologically addictive*. They are classified as C-II and C-III.

Drugs Used for Anxiety

Most drugs used for anxiety (**anxiolytics**) are of the benzodiazepine class. It should be noted that, although these drugs are efficacious in the treatment of anxiety, a "rebound" effect (rebound anxiety) may be seen upon withdrawal of the drug. It should also be noted that these drugs are not to be used for the occasional anxiety attack. They are psychologically addictive and are classified under the Controlled Substance Act as C-III and C-IV. Newer nonbenzodiazepine agents have also been developed for use in the therapy of anxiety (e.g., buspirone).

Alprazolam

Brand name: Xanax, Xanax XR

Available as: 0.25 mg, 0.5 mg, 1 mg, and 2 mg tablets: 0.5 mg, 1 mg, 2 mg, and 3 mg extended-release tablets; 1 mg/mL intensol solution.

Dosage: 0.25–0.5 mg three times daily. Maximum daily dose: 4 mg geriatric or hepatically compromised dosage: 0.25 mg two to three times daily.

Special notes:
- Has a short half-life, as compared with other benzodiazepines.
- Has antimuscarinic effects and so is contraindicated in patients with narrow angle glaucoma or myasthenia gravis.
- Contraindicated in pregnancy.
- Not recommended for use in patients whose primary diagnosis is psychosis or depression.

Lorazepam

Brand name: Ativan

Available: 0.5 mg, 1 mg, and 2 mg tablets; 2 mg/mL and 4 mg/mL injection; 2 mg/mL oral solution.

Dosage: Oral: 2–6 mg/day in divided doses. Geriatric dose: 1–2 mg/day.

Intramuscular: 0.05 mg/kg up to a maximum dose of 4 mg. Intravenous: 0.02 mg/lb, up to 2 mg total dose.

Storage: Solutions for injection and oral administration: store refrigerated, protect from light.

Special notes:

- Intravenous administration of lorezepam could cause respiratory impairment.
- Lorazepam has an extremely long half-life (approximately three to four days), making it useful in the therapy of anxiety, seizures, and certain types of insomnia.
- When administered IV, infusion must be slow and care must be taken to avoid extravasation into tissues.

Buspirone

Brand name: BuSpar

Available as: 5 mg, 7.5 mg, 10 mg, 15 mg, and 30 mg tablets.

Dosage: 5 mg tid up to 60 mg/day

Dispensing: Dispense in a tight, light-resistant container.

Special notes:

- Buspirone is a partial agonist at certain dopamine (D_2) receptors and an agonist at certain serotonin receptors ($5HT_1$). The exact mechanism of action of this drug is unclear.
- Buspirone is contraindicated in patients with severe hepatic or severe renal impairment.

Drugs Used in the Therapy of Insomnia and Sleep Disorders

Two classes of drugs are used in the therapy of insomnia. These are benzo-diazepines (obtained by prescription) and certain antihistamines (obtained by prescription or over the counter). In addition, the new hypnotic agent, *zolpidem,* is very effective.

Drugs Available

Temazepam

Brand name: Restoril

Classification: Benzodiazepine

Available as: 7.5 mg, 15 mg, 22.5 mg, and 30 mg capsules

Dosage: 15 mg (range = 7.5–30 mg)

Special notes:

- Has a serum half-life is 8 to 10 hours.
- Is useful in "premature awakening" insomnia.
- Does not decrease sleep latency, so is not useful in the "delayed sleep" type of insomnia.
- Does not affect REM sleep—no decrease in REM sleep or rebound insomnia is seen.

Triazolam

Brand name: Halcion

Classification: Benzodiazepine

Available as: 0.125 mg and 0.25 mg tablets

Dosage: 2.5 mg (range 1.25 mg–0.5 mg). Maximum dose: 2.5 mg; geriatric dose: 0.125 mg.

Special notes:

- Triazolam is for short-term use only. Prescriptions should be written for a 7 to 10 day course of therapy. No more than a one-month supply should be dispensed.
- Short serum half-life—approximately three hours.
- Significant tolerance effect—after two weeks of consecutive nightly administration, the drug's effect on total wake time is decreased.
- Significant rebound insomnia and shortening of REM sleep are seen.
- A significant amount of anterograde amnesia is seen—next-day memory loss can occur, particularly in the elderly.
- Daytime anxiety and depression may be seen with users of this drug.
- This drug is metabolized by the liver, so dosage adjustments are required in the elderly.

Zolpidem

Brand name: Ambien, Ambien CR

Available as: 5 mg and 10 mg tablets; 6.25 mg and 12.5 mg extended-release tablets.

Dosage: 10 mg; geriatric dose: 5 mg.

Storage: Below 30°C

Mechanism of action: This drug is similar in structure to the benzodiazepines, and, like the benzodiazepines, binds to a receptor (the omega-3 receptor) on the chloride channel, causing a decrease in sensitivity of neuronal membranes to stimulus. It is *not* considered to be a benzodiazepine, however, and has therefore been termed the "non-benzodiazepine benzodiazepine."

Types of Insomnia

There are two general classifications of insomnia, which require different therapies. The most common type is the delayed sleep type of insomnia, where the person cannot get to sleep. Most hypnotic agents are oriented toward this type of insomnia. The second type is the *premature awakening* type of insomnia, where the person falls asleep normally, but wakes up early in the morning hours and is unable to get back to sleep. This type of insomnia is more difficult to treat.

These agents are meant for short-term therapy only.

Special notes:

- Zolpidem has a rapid onset and short duration (approximately four hours), making it useful in the delayed sleep onset type of insomnia.

- Instances of sleep walking and amnesia have been noted with the use of zolpidem.

- Like the benzodiazepines, this drug:
  - exhibits tolerance.
  - shortens REM sleep.
  - may cause rebound insomnia.

Antihistamines: Antihistamines with a high degree of antimuscarinic effect are useful in the therapy of insomnia (e.g., diphenhydramine [Benadryl]).

Drugs Used in the Therapy of Seizures

Seizure Formation—What Exactly Causes Seizures?

Every function of the body is regulated by some portion of the nervous system. Information moves along specific neuronal *pathways*—formed of a number of neurons in sequence. A neuronal pathway that regulates one function may lie very close to other pathways that regulate other functions. Since the neuronal membranes are excitable, "overexcitation" of a neuron in one pathway may cause an electrical "spike," which, if it is powerful enough, excites a neuron in an adjacent pathway. This adjacent pathway is now activated and whatever function it regulates is stimulated (e.g., muscle contraction), even though it is not needed. Seizures may exist in almost any pathway, and in any part of the brain, so the visible results of seizures are varied. Some seizures involve memory and learning, while others manifest as convulsions or abnormal movements. Small seizures are called *petit mal* seizures, and are usually associated with abnormal small movements or memory. Seizures that involve the whole body are termed *grand mal* seizures. Those that involve either muscle contraction or memory loss are termed *"partial"* seizures.

Drugs used in the therapy of seizures are correctly termed anticonvulsants. The function of these drugs is to decrease the excitability of neuronal membranes, so that aberrant electrical "spikes" will not be formed. This may be done by:

- reducing the conductance of sodium into the cell.

- reducing the conductance of potassium out of the cell.

- increasing the conductance of chloride into the cell (i.e., mimicking the effects of GABA).

- decreasing the amount of excitatory neurotransmitter released, or blocking receptors for excitatory neurotransmitters.

General contraindications: Alcohol is contraindicated with any antiseizure agent, as the effect of alcohol lowers the threshold for seizure activity and potentiates adverse effects of anticonvulsants (e.g., sedation). Alcohol can also interfere with the metabolism of anticonvulsants.

Tolerance and addiction: Physical dependence is a consequence of anticonvulsant therapy. The effects of anticonvulsants may also decrease over time, as a tolerance effect may be seen. This varies with the individual drug.

Withdrawal of the drug: *Withdrawal of any antiseizure agent must be done gradually.* Abrupt withdrawal may lead to a life-threatening seizure condition called **status epilepticus.** If a patient is changed from one anticonvulsant drug to another, it is wise to start the new medication concurrently with the existing medication, and then gradually increase the dose of the new drug while decreasing the dose of the existing drug. As the two drugs have different mechanisms, physical addiction to the first will not be changed by therapy with the second drug, so the possibility of the patient going into status epilepticus still exists.

Therapy of status epilepticus: Drugs effective for this condition are intravenous benzodiazepines—the drug of choice is diazepam; however, clonazepam is also effective. These drugs are administered by intravenous bolus, followed by intravenous drip.

Choice of drug: Most drugs available for the therapy of seizures are most useful in the therapy of partial seizures. The *absence* (ahb-SOHNS) seizure is a peculiar type of seizure involving short-term memory and is only seen in children. These conditions require therapy with specific agents, such as valproic acid and its derivatives. The choice of drug is based not only on the type of seizure and the apparent location of seizure activity, but also considers the degree of sedation, sensitivities, and other effects.

> *Withdrawal of any antiseizure agent must be done gradually. Abrupt withdrawal may lead to a life-threatening seizure condition called status epilepticus.*

Drugs Available: Sodium Channel Blockers

Carbamazepine

Brand name: Tegretol, Tegretol XR, and Carbatrol

Available as: 100 mg (chewable) and 200 mg tablets; 20 mg/mL suspension; 200 mg and 400 mg extended-release tablets (Tegretol XR); 200 mg and 300 mg capsules (Carbatrol)

Dosage: 200 mg bid for seizures, 200 mg per day for trigeminal neuralgia; pediatric: 100 mg bid

Storage: Store below 30°C

Dispensing: Dispense in a tightly closed, light-resistant container.

Special notes:

- Effective in the therapy of partial seizures, including memory.

- Carbamazepine can cause aplastic anemia, which is irreversible and fatal—regular blood analysis is therefore necessary.

- Highly plasma protein bound, so interactions may be seen with other drugs that have a high degree of protein binding.

- Carbamazepine has antimuscarinic actions (blocks muscarinic receptors for acetylcholine). This effect results in effects on the heart, added to the sodium-blocking effect, results in effects on the heart and cardiovascular system. Saliva is also decreased and changes in bowl and bladder function.

- The negative inotropic effects of the drug, as well as the changes in salt balance, result in decreased blood flow and the formation of edema, particularly in the extremities.

- This drug causes effects on salt and water balance, because of its effects on sodium.

- This drug causes a sensitivity to sun—severe sunburn may result from relatively mild sun exposure.

Phenytoin sodium

Brand names: Dilantin, Dilantin-125

Available as: 50 mg chewable tablet (Infatab); 125-mg/5 mL suspension; 30 mg or 100 mg extended-release capsules.

Dosage: Adult dose: 100 mg tid, or a single dose of 300 mg in the extended-release formulation. A loading dose may be necessary, to achieve therapeutic plasma levels quickly. A typical loading dose would be 1,000 mg administered in six hours (e.g., a 400 mg dose and two 300 mg doses administered three hours apart). Pediatric dose: 5 mg kg/day in two to three divided doses. Maximum dose: 300 mg/day.

Adverse effects:

- **Osteomalacia,** due to the effects of the drug on vitamin D.
- **Hypoglycemia,** due to inhibition of insulin release.
- **Gingival hyperplasia** (swelling of the gums).
- CNS effects: nystagmus, ataxia, slurred speech, decreased coordination, and mental confusion.
- Bone marrow suppression and blood dyscrasias.
- Phenytoin is contraindicated in pregnancy, as severe fetal malformations have been shown to occur. These are collectively termed *fetal hydantoin*

syndrome and also occur with chronic administration of barbiturates or alcohol during pregnancy.

- Phenytoin has been associated with the development of certain lymphoid cancers.

- Phenytoin may produce a characteristic urticaria ("phenytoin rash"). Should this occur, therapy should be discontinued, and reinstated at a later date. Should the rash again occur, therapy should be discontinued permanently.

- Phenytoin is not administered by rapid injection—because of its low solubility in water the drug must first be dissolved in other chemicals. These chemicals will cause toxic cardiovascular effects (e.g., hypotension, arrhythmias) if administered quickly. Thus, IV forms of phenytoin must be administered slowly. This makes it less useful in the therapy of status epilepticus.

Special notes:
- Phenytoin produces a blockade of both sodium and potassium channels.

- The primary site of action appears to be the motor cortex, making the drug useful in the tonic phase of grand mal seizures.

- Phenytoin is not effective against petit mal seizures, and should not be used in the therapy of seizures due to metabolic origin (such as those produced by hypoglycemia).

- Phenytoin is metabolized by the liver. The enzymes involved in the pathway are saturable—that is, the enzymes involved can only metabolize a certain amount of drug at one time. This means that small increases in dose can produce a large increase in physiological effects, or even produce toxicity.

- Metabolism of phenytoin involves the enzyme aldehyde dehydrogenase, so it may produce "disulfiram-like" reactions, particularly with the concurrent administration of ethanol. Recall that the metabolism of ethanol is a two-step process—the product of the first step is toxic substances, which may cause discomfort. These toxic substances are quickly inactivated and converted to less toxic substances by an enzyme in the liver called *aldehyde dehydrogenase*. If the actions of aldehyde dehydrogenase are inhibited (or if the enzyme is busy doing something else, like metabolizing phenytoin), the toxic metabolites will accumulate; inhibition of the second step (involving aldehyde dehydrogenase) results in the accumulation of the toxic metabolite, and uncomfortable effects, such as nausea and vomiting, will occur. Disulfiram is a drug used in the therapy of alcoholism, which inhibits this enzyme and thus discourages the patient from drinking. Thus, these events are termed *disulfiram-like reactions.*

Fosphenytoin

Brand name: Cerebyx

Available as: 75 mg/mL solution for injection, equivalent to 50 mg/mL of phenytoin.

Dosage: Emergent dosage: A loading dose of 15–20 PE/kg, followed by an infusion of 100–150 PE/min. Infusion at a rate greater than 150 PE/min can cause severe hypotension, and is not recommended. Nonemergent dosage: 10–20 PE administered IV or IM, followed by an infusion. Total daily maintenance dose is 4–6 PE/kg. (Note: PE = phenytoin equivalent.)

Storage: Vials should be stored refrigerated at 2–8°C. Vials should not be exposed to room temperature for longer than 48 hours.

Special notes:
- Fosphenytoin is a prodrug of phenytoin—it is rapidly converted to phenytoin after IV administration.
- May be administered by rapid injection, making it useful in the therapy of status epilepticus.
- Dose and rate of infusion are expressed as "phenytoin equivalents" (PE), as the conversion to phenytoin is 1.5:1.

Drugs That Mimic the Effects of GABA

Gabapentin

Brand name: Neurontin

Available as: 100 mg, 300 mg, and 400 mg capsules; 600 mg and 800 mg filmtabs; 50 mg/mL oral solution.

Primary Uses: Supplemental (adjunct) therapy in control of seizures, and in the therapy of bipolar disorder.

Dosage: 900–1,800 mg/day in divided doses, starting with 300-mg capsules taken three times a day.

Special notes:
- Structurally related to GABA, but the exact mechanism of action is unknown.
- Gabapentin does not bind significantly to other receptors (e.g., muscarinic, adrenergic), so adverse effects, such as sedation, dry mouth, etc., are less.

- Absorption is dose-dependent and decreases with increasing dose (e.g., a larger fraction of a 100 mg dose will be absorbed than a 400 mg dose).
- Large volume of distribution.
- Renal excretion—dosage adjustment in the elderly and renally compromised patients is necessary.

Pregabalin

Brand name: Lyrica

Available as: 25 mg, 50 mg, 75 mg, 100 mg, 150 mg, 200 mg, 225 mg, and 300 mg capsules.

Special notes:

- Binds to calcium channels and modulates calcium influx.
- Is structurally similar to gabapentin, but more potent.
- Has few known interactions.
- Is an adjunct use only for partial seizures.
- Can be used for diabetic neuropathy.
- Used into treat fibromyalgia.

Vigabatrin

Brand name: Sabril

Available as: 500 mg tablets; 500 mg oral solution powder packets.

Dosage: Maximum dosage is 4 g/day. Starting dose is 1 to 2 g/day.

Mechanism of action: Vigabatrin increases the amount of available GABA. It is similar in structure to GABA (it is a "structural analog" of GABA), and competes with GABA for binding sites on the enzyme (GABA transaminase) that metabolizes GABA. Thus, it interferes with the metabolism of GABA, resulting in increased levels of available GABA.

Special notes:

- Considered in monotherapy for infantile spasms in patients 1 month – 2 years.
- Loss of vision is possible.
- Used in the therapy of partial seizures that do not respond to other agents.
- Primarily used as adjunct therapy, not used alone (e.g., as monotherapy).
- Could possibly increase seizure frequency in certain patients.

Tiagabine

Brand name: Gabatril

Available as: 2 mg, 4 mg, 12 mg, and 16 mg tablets.

Dosage: 32–64 mg/day in divided doses.

Mechanism of action: Tiagabine selectively inhibits the neuronal reuptake of GABA. This results in increased levels of GABA available to bind to the GABA receptor.

Special notes:

- Is used as adjunct therapy for simple or complex seizures.
- Effective against a broad spectrum of seizure types, including electro-shock-induced and drug-induced seizures.
- Extensively bound to plasma proteins.

Drugs That Affect Excitatory Neurotransmitter Levels

Valproic acid

Brand names: Depakene (valproic acid), Depakote (sodium divalproex), Depakote ER, Depacon (injection form), Stavzor (valproic acid)

Available as: Depakote = 125 mg, 250 mg tablets, and 500 mg; 250 mg and 500 mg sustained-release tablets and 125 mg sprinkles; Depakene = 250 mg capsule; and 250 mg/5 mL syrup (valproate); 250 mg/5 mL syrup (sodium salt); 500 mg tablets (SR); Depacon = 100 mg/mL injection.

Special notes:

- Drug of choice for absence seizures.
- Extremely sedating. Tolerance may develop to the sedation, with time.
- Potent liver toxicity—liver function tests must be run routinely during therapy.
- The sodium salt (divalproex Na) causes significant edema, due to the increased sodium load.
- Highly plasma protein bound (> 99%), causing potential drug interactions.
- Concurrent administration with clonazepam may result in status epilepticus.
- Alteration in thyroid function (hypothyroidism) may be caused by these drugs.
- Highly teratogenic; is contraindicated in pregnancy.

Topiramate

Brand name: Topamax

Available as: 25-mg, 50-mg, 100-mg, and 200-mg tablets; 15-mg and 25-mg sprinkle caps.

Special notes:

- Use as an add-on therapy to carbamazepine or phenytoin.

- Decreases craving for alcohol but takes six weeks to see effectiveness.

- Effective for partial onset adult seizures.

Lamotrigine

Brand name: Lamictal

Available as: 25 mg, 100 mg, 150 mg, and 200 mg tablets; 2 mg, 5 mg, and 25 mg chewable tablets.

Dosage: 50 mg qd for two weeks, increasing to 100 mg/day in divided doses for an additional two weeks, and 100 to 150 mg/day, thereafter, in divided doses. The clearance of lamotrigine is substantially decreased with concurrent valproic acid therapy. Dosage should be reduced by 50%.

Special notes:

- Useful as adjunct therapy in the management of seizures.

- May cause severe, potentially life-threatening skin rashes, particularly in children (incidence = 1:50 to 1:100). These appear to be dose related incidence also increases with concurrent administration of valproic acid, or when the drug is administered rapidly or in large doses. These can be simple skin rashes, but may be life-threatening, including serious conditions such as Stevens-Johnson syndrome and epidermal necrolysis. If a skin rash develops, the drug should be withdrawn.

- Adverse effects are mainly of CNS origin and include dizziness, diplopia, ataxia, and blurred vision. These are dose-related and appear to occur more commonly in patients on concurrent therapy with carbamazepine, in combination with lamotrigine.

Barbiturates and Benzodiazepines as Anticonvulsants

Certain benzodiazepines are used as anticonvulsants. However, the use of barbiturates as anticonvulsants is not routine, as the action of these drugs is too nonspecific. The following barbiturates are used clinically as anticonvulsants:

Phenobarbital

Available as: 15 mg, 30 mg, 32 mg, 60 mg, and 100 mg tablets; 16 mg capsule; 15 mg/5 mL and 20 mg/5 mL oral liquid; 30 mg/mL, 60 mg/mL, 65 mg/mL, and 130 mg/mL injection

Administration: Oral or intravenous

Special notes:

Phenobarbital is mainly used in the therapy of pediatric epilepsy. It is also used in combination therapy in adults.

Butabarbital

Brand name: Butisol

Available as: 30 mg and 50 mg tablets; 30 mg/5 mL oral solution.

Special notes:

Butabarbital is useful in suppression of the spread of seizure activity in the cortex, thalamus, and limbic systems.

Secobarbital

Brand name: Seconal

Available as: 100 mg capsule

Special notes:

- Secobarbital is a short-acting barbiturate, used in the therapy of status epilepticus.
- Secobarbital increases the threshold for electrical stimulation in the motor cortex, which contributes to its use in the therapy of status epilepticus.
- *Protective effects:* Secobarbital has protective effects on brain tissue—it decreases damage due to lack of oxygen.

Benzodiazepines

Benzodiazepines, such as clonazepam and diazepam, are used in the therapy of status epilepticus. Clonazepam is also used as adjunct or monotherapy in the prevention (prophylaxis) of seizures.

Diazepam

Brand name: Valium, Diastat

Available as: Injectable solution, 5 mg/mL; 2 mg, 5 mg and 10 mg tablets; 5 mg/5 mL oral solution; 5 mg/mL oral concentrate; 2.5 mg, 5 mg, 15 mg, and 20 mg rectal (Diastat).

Uses: Anxiety disorders, also used in endoscopic surgery as a muscle relaxant. It is of particular use due to its tendency to cause anterograde amnesia. Drug of choice for the therapy of status epilepticus.

Dosage: 2 to 10 mg IV

Special notes:

- Diazepam possesses all of the properties of the benzodiazepine class. It is a(n):
  - anticonvulsant.
  - hypnotic agent and anxiolytic agent (low doses).
  - skeletal muscle relaxant.
- Diazepam is metabolized by the liver to active metabolites desmethyldiazepam and oxazepam. Both of these have pharmacological activity.

Therapy of Status Epilepticus

> Remember: Abrupt discontinuation of any anticonvulsant drug therapy can precipitate status epilepticus!

Status epilepticus is a life-threatening condition that can cause death in a matter of minutes, if not seconds. Agents administered for this condition must have a very fast onset. Thus, agents for the therapy of status epilepticus are *administered intravenously*, as a bolus, normally followed by an IV drip.

Drugs Used in the Therapy of Status Epilepticus

- IV diazepam is the drug of choice.
- IV clonezepam or secobarbital may be used.
- IV fosphenytoin is useful, as it can be rapidly administered IV or IM.

Therapy of ADHD

Attention deficit hyperactivity disorder (ADHD) is commonly seen among children. The children are overactive, difficult to control, and have difficulty in learning and comprehension. The condition is treated by increasing dopamine levels and activity in certain parts of the brain. Oddly enough, the drugs used to treat this disorder are stimulants (not the first thing that one would think of for an overactive child)—*neurostimulants*, to be exact. Drugs that may be used are:

- Tricyclic antidepressants: These increase available norepinephrine, serotonin, and dopamine. Increased levels of these transmitters help to increase concentration and elevate mood.
- Amphetamines: These drugs have a low margin of safety, and are no longer drugs of first choice. Amphetamines also increase circulating levels of norepinephrine and dopamine in the CNS.

The drugs of choice are the following:

Methylphenidate

Brand names: Ritalin, Concerta (methyphenidate XR), Daytrana

Available as: 5 mg, 10 mg, and 20 mg tablets; 20 mg extended-release tablet (Ritalin) 18 mg, 27 mg, 36 mg, and 54 mg tablets (Concerta), patch (Daytrana).

Dosage: 20–30 mg daily. Pediatric dosage: 10 mg bid. Maximum dose in children is 60 mg/day.

Dispensing: Dispense in a light-proof, tightly sealed container.

Mechanism of action: Methylphenidate selectively blocks neuronal reuptake of dopamine in the central nervous system. This results in an increase in central levels of dopamine in the brain stem, which regulates arousal, and the cerebral cortex, which regulates cognitive ability. Levels may also be increased in the nigrostriatal tract and limbic system, which are involved in the regulation of movement and learning/memory/behavior, respectively.

Special notes:
- The drug should be administered 25 to 45 minutes before meals.
- Physical dependence is not considered to be a characteristic of methylphenidate; however, it is considered *psychologically* addictive. Psychological addiction is more likely to occur with parenteral administration, such as would be seen when the drug is abused.
- Peripheral effects of increased dopamine (e.g., cardiovascular effects) are negligible.

Atomoxetine

Brand name: Strattera

Available as: 10 mg, 18 mg, 25 mg, 40 mg, and 60 mg tablets

Special notes:
- It is primarily used for ADHD.

Modafinil

Brand name: Provigil

Available as: 100 mg and 200 mg tablets

Special notes:
- Is a nonamphetamine stimulant.
- Effective for ADHD in adults.
- Effective for narcolepsy.

Parkinson's Disease

Parkinson's disease results from an imbalance of dopamine and acetylcholine in an area of the brain called the *substantia nigra*. Dopaminergic neurons begin to degenerate and die, due to old age, drug use, or infectious disease (e.g., encephalitis). This leaves the area with too many neurons that make acetylcholine and too few that make dopamine. Since dopamine acts as an inhibitory neurotransmitter and acetylcholine is excitatory, an imbalance between excitatory and inhibitory actions is seen, which produces things like unnecessary or uncontrolled muscle contractions, excess salivation, and so on. Therefore, alterations in movement are seen, followed by facial paralysis and, eventually, total incapacitation. The disease is progressive, so medications available only treat the symptoms and attempt to give the patient a better quality of life. In addition, because the disease is progressive, the majority of medications available will not be effective after a certain point in the progression of the disease.

Drugs That Increase the Level or Activity of Dopamine

> Remember: The objective in the therapy of Parkinson's disease is to normalize the balance between dopamine and acetylcholine!

The drug of choice in the therapy of Parkinson's disease is L-dopa. A dopaminergic agonist, such as *bromocriptine*, may also be used. Bromocriptine is considered a first-line drug for the therapy of Parkinson's disease.

- Effective drug therapies attempt to normalize the balance between dopamine and acetylcholine—either by increasing dopamine levels or decreasing levels of acetylcholine.
- It should be noted that dopamine administration is not effective in Parkinson's disease, as dopamine does not cross the blood-brain barrier and will not enter the CNS!

Drugs Prescribed

L-dopa (levodopa)

Levodopa is a brain chemical found in dopaminergic neurons, which is converted to dopamine by enzymes in the dopaminergic neuron. It is also called levodopa.

Brand names: Dopar, Larodopa

Available as: 100 mg, 250 mg, and 500 mg tablets and capsules

Special notes:

Levodopa has a variety of adverse effects, which are related to the increased levels of dopamine in certain parts of the brain. Increased dopamine in the striatal tract can produce psychiatric symptoms, such as hallucinations and behavioral changes. Changes in learning and memory may be seen, as well. The major adverse effects seen with L-dopa therapy are extrapyramidal effects, in which changes in autonomic function may be seen.

A major problem with the use of L-dopa is that it can be converted to dopamine in *any dopaminergic* nerve terminal. This includes dopaminergic neurons in the body (peripheral), as well as the brain (central). Increased production of peripheral dopamine results in a tremendous number of adverse effects, such as unwanted changes in cardiovascular and renal activity. In addition, the peripheral nerve terminals will remove the L-dopa from the bloodstream, *before* it can get to the brain where it is needed, resulting in less drug available to be converted to dopamine in the CNS. To avoid this problem, we give a second drug that inhibits the neuronal conversion of L-dopa into dopamine. This drug is called carbidopa and inhibits the enzyme (dopa decarboxylase), which is necessary for the conversion. This drug may be incorporated with L-dopa into one tablet (e.g., *Sinemet*).

> Carbidopa is useful, as it does not cross the blood-brain barrier! Thus, it acts only on peripheral neurons and decreases the amount of dopamine made in the body. It does not decrease the amount of dopamine made in the CNS!

Levodopa with Carbidopa

Brand name: Sinemet, Sinemet CR

Available as: Sinemet tablets containing 100 mg levodopa with 10 mg Carbidopa (10/100), 25 mg Carbidopa with 100 mg levodopa (25/100), or 25 mg Carbidopa with 250 mg levodopa (25/250), Sinemet CR tablets containing 25 mg Carbidopa and 100 mg levodopa (25/100) or 50 mg Carbidopa and 200 mg levodopa (50/200).

The effects of L-dopa wear off after a period of time. Therapy must then be stopped, and reinstated at a later date. The period of time between therapies is called a *drug holiday* and gives the tissue time to return to a responsive state. During this time, other agents, such as bromocriptine, are substituted.

Levodopa/Carbidopa/Entacapone

Brand name: Stalevo

Available as: Carbidopa 12.5 mg/Entacapone 200 mg/Levodopa 50 mg; Carbidopa 25 mg/Entacapone 200 mg/Levodopa 100 mg; Carbidopa 37.5 mg/Entacapone 200 mg/Levodopa 150 mg.

Special notes:
- It is used in patients with "wearing off" effect of levodopa.
- Entacapone boosts the efficacy.
- It is cost effective.

Bromocriptine

Brand name: Parlodel

Available as: 2.5 mg tablet; 5 mg capsule.

Dosage: 1.25 mg bid with meals, increasing every 2 to 3 weeks in 2.5 mg intervals.

Storage: Below room temperature (< 25°C)

Mechanism of action: Bromocriptine is an agonist at dopamine receptors. It therefore stimulates the receptor and mimics the effects of dopamine.

Special notes:

- Inhibits prolactin secretion so it can be used to dry up breast milk in nursing mothers.

- Bromocriptine can cause a high degree of psychiatric effects, mimicking schizophrenia. The autonomic (e.g., cardiovascular) effects of the drug are minimal. Bromocriptine is used during the "drug holiday" from L-dopa, and is also used in conjunction with L-dopa.

- Using bromocriptine and L-dopa together allows control of the disease symptoms and reduction of dosage of both drugs. This reduces the number and severity of adverse effects, as these effects are dose-related.

Physiology Review—The Metabolism of Catecholamines

There are two major ways that catecholamines, such as norepinephrine and dopamine, are metabolized:

- A mitochondrial enzyme, monoamine oxidase, or MAO breaks down these transmitters as they are taken back up into the neuronal ending from the synaptic cleft. MAO_A breaks down norepinephrine, while another MAO, MAO_B metabolizes dopamine.
- Neurotransmitter released into the synaptic cleft is broken down and inactivated by a tissue enzyme called catechol-O-methyl transferase or COMT.

Tolcapone

Brand name: Tasmar

Available as: 100 mg or 200 mg tablets

Dosage: 100 mg tid, always as adjunct therapy to L-dopa. At doses approaching 600 mg/day, the risk of liver failure increases.

Mechanism of action: Tolcapone is an inhibitor of COMT. It thus:

- decreases the metabolism of dopamine in the synaptic cleft, resulting in increased levels of available dopamine.

- decreases tissue metabolism of L-dopa, so when tolcapone and L-dopa are given concurrently, greater amounts of L-dopa are presented to the neuron and drug potency is increased.

Special notes:

- Because of the risk of severe liver injury, tolcapone should not be used as a first-line drug. In addition, if a patient does not show significant improvement with tolcapone therapy, the drug should be withdrawn.

> Dopaminergic nerve terminals are required in order to convert the L-dopa into dopamine, and these nerve terminals are progressively degenerating, due to the disease. Therefore, L-dopa is only going to be effective in the first stages of the disease. After that, the drug becomes progressively less effective as there are fewer terminals present to convert it to dopamine!

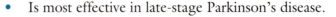

- Is most effective in late-stage Parkinson's disease.
- Potentiates the actions of L-dopa (a drug synergism).
- May cause extreme liver toxicity, and should be given only to patients not responding to other therapies.
- Patients who fail to show clinical benefit within three weeks should be taken off of the drug.
- Patients must be advised of the risks of taking the drug, and, if appropriate, written release should be obtained.
- Patients must be educated as to self-monitoring techniques for the symptoms of impending liver failure (e.g., jaundice, grayish stools, a persistent feeling of nausea) and made aware of the importance of regular and frequent liver function tests.
- Liver enzyme levels (e.g., SGPT and SGOT) must be determined at the onset of therapy to establish baseline liver function, and monitored every 2 weeks thereafter for the first year of therapy, then every 4 to 6 weeks thereafter.
- Tolcapone should be withdrawn gradually, as Parkinson's symptoms may reappear.

Pramipexole
Brand name: Mirapex

Available as: 0.125 mg, 0.25 mg, 0.5 mg, 1 mg, and 1.5 mg tablets

Special notes:
Commonly used for Restless Leg Syndrome (RLS).

Ropinirole
Brand name: ReQuip

Available as: 0.25 mg, 0.5 mg, 1 mg, 2 mg, and 5 mg tablets

Special notes:
- It is a dopamine agonist.
- Hypotension is often seen at the start of therapy.
- Can be used in RLS.

Selegiline
Brand names: Eldepryl, Zelapar, Emsam

Available as: 5 mg tablets or capsules; 1.25 mg disintegrating tablets (Zelapar); transdermal patch (Emsam).

Dosage: 10 mg/day in divided doses (taken at breakfast and lunch).

Mechanism of action: Irreversibly inhibits MAO_B, resulting in decreased rate of dopamine breakdown within the neuron.

Special notes:

- Selegiline is otherwise known as *l-deprenyl*.

- *Dietary restrictions are not necessary in the low dosage range*: At doses 10 mg/day, the drug selectively inhibits MAO_B, so no dietary restrictions are necessary. At higher doses, MAO_A is also inhibited, so ingestion of foods containing tyramine may cause an increase in norepinephrine levels and may precipitate a hypertensive crisis, just as with MAO inhibitors.

- Emsam is used for depression.

- Zelapar requires a decreased dosage.

Agents That Decrease Levels or Activity of Acetylcholine (Antimuscarinic Agents)

Mechanism of action: These drugs block muscarinic receptors and decrease cholinergic activity.

Therapeutic effects: Blockade of muscarinic effects in the nigrostriatal tract, resulting in normalization of acetylcholine/dopamine activity ratio.

Adverse effects: Increased intraocular pressure, urinary retention, cardiac dysfunction, xerostomia (lack of stomach fluid), blurred vision, nausea/vomiting, drowsiness, dizziness, and mental confusion. Adverse effects seen with parenteral administration may include transient hypotension, coordination disturbances, and temporary euphoria.

Contraindications: Glaucoma (the "angle-closure" type, in particular), obstruction of the lower stomach (pyloric) valve or duodenum, enlarged prostate, obstructed bladder, myasthenia gravis, and megacolon.

Drugs Prescribed

Procyclidine

Brand name: Kemadrin

Available as: 5 mg tablets

Dosage: 30 mg/day

Special notes:
- Pregnancy category C—may pose a risk to the developing fetus.

Biperiden

Brand name: Akineton

Available as: 2 mg tablets; 5 mg/mL ampule—solution for injection.

Adverse effects: The antimuscarinic activity relieves muscle rigidity, fatigue, weakness, and sluggishness and decreases tremor activity.

Special notes:

- Oral and parenteral antimuscarinic agent.
- Used as adjunct treatment for Parkinson's disease.
- Also used for the relief of extrapyramidal symptoms associated with antipsychotic agents.

Amantadine HCl

Brand name: Symmetrel

Available as: 100 mg capsules; 10 mg/mL syrup.

Amantadine is an antiviral agent that has anticholinergic properties. It decreases the activity of acetylcholine in the nigrostriatal tract. Recently, amantadine has been shown to increase dopamine secretion, as well, making it a useful, though second-line, drug in the therapy of Parkinson's disease.

Drugs Used in the Therapy of Alzheimer's Disease

Drugs used in the therapy of *Alzheimer's* disease are inhibitors of acetylcholinesterase, the enzyme that breaks down acetylcholine (ACh). Inhibition of the breakdown of ACh results in more ACh present in areas of the brain, such as the forebrain, cortex, and limbic system, that are involved in memory. The effects of these drugs are only symptomatic—the progression of the disease is not affected!

Alzheimer's disease is a progressive disorder involving changes in neuronal pathways and formation of neurofibrillary tangles in brain tissue. The primary areas affected are the cerebral cortex, forebrain, and limbic system, which regulate coherent thought, reasoning, and memory/emotion, respectively. Since acetylcholine is a primary excitatory neurotransmitter in these areas, it is thought that raising available levels of acetylcholine will provide symptomatic relief. Thus, drugs currently useful in the therapy of Alzheimer's are targeted to raise levels of acetylcholine in these portions of the brain. There are presently two agents in use, chosen for particular chemical properties (since these agents must cross into the brain to have an effect, they cannot be charged or ionized in the plasma, must be fat soluble, and have a relatively long duration of action).

Why not just administer acetylcholine in the therapy of Alzheimer's? Acetylcholine has a very brief half-life, as it is metabolized almost immediately by enzymes in the plasma (*plasma cholinesterases*, or *pseudocholinesterases*). It would also not cross into the brain, as the molecule carries a charge at physiological pH.

Mechanism of action: These drugs bind to the enzyme acetylcholinesterase. Binding occurs at the site where the enzyme normally binds acetylcholine, and destroys it. The result is more available acetylcholine. Since there are slight differences in structure between acetylcholinesterase in the CNS and the periphery, these drugs are targeted to selectively inhibit CNS cholinesterase, resulting in decreased adverse effects. Nevertheless, in high doses, toxicity may be seen. Toxicity of cholinesterase inhibitors usually shows up as one or more of the following:

- Bradycardia (slow heart rate)
- Hypotension (low blood pressure)

- Bowel and/or bladder dysfunction
- Miosis (pinpoint pupils)
- Dyspepsia (upset stomach)
- Difficulty in breathing, muscle weakness, and confusion may also be present

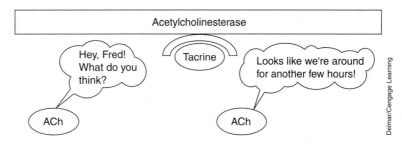

Tacrine

Brand name: Cognex

Available as: 10 mg, 20 mg, 30 mg, and 40 mg tablets

Special notes:
- The mechanism of action and clinical actions are not fully understood.
- Because the effects of the drug rely on the presence of acetylcholine, the effects of the drug decrease with progression of the disease, as cholinergic neurons degenerate.
- This drug may be toxic to the liver.
- *Liver transaminase levels must be monitored* every two weeks for the first four months, and every three months thereafter. Significantly elevated transaminase levels (> 8 × normal) necessitate withdrawal of the drug. Treatment may be reinstated after transaminase levels return to normal, unless hypersensitivity reactions (e.g., rash, fever) are present.

Donezepil

Brand name: Aricept

Available as: 5 mg, 10 mg tablets

Special notes:
- Donezepil is a piperadine-type inhibitor of acetylcholinesterase.
- Adverse effects commonly seen include nausea, diarrhea, vomiting, muscle cramps, insomnia, and anorexia.
- Donezepil is not associated with hepatotoxicity.
- The drug has a high degree of binding to plasma proteins (96%).
- Metabolism by the liver produces active metabolites. Thus, both the elimination and the clinical duration of action are influenced by the patient's liver function (normally decreased in the elderly, who are the primary target for the drug).

Rivastigmine

Brand name: Exelon

Available as: 1.5 mg, 3 mg, 4.5 mg, and 6 mg tablets; 2 mg/mL oral solution; transdermal patch.

Special notes:

- The patch can be used for parkinsonism or Alzheimer's disease; it is in a matrix formulation.
- Similar to donezepil with fewer interactions.

Drugs Used in the Therapy of Schizophrenia (Antipsychotics)

Schizophrenia is thought to be due to increased levels of dopamine in an area of the brain called the *striatum*. This increased dopamine activity results in behavioral abnormalities, such as delusions, withdrawal from reality, and altered mental perceptions. *Note that schizophrenia and multiple personality disorder ("split personality") are very dissimilar conditions. They are not the same thing at all.*

Treatment of Schizophrenia

Schizophrenia is treated with agents that block dopamine receptors (dopamine antagonists). This helps to bring the symptoms of the condition under control. As with the other neurotransmitter-based conditions that we have discussed, *therapy is not curative*—the underlying basis of the condition still remains. *Once the drug is withdrawn, psychosis will again develop.*

Dopamine receptor antagonists useful in schizophrenia block the "D_2" type of dopamine receptor. This entire mechanism of action of these drugs in the treatment of schizophrenia is not yet clear. These agents are relatively nonspecific and may block muscarinic receptors or histamine receptors, as well.

These drugs have a wide variety of undesirable effects, and *patient compliance is poor*. These agents can cause:

> **Neuroleptic malignant syndrome**: a life-threatening condition that can be caused by antipsychotic agents. It is treated by administration of the skeletal muscle relaxant dantrolene, in combination with anti-Parkinson drugs.

- Increased prolactin secretion and milk production (in both men and women), due to the inhibition of dopamine actions at the pituitary.
- Gynecomastia (enlarged breasts), particularly in men.
- Cardiodepressant actions, due to their antimuscarinic effects.
- Parkinson-like symptoms, due to blockade of dopamine receptors in the substantia nigra.
- **Neuroleptic malignant syndrome**, characterized by severe fever, muscle rigidity, altered mental status (e.g., catatonia), and cardiovascular instability (e.g., unstable heart rate and blood pressure). This syndrome is similar to the malignant hyperthermia seen with inhalation anesthetics, and is a life-threatening condition.

Symptoms of overdose of antipsychotic drugs include:

- Parkinson-like effects.
- CNS effects, such as sleepiness, seizures, inability to adjust to changes in temperature.
- Anticholinergic effects, such as dry mouth, blurred vision, and urinary retention.
- Cardiovascular effects, such as rapid heart rate, cardiac arrhythmias, and decreased blood pressure.

There are many classes of antipsychotic drugs. The oldest, and still widely used, class is the phenothiazine antipsychotics, named for their unique chemical ring structure. Characteristics of the phenothiazine antipsychotics include:

- A high "first-pass" effect through the liver—a large amount of the drug is destroyed immediately after absorption.
- A high incidence of **postural hypotension** (a drop in blood pressure upon standing), due to the blockade of alpha receptors (α_1) by the drug.
- *Antipsychotics of the phenothiazine class should never be administered concurrently with epinephrine. To do so can cause an extreme loss of blood pressure!*

Phenothiazine antipsychotics are classified into three groups. Classification is done by the type of "side chain," or chemical group that is present on the structure. The type of side chain present determines the properties of the drug. The three groups are:

- Aliphatic side chain phenothiazines (e.g., chlorpromazine). These are the *least potent* class, and have a lot of adverse effects, particularly anticholinergic effects. These drugs affect several types of receptors, including receptors for serotonin, acetylcholine, and histamine. Adverse effects are therefore varied, and include sedation, dry mouth, hypotension, and autonomic (extrapyramidal) effects. These effects are dose-related (so a more potent drug will show less adverse effects). The most serious adverse effect is **tardive dyskinesia**—a motor disorder characterized by lip-smacking. It is irreversible, once established. Tardive dyskinesia is the dose-limiting factor in the administration of these drugs. *If this condition develops, therapy must be stopped immediately!*

- The piperadine side chain antipsychotics (e.g., thioridizine):
  - These drugs are less selective for the D_2 subtype of dopamine receptor—they also block the D_1 receptor, causing a high degree of undesirable autonomic effects.
  - These drugs produce a higher degree of tardive dyskinesia.
  - Potency is low, so higher dosages must be used for therapeutic effect.

> Phenothiazine antipsychotics can have severe autonomic effects, such as tardive dyskinesia, an irreversible motor disorder characterized by smacking of the lips.

> Antipsychotics act at a central level to reduce nausea and vomiting. They are thus useful as antiemetics!

- The piperazine side chain phenothiazine antipsychotics (e.g., fluphenazine):
  - These drugs have the highest potency of the phenothiazines (but are still classified as intermediate potency as compared with all classes) and least amount of adverse effects.
  - Sedation is low.
  - Hypotensive effects are decreased.

Antipsychotic Drugs

Drug Class	Prototype(s)	Potency	Degree of Adverse Effects
Phenothiazines:			
Aliphatic side chain:	promazine, chlorpromazine	low	autonomic effects, sedation, cardiovascular, extrapyramidal effects
Piperadine side chain:	thioridazine, mesoridazine	low	cardiotoxicity, fewer extrapyramidal effects
Piperazine side chain:	fluphenazine	intermediate	low sedation, decreased hypotensive effects
Dibenzoxapines:	loxapine clozapine	low	agranulocytosis, seizures; low extrapyramidal effects, low sedation/ hypotension
Thioxanthines:	thiothixine chlorprothixine	intermediate	less sedation, extra-pyramidal effects, decreased risk of tardive dyskinesia
Buterophenones:	haloperidol	high	fewer autonomic effects, low sedation, severe extrapyramidal effects
Benzisoxazoles:	risperidone	high	low extrapyramidal effects, low sedation/ hypotension
Thienobenzodiazepines:	olanzepine	high	sedation, low hypotension, low extrapyramidal effects
Floourophenylindoles:	sertindole	high	low extrapyramidal effects, low sedation/ hypotension

Frequently Prescribed Drugs

Chlorpromazine

Brand name: Thorazine

Available as: 10-mg, 25-mg, 50-mg tablets. Also available in 100 mg and 200 mg strengths. Also in 30 mg, 75 mg, and 150 mg sustained-release capsules; 25 mg and 100 mg suppositories; 30 mg/mL and 100 mg/mL concentrated syrup; 10 mg/5 mL oral syrup; and 25 mg/mL injection.

Dosage: 25 to 75 mg (mild cases) or 75 to 150 mg (more severe cases) in two to four divided doses; rectal: 100 to 300 mg/day. Maximum dose: 900 mg/day.

Special notes:

- Clinical Effects Delayed—effects may not be seen for several weeks, even months.

- May be given IM for therapy of acute attacks. Parenteral therapy is not used in the normal course of therapy.

- Intramuscular injection (rapid infusion) is associated with severe hypotension, so the patient should be lying down and remain there for at least hour.

- The drug should be protected from light. *Pink or discolored solutions should be discarded*.

- Used as an antiemetic.

- Used for relief of uncontrolled hiccups.

- *Toxicity*: Parkinson-like symptoms, abnormal muscle movements, sleepiness, and seizures may be seen. Other effects may be anticholinergic effects, such as dry mouth, blurred vision, urinary retention, tachycardia, cardiac arrhythmias, hypotension, and, in more severe toxicity, hypothermia or hyperthermia.

- Liver problems (e.g., cholestatic jaundice), sensitivity to light and severe allergic reactions (anaphylaxis) may occur and are classified as hypersensitivity reactions.

- Skin abnormalities: A peculiar skin-eye condition has been correlated with the long-term administration of phenothiazines. This consists of a progressive pigmentation of areas of skin or conjunctiva and/or discoloration of the eye.

Thioridazine

Brand name: Mellaril

Available as: 10 mg, 15 mg, 25 mg, 50 mg, 100 mg, 150 mg, and 200 mg tablets; 30 mg/mL solution; 10 mg/5 mL oral suspension.

> Patients on long-term therapy with phenothiazine-type antipsychotics need regular complete eye examinations!

Special notes:

- Thioridazine is not useful as an antiemetic.

- May produce adverse cardiovascular effects.

- May produce **paradoxical** behavioral symptoms, such as agitation, excitement, insomnia, and nightmares, and may paradoxically aggravate psychotic symptoms.

- May produce adverse effects on blood and GI.

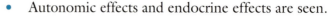

- Autonomic effects and endocrine effects are seen.
- Maximum dose of 1000 mg/day.

Risperidone

Brand names: Risperdal, Risperdal-M, Risperdal Consta

Available as: 0.25 mg, 0.5 mg, 1 mg, 2 mg, 3 mg, and 4 mg tablets; 1 mg/mL oral solution; 0.5 mg, 1 mg, 2 mg, 3 mg, and 4 mg disintegrating tablets; 12.5 mg, 25 mg, 37.5 mg, and 50 mg for injection.

Special notes:
- Used for bipolar disorders.

Haloperidol

Brand name: Haldol

Available as: 0.5 mg, 1 mg, 2 mg, 5 mg, 10 mg, and 20 mg tablets; 2 mg/mL concentrate; 5 mg/mL solution for IM injection; 50 mg/mL and 100 mg/mL for long-acting decanoate.

Special notes:
- Haloperidol blocks dopamine receptors, which effectively decreases dopaminergic activity. It also may decrease dopamine release.
- Is useful in the treatment of Tourette's syndrome, and in therapy of mania.
- May potentiate the action of barbiturates, general anesthetics, and other CNS depressant drugs.

Olanzapine

Brand name: Zyprexa

Available as: 2.5 mg, 5 mg, 7.5 mg, 10 mg, 15 mg, and 20 mg tablets; 5 mg, 10 mg, 15 mg, and 20 mg disintegrating tablets; 10 mg powder for injection.

Mechanism of action: Affects serotonin as well as dopamine activity.

Special notes:
- Risk of the development of tardive dyskinesia increases with dose.
- May increase a patient's risk for diabetes due to the potential for weight gain.
- Tablets contain lactose and are contraindicated with lactose-intolerant patients.
- May induce orthostatic hypotension, tachycardia, dizziness, and sometimes syncope, especially at the initiation of treatment.
- May promote seizures.
- May promote liver damage—liver function tests should be done routinely, to check for elevated liver transaminase (SGPT).

Clozapine

Brand name: Clozaril

Available as: 12.5 mg, 25 mg, and 100 mg tablets; 25 mg and 100 mg disintegrating tablets.

Special notes:

- Useful in patients not responsive to other therapies.
- May reduce behavioral symptoms, such as withdrawal and antisocial behavior.
- Not a first-line drug.
- Pharmacy must maintain leukocyte and neutrophil counts.
- Prescriptions are limited to 7–28 days.

Fluphenazine

Brand name: Prolixin

Available as: 1 mg, 2.5 mg, 5 mg, and 10 mg tablets; 2.5 mg/5 mL elixir; 5 mg/mL concentrate; 2.5 mg/mL IM injection.

Special notes:

Clinical effects of fluphenazine are seen in two to four days, and effects may last up to eight weeks.

- Fluphenazine decanoate is more slowly released from the injection site than fluphenazine HCl. It thus is used as a sustained-release form.
- This drug has considerable interpatient variation, so careful supervision is required.
- Fluphenazine is less sedating than other phenothiazines. Fewer interactions are seen with anticonvulsant agents, anesthetics, etc.
- Hypotension is less frequently caused by fluphenazine vs. other phenothiazines—a good choice for the psychotic patient who is hypotensive or has congestive heart failure.

Effects of fluphenazine are not predictable from patient to patient! Careful patient monitoring is required!

- This drug has a high degree of extrapyramidal effects (e.g., tardive dyskinesia), particularly in older patients and women.
- Should not be used when confusion and/or agitation are present, particularly in the elderly.
- Fluphenazine decanoate has an increased potential for causing hypersensitivity reactions.

Loxapine

Brand name: Loxitane

Available as: 5 mg, 10 mg, 25 mg, and 50 mg capsules; 25 mg/mL concentrate.

Special notes:

- Administration results in strong inhibition of spontaneous motor activity.
- Contraindicated if CNS depression, such as alcohol induced, etc., is present.
- Contraindicated in a comatose patient.

- Contraindicated with seizures, or the potential for seizures, as the drug lowers seizure threshold.
- Use with caution in patients with cardiovascular disease. Increased pulse rate and transient hypotension have both been reported.

Quetiapine

Brand name: Seroquel, Seroquel XR

Available as: 25 mg, 100 mg, 200 mg, 300 mg, and 400 mg tablets; XR, 50 mg, 150 mg, and 200 mg tablets.

Dosage: Initial dose of 25 mg bid, increasing to a target dose of 300 to 400 mg/day.

Special notes:

- Has a low incidence of extrapyramidal symptoms.
- Blocks both serotonin and dopamine receptors.
- Blocks histamine receptors, which accounts for some adverse effects.
- Does not block muscarinic receptors, so no anticholinergic effects (e.g., dry mouth, sedation) are seen.
- Blocks α_1 receptors, so may cause postural hypotension.
- May decrease circulating thyroid hormone levels (T_4).
- May increase blood cholesterol and triglyceride levels.
- Quetiapine is metabolized by an isoenzyme of liver cytochrome P_{450}, which also metabolizes several other drugs. Drug interactions are thus possible, as other drugs will compete for metabolism, causing altered or unpredictable drug levels.
- Because of the alpha receptor blockade, the drug should not be administered to a patient who is hypotensive, has fainting spells, or has cardiovascular disease (e.g., CHF, angina).
- Phenytoin and thioridazine will both increase quetiapine clearance, due to actions on cytochrome P_{450}.
- This drug may cause liver damage—liver transaminase levels (SGPT) should be monitored regularly.

Aripiprazole

Brand name: Abilify

Available as: 2 mg, 5 mg, 10 mg, 15 mg, 20 mg, and 30 mg tablets; 1 mg/mL oral solution; 10 mg and 15 mg disintegrating tablets; 9.75 mg/1.3 mL injection.

Special notes:

- Used in schizophrenia for both acute and maintenance treatment.
- Adjunct to lithium and valproate.
- Common side effects include: nausea/vomiting, constipation, headache, dizziness, and insomnia.

Chapter Review Questions

1. Fluoxetine and fluvoxamine:
   a. are antidepressant agents
   b. are monoamine oxidase inhibitors
   c. may be safely used together
   d. are anticonvulsant agents

2. Valium and alcohol:
   a. may safely be used together
   b. are not sedative hypnotic drugs
   c. will cause seizures if used together
   d. will cause excessive sedation if used together

3. Phenobarbital:
   a. is a first-line anticonvulsant agent
   b. is a short-acting drug
   c. is a barbiturate
   d. is a completely safe drug

4. An appropriate therapy for the "premature awakening" type of insomnia might be:
   a. Diazepam
   b. Zolpidem
   c. Lorazepam
   d. Carbamazepine

5. An appropriate anxiolytic might be:
   a. Zolpidem
   b. Secobarbital
   c. Depakote
   d. Alprazolam

6. Paxil is to paroxetine as Lamictal is to:
   a. Zolpidem
   b. Phenobarbital
   c. Carbamazepine
   d. Lamotrigine

Questions 7-10 refer to the profile below.

The patient profile for John Hill contains the following drugs:

Tegetrol

Nardil

Aspirin

Alprazolam

7. Mr. Hill is flushed, and his blood pressure is elevated. The cause of this might be that:
   a. the Tegretol raised his heart rate
   b. the alprazolam caused an anxiety attack, which raised his blood pressure
   c. he attended a wine and cheese party while taking Nardil
   d. he just ran from the parking lot into the pharmacy

8. From his profile, you infer that Mr. Hill probably has:
   a. trouble sleeping
   b. chronic anxiety
   c. a seizure disorder
   d. both b and c

9. Drug interactions would most likely be seen with which two of Mr. Hill's drugs?
   a. Alprazolam and Aspirin
   b. Alprazolam and Nardil
   c. Tegretol and alprazolam
   d. Aspirin and Nardil

10. It is found that Mr. Hill is hyperthyroid. Which medication should be eliminated?
    a. Dilantin
    b. Alprazolam
    c. Nardil
    d. Aspirin

11. Which of these drugs is an antipsychotic?
    a. Ambien
    b. Wellbutrin
    c. Paxil
    d. Thorazine

12. Which of these drugs is contraindicated with L-dopa therapy?
    a. Carbamazepine
    b. Phenytoin
    c. Haldol
    d. Neurontin

13. Which of the following should not be stored at room temperature?
    a. Tolcapone
    b. Bromocriptine
    c. Xanax
    d. Halcion

14. Which of the following can cause liver failure?
    a. Tolcapone
    b. Tacrine
    c. Ritalin
    d. Elavil

15. Abilify is the brand name for:
    a. Duloxetine
    b. Aripiprazole
    c. Nefazadone
    d. Amoxapine

16. A patient is prescribed Paxil. Which of the following drugs in his patient profile could be an example of a therapeutic duplication?
    a. Xanax
    b. Tegretol
    c. Zoloft
    d. Zocor

17. Which of these drugs is prescribed in overdose?
    a. citalopram 10 mg hs
    b. Pamelor, 25 mg tabs i qid, for a 75-year-old man
    c. Tegretol 200 mg qid
    d. Desyrel 100 mg qid

18. Which of the following drugs must be stored in the refrigerator?
    a. Xanax tablets
    b. Zyban transdermal patch
    c. Ativan solution for injection
    d. BuSpar solution for injection

19. Valproic acid is a generic name for:
    a. Depakene
    b. Abilify
    c. Xanax
    d. Symmetrel

20. Citalopram and Sertraline are both:
    a. Tricyclic antidepressants
    b. Axiolytics
    c. SSRIs
    d. MAOIs

CHAPTER 23

Pain Management Agents: Nonsteroidal Anti-Inflammatory Drugs and Narcotics

Quick Study

I. General mechanism of action of NSAIDS

II. General categories of NSAIDS and their adverse effects

- Nonsteroidal pain relievers (e.g., acetaminophen)
- NSAIDS—Inhibition of prostanoid synthesis:
  1. Prostaglandins
  2. Prostacyclins
  3. Thromboxanes
- Nonsteroidal anti-inflammatory drugs available
  1. Aspirin (ASA)
  2. Ibuprofen and related drugs
  3. Naproxen and related drugs
  4. Indomethacin
  5. Prodrugs (e.g., sulindac)
  6. Other NSAIDS

III. Mechanisms of action and adverse effects of various NSAIDS and nonsteroidal pain relievers

1. Cyclooxygenase inhibitors—COX-1 vs. COX-2
2. Non-cyclooxygenase inhibitors
3. Physiological effects and interactions of COX-1 inhibitors vs. COX-2

IV. Narcotic analgesics

V. Drug interactions—due to pharmacokinetics or drug mechanism

Drugs Used in the Therapy of Pain and Inflammation

The therapy of pain and anti-inflammatory effects often go hand in hand. The nonsteroidal anti-inflammatory agents decrease both pain and inflammation, while nonsteroidal pain relievers, such as acetaminophen, decrease only pain and not inflammation. In the same way, narcotic drugs decrease only pain, so may be combined with an anti-inflammatory pain reliever.

Nonsteroidal Anti-Inflammatory Drugs

The nonsteroidal anti-inflammatory drugs (NSAIDS) work by inhibition of prostanoid synthesis. Prostanoids, such as prostaglandins, prostacyclins, and thromboxanes, are products of the metabolism of a fatty acid found in cell membranes, called *arachidonic acid*. NSAIDS inhibit the first step in this metabolism, by inhibiting an enzyme called *cyclooxygenase* (*COX*). A schematic of the large number of prostanoids that come from cyclooxygenase metabolism is shown in Figure 23-1.

These substances have many functions within the body, and not all are well understood as yet. You should know that:

- Thromboxanes (thromboxane A_2 or TXA_2, for short) are found in the platelet and facilitate platelet aggregation, which eventually leads to clot formation. Thromboxanes also cause vessels to constrict.
- Prostacyclins are found in the cells lining blood vessels (vascular endothelial cells) and inhibit platelet aggregation. They also cause vasodilation.
- Prostanoids in the bronchioles of the lung have a protective function, and keep the airways open. They are bronchodilatory.
- Prostanoids in the cells lining the stomach are **cytoprotective**—they protect the stomach lining from gastric acid.

Other prostanoids cause:
- increased body temperature.
- edema and inflammation.
- increased sensitivity of pain fibers.

> You should memorize the actions of these prostanoids and think about what would happen if they were inhibited!

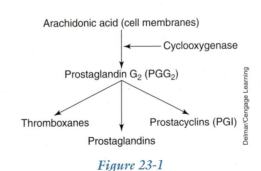

Figure 23-1

COX-1 and COX-2

> Only COX-1 is responsible for platelet aggregation and the cytoprotective effect in the stomach.

There are two isoenzymes of cyclooxygenase, abbreviated COX-1 and COX-2. The distinctions are important, as they have different functions. Although both are anti-inflammatory, only COX-1 is responsible for platelet aggregation and the cytoprotective effect in the stomach. Why is this important? Different drugs have different selectivities for the two isoenzymes. Those that affect COX-1 will promote ulcers and have an **antithrombotic** (inhibitory action toward platelets) action, and will prolong bleeding time.

Choice of Drug

> All NSAIDS are reversible inhibitors of cyclooxygenase, with the exception of aspirin, *which is* irreversible.

The choice of drug is based on many factors. First is the enzyme specificity, as mentioned above. Also:

- Where the drug is absorbed—a patient with a duodenal ulcer should not take ibuprofen, for example, as it is absorbed in the duodenum and may worsen the ulcer.
- The duration of action of the drug.
- The adverse effect profile.
- The condition of the patient—drugs that inhibit COX-1 decrease levels of prostacyclins. Prolonged therapy, in doses therapeutic for pain and inflammation, could result in decreased blood flow to organs, such as the kidney and heart.
- The route of elimination of the drug—some drugs are eliminated entirely by the liver. These would not be a good choice for a neonate or patients with liver damage.
- Anti-inflammatory effects—some drugs have delayed effects or decreased effects on inflammation.

Drugs Available

Aspirin (ASA) (acetylsalicylic acid)

Available as: 300 mg (gr v) tablet; 300 mg enteric-coated tablet, granules; 325 mg and 81 mg tablets.

Special notes:

- An *irreversible* acetylator of the cyclooxygenase enzyme. The cell must synthesize more enzyme to resume function.
- Has a high degree of action against COX-1. It therefore has potent antithrombotic effects, and may promote ulcers in high doses.
- May prolong bleeding time due to its effects on platelets.

"Aspirin allergy"—a potential adverse effect of NSAIDS. NSAIDS can cause inhibition of the protective (bronchodilatory) prostanoids in the lung. This can result in severe bronchoconstriction.

- Is metabolized by the liver and eliminated by the kidney. It is metabolized by glucuronidation. (Enzymes are decreased in neonates and geriatric patients, so the dose should be reduced in the elderly.) A small amount is secreted directly into the kidney tubules and eliminated.

- Is beneficial in low doses as an antithrombotic agent, decreasing the formation of small clots. In low doses (85 mg or less), aspirin has a potent antithrombotic effect, but does not cause vasoconstriction (e.g., prostacyclins are not significantly affected).

- Aspirin is a potent anti-inflammatory agent with immediate effects.

- Because of aspirin's effect on platelets, it has synergystic effects with anticoagulants (e.g., warfarin) and additive effects with other antithrombotic agents.

- Patients who are "aspirin allergic" should not be given other NSAIDS, as there is cross-sensitivity.

Ibuprofen

Brand names: IBU, Motrin, Advil

Available as: 100 mg and 200 mg tablets OTC; 400 mg, 600 mg, and 800 mg tablets; 50 mg and 100 mg chewable tablets; 40 mg/mL oral drops and 100 mg/5 mL oral suspension.

Special notes:
- Related to ketoprofen, fenoprofen, and flurbiprofen.
- A competitive antagonist of cyclooxygenase.
- A nonspecific agent—it acts on both COX enzymes equally.
- Is generally less potent than other drugs of the class.
- Useful in inflammation, as it stabilizes lysosomal membranes.
- Has a half-life of two to four hours; the drug is completely eliminated in 24 hours.

Ketoprofen

Brand names: Oruvail, Orudis

Available as: 50 mg and 75 mg tablets (Orudis); or 100 mg, 150 mg, or 200 mg capsule (Oruvail).

Special note:
- Similar to ibuprofen but increased potency (more than fivefold).

Flurbiprofen

Brand names: Ansaid, Ocufen (ophthalmic)

Available as: Ophthalmic solution (Ocufen); 100-mg tablets (Ansaid).

Special notes:
- Similar to ibuprofen but with a longer half-life (three to nine hours).
- May be taken orally or used in the eye (e.g., ophthalmic surgery).
- Has a higher risk of GI bleed than other NSAIDs.

Indomethacin

Brand name: Indocin

Available as: 25 mg and 50 mg capsules; 25 mg/5 mL oral suspension; 50 mg suppository; 75 mg SR capsule; 1 mg injection.

Special notes:
- Has a selective and potent activity against COX-1.
- Potent anti-inflammatory agent.
- Used in closure of ductus arteriosus.

Ketorolac

Brand name: Toradol, Acular OPHT

Available as: 10 mg tablets for oral administration; ophthalmic solution: 0.5% sterile isotonic solution; 15 mg/mL, 30 mg/mL, or 60 mg/2 mL solution for intravenous or IM administration.

Special notes:
- Is a selective inhibitor of COX-1.
- Can be used orally, parenterally, or in the eye.
- Indicated for the *short-term* management of moderately severe pain that requires analgesia at the opiate level. It is not used for routine pain (e.g., headaches, arthritis).
- Is contraindicated in patients with peptic ulcers.
- Has a large number of adverse effects, including renal toxicity, anaphylaxis (a life-threatening allergic reaction), and increased risk of bleeding.
- The intravenous drug preparation is alcohol-based and is thus contraindicated for epidural anesthesia, and use in nursing mothers.

Sulindac

Brand name: Clinoril

Available as: 150 mg and 200 mg tablets.

Special notes:
- Inhibitor of both COX-1 and COX-2.
- Does not promote ulcers—sulindac is a **prodrug** that is converted to the active form *after* absorption. It therefore does not disrupt prostanoid synthesis by the gastric epithelium.
- Effects and pharmacology are similar to indomethacin.

Nabumetone
Brand name: Relafen

Available as: 500 mg and 750 mg tablets.

Naproxen
Brand names: Naprosyn, EC-Naprosyn, Naprelan

Available as: 375 mg and 500 mg enteric-coated tablets; 250 mg, 375 mg, and 500 mg tablets; 25 mg/mL suspension.

Special notes:
- Related to ibuprofen, ketoprofen, flurbiprofen, and fenoprofen.
- Less rapidly absorbed than naproxen sodium.
- Has a long half-life of up to 10 hours.
- Delayed anti-inflammatory effects—up to two weeks.

Naproxen sodium
Brand names: Anaprox, Naprelan, Aleve (OTC)

Available as: 220 mg (OTC); 375 mg and 500 mg tablets; 375 mg and 500 mg extended-release tablets.

Special note:
- Similar in character to naproxen, but more rapid absorption.

Celecoxib
Brand name: Celebrex

Available: 100 mg, 200 mg, 400 mg capsules.

Special notes:
- Used for osteoarthritis.
- Used in rheumatoid arthritis.
- Can cause GI bleeding.
- Should be taken with food or milk to decrease GI distress.

Nonsteroidal Pain Relievers

Acetaminophen(APAP)
Brand name: Tylenol

Available as: 325 mg, 500 mg, and 650 mg tablets; multiple formulations, and in combination with other drugs (e.g., Vicodin, Tylenol #2–4) 325 mg tablets; 160 mg per tsp.; 80 mL/0.8 mLs; 80 mg and 160 mg chewable tablets; 120 mg, 300 mg, and 600 mg suppositories.

> Metabolism of acetaminophen is a two-step process in which a toxic intermediate is formed. This intermediate is neutralized by reduced glutathione stored in the liver. Stores of reduced glutathione are limited, so, with large or frequent dosing, toxic intermediates can cause liver damage.

Mechanism of action: Direct suppression of cortical and thalamic centers. Acetaminophen is not a cyclooxygenase inhibitor, and it is not an anti-inflammatory agent.

Special notes:

- Abbreviated as *APAP*.
- Eliminated by hepatic metabolism—not suitable for liver-compromised patients; causes extreme liver toxicity with large or frequent doses.
- The antidote for overdose—reduced glutathione.
- *No anti-inflammatory action*—acetaminophen is not an NSAID.
- Mucomyst (N-acetylcystein) is used as an antidote for acetaminophen overdose.

Narcotic Analgesics

> Because narcotic opiates slow the rate of breathing, the patient becomes acidotic, due to the retention of carbon dioxide. The change in pH causes dilation of vessels in the brain, which may increase intracranial pressure. Opiates are therefore contraindicated with a head injury!

Narcotic analgesics act at the level of the spinal cord to relieve pain. These agents also act at sites in the central nervous system to reduce the *perception* of pain. Opiate analgesics have the following physiological actions:

- Analgesia
- Anesthesia
- Euphoria
- Antitussive effects
- Nausea and vomiting (emesis)
- Miosis
- Antidiarrheal effects (slows peristalsis in the bowel)
- Respiratory depression

Opiate Addiction

> The dose-limiting effect in the administration of narcotic opiates is respiratory depression!

- Narcotic opiates are both physically and psychologically addictive. The degree of addiction to a particular drug is related to how well the drug crosses into the brain.
- Psychological addiction—related to the amount of euphoria produced.
- Physical addiction—related to receptor sensitivity.
- Opiates that cross into the brain will inhibit sympathetic activity, resulting in a calming effect.
- Opiates are classified as *strong*, *intermediate*, or *weak agonists*.

Adverse effects:
Adverse effects are related to the physiological effects of the drugs:

- **Hypotension** occurs due to muscarinic cholinergic effects.
- The decrease in bowel movement produces constipation.
- Pinpoint pupils, or **miosis**, is seen due to muscarinic cholinergic effects.
- Respiratory depression—this is the dose-limiting adverse effect. Respiratory depression is intensified by concurrent administration of other respiratory depressants (e.g., barbiturates).

Interactions:
- *Antipsychotics*: Synergism—severe hypotension and sedation are produced.
- *Sedative-hypnotics*: Synergism—extreme sedation.
- Elevated body temperature produced by opiates may combine with the effects of MAO inhibitors to produce a hyperpyrexic coma.

Morphine sulfate

Brand name: Morph Sul, MSIR, RMS, Roxanol. Preservative free injections: Astromorph PF, Duramorph PF, Infumorph. Oral formulations: MS Contin, Avinza (extended release), Oromorph, Kadian.

Classified as: Strong agonist (C-II)

Available as: 15 mg, 30 mg, 60 mg, 100 mg tablets (morphine sulfate); 30 mg, 60 mg, 90 mg, and 120 mg extended-release tablets; 0.5 mg/mL or 1 mg/mL solution for injection, preservative free; single-use 10 mL dosettes containing 0.5 mg/mL or 1 mg/mL morphine sulfate.

Special notes:
- Morphine is the most potent of the opiate analgesics.
- Administered orally, epidurally, intramuscularly, or intravenously (IV drip).
- Rapid intravenous bolus may cause increased respiratory depression.
- Morphine is poorly bioavailable due to extensive liver metabolism.
- Parenteral injection is more effective.
- Morphine produces a strong sedative effect, particularly in the elderly. This effect may synergize with sedation produced by other drugs (e.g., antidepressants, antihistamines).

Meperidine hydrochloride

Brand name: Demerol

Classified as: Strong agonist (C-II)

Available as: 50 mg and 100 mg tablets; 50 mg/5 mL oral suspension; 10 mg/mL, 50 mg/mL, and 100 mg/mL sterile solution for injection; 25 mg, 50 mg, 75 mg, and 100 mg dosettes.

Special notes:
- Extremely potent euphoric effects—produces the greatest euphoria of the opiates.
- Has an increased potential for psychological addiction.
- It is less effective as an analgesic than morphine.

Hydromorphone hydrochloride

Brand name: Dilaudid

Classified as: Strong agonist (C-II)

Available as: 1 mg, 2 mg, 3 mg, and 4 mg tablets; 3 mg suppositories; 1 mg/mL, 2 mg/mL, 3 mg/mL, 4 mg/mL, and 10 mg/mL solution for injection.

Special notes:
- Has a greater potency than hydrocodone.
- Has a greater potential for euphoria, addiction, and abuse.

Fentanyl (fentanyl base)

Brand name: Actiq

Classified as: Strong agonist (C-II)

Available as: Buccal tablet in 200 mcg, 400 mcg, 600 mcg, 800 mcg, 1200 mcg, and 1600 mcg.

Fentanyl citrate

Brand name: Duragesic transdermal patch, Sublimaze injection

Classified as: Strong agonist (C-II)

Available as: 10 cm (25 mcg), 20 cm (50 mcg), 30 cm (75 mcg), and 40 cm (100 mcg) patches, .05 mg/mL injection (2 mL, 5 mL, 10 mL, 20 mL).

Special notes:
- Used in combination with droperidol to produce dissociative analgesia (*neuroleptanalgesia*).
- Less stimulation of histamine release with intravenous administration of fentanyl than with other opiates.
- May cause skeletal muscle rigidity, resulting in chest compression and impaired breathing.
- Can be used epidurally.

Methadone

Brand name: Dolophine

Classified as: Strong agonist (C-II)

Available as: 5 mg and 10 mg tablets.

Special notes:

- Has a long duration of action.

- Used in the therapy of opiate addiction.

- When prescribed for the therapy of narcotic addiction, methadone may only be dispensed by pharmacies approved to do so. When dispensed as an analgesic, it may be dispensed by any licensed pharmacy.

- Does not produce euphoria, so it should not be psychologically addictive.

Codeine and acetaminophen

Brand names: Tylenol #2, #3, or #4

Classified as: Intermediate agonist (C-III)

Available as: 15 mg codeine (Tylenol #2); 30 mg codeine (Tylenol #3); or 60 mg codeine (Tylenol #4), with 300 mg acetaminophen (tablets).

Special notes:

- Codeine crosses the blood-brain barrier only weakly, so potency is less than other opiates.

- Abuse is somewhat limited, as large doses are needed to produce euphoria.

- Acetaminophen is added as an additional analgesic, but primarily to discourage abuse.

- Causes more nausea than other opiates.

Hydrocodone and acetaminophen

Brand names: Anexia, Lorcet, Vicodin, Lortab, Zydone

Classified as: Controlled substance (C-III)

Available as: 2.5 mg/500 mg, 5 mg/325 mg, 5 mg/500 mg, 7.5 mg/325 mg, 7.5 mg/500 mg, 7.5 mg/650 mg, 7.5 mg/750 mg, 10 mg/325 mg, 10 mg/500 mg, 10 mg/650 mg combinations; oral liquid in 2.5 mg/167 mg per teaspoon (5 mL).

> The addition of acetaminophen to opiate preparations discourages abuse! Large doses of the opiate large doses of acetaminophen, which will cause liver toxicity!

Special notes:

- Hydrocodone is a derivative of codeine and thus has similar properties.

- Hydrocodone is an intermediate agonist.

Oxycodone

Brand names: Percocet, Tylox (with acetaminophen), Percodan (with aspirin)

Classified as: C-II

Available as: 4.9 mg oxycodone with 325 mg aspirin (Percodan); 5 mg oxycodone with 325 mg or 500 mg APAP (Percocet); Percocet—2.5 mg/325 mg, 5 mg/325 mg, 7.5 mg/500 mg, 7.5 mg/325 mg, 10 mg/325 mg, 10 mg/650 mg tablets; Percodan = 2.5 mg/325 mg, 5 mg/325 mg tablets, Tylox = 5 mg oxycodone with 500 mg APAP capsule.

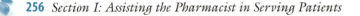

Special notes:
- A derivative of codeine and thus has similar properties.
- Is an intermediate agonist.

Opiates with Low Abuse Potential

Propoxyphene hydrochloride
Propoxyphene hydrochloride with aspirin

Brand names: Darvon, Darvon Compound

Classified as: Controlled substance (C-IV)

Available as: Darvon 65 mg capsules; Darvon Compound = 32 mg or 65 mg propoxyphene, 389 mg aspirin, 32.4 mg caffeine.

Propoxyphene napsylate
Propoxyphene napsylate with acetaminophen

Brand name: Darvon-N, Darvocet-N

Available as: Darvon-N 100 mg tablet; Darvocet-N = 50 mg/325 mg, 100 mg/650 mg.

Special notes:
- Propoxyphene does not cross into the brain very well, unless high doses are taken or the patient has a compromised blood-brain barrier (e.g., stroke victim, brain injury, or an elderly person). This drug can be abused, as the effects are dose-dependent (e.g., if only a small fraction of the drug crosses into the brain, the abuser simply needs to take a larger dose).

> **NOTE**
>
> The FDA is considering the removal of propoxyphene from the U.S. Market.

Partial Agonists and Antagonists

> Partial opiate agonists, or "mixed agonist/antagonist drugs" are useful in recovery from opiate addiction!

Partial agonists are weak agonists that, because of their low level of activity, can act as antagonists in certain situations. Partial opiate agonists are useful in the therapy of opiate addiction.

Adverse reactions of partial opiate agonists include sedation, dizziness, vertigo, headache, hypotension, nausea/vomiting, hypoventilation, miosis, and sweating.

Drugs Prescribed

Butorphanol

Brand names: Stadol, Stadol NS

Classified as: Controlled substance (C-IV)

Available as: 1 mg/mL, 2 mg/mL solution for injection; Stadol NS: 2.5 mL of a 10 mg/5 mL solution.

- Butorphanol is a typical mixed agonist/antagonist in that it is a weak agonist at the "mu" opiate receptor.
- Effects are similar to those of morphine, including withdrawal symptoms (less severe with butorphanol).
- Respiratory depressant effects and sedative effects of barbiturates and benzodiazepines may be increased by concurrent administration of butorphanol.

Buprenorphine
Brand name: Buprenex (C-IV), Subutex (C-III)
Available as: 0.3 mg/mL injection; 2 mg and 8 mg SL tablets.

Special note:
- A dose of 0.4 mg is equivalent to 10 mg of morphine or 75 mg of meperidine.
- Tablets are used to treat opiate dependence.
- Injection is used for moderate to severe pain.

Tramadol
Brand name: Ultram, Ultracet (with acetaminophen)
Available as: 50 mg tablet (Ultram); 37.5 mg/325 mg tablet (Ultracet).

Special notes:
- Is a nonnarcotic analgesic.
- Used for pain control for osteoarthritis and rheumatoid arthritis.
- Used for pain management in fibromyalgia.
- Dosing adjustment needed for impaired renal or hepatic function.

Pentazocine
Brand name: Talwin and Talwin NX
Classified as: Mixed agonist/antagonist opiate, control substance (C-IV)
Available as: Talwin 30 mg/mL solution (pentazocine lactate), Talwin NX tablets

Special notes:
- High degree of psychiatric effects produced by pentazocine, including anxiety, nightmares, and hallucinations.
- Parenteral administration is utilized. Although, Talwin NX is oral administration.
- Also used as an analgesic.

Opiate Antagonists

Opiate antagonists are used in the therapy of opiate addiction (e.g., naltrexone) and in short-term diagnosis of opiate intoxication (e.g., naloxone). They are also useful in partial reversal of the respiratory depression caused by opiates.

Naloxone

Brand name: Narcan

Available as: 400 mcg/mL solution for injection

Special notes:
- IM, IV, or subcutaneous administration.
- Besides treatment of opiate overdose, it has been used to reverse the effects of ethanol and benzodiazepines, to reverse hypotension associated with spinal injury, to improve neurologic recovery after ischemic stroke, and to treat hypercapnic COPD.
- Multiple doses may be required in treatment of opiate overdose, due to the short half-life.
- Naloxone is very short-acting, with reversal of effects seen in a matter of minutes.

Nalmefene

Brand name: Revex

Available as: Solution for injection as 100 mcg/mL or 1000 mcg/mL concentrations.

Special notes:
- Administered intravenously, subcutaneously, or intramuscularly.
- Has a long duration of action.

Naltrexone

Brand name: ReVia, Vivitrol

Available as: 50 mg tablets (ReVia); solution for injection 380 mg vial (Vivitrol).

Special notes:
- Naltrexone has a *three-day half-life,* making it useful in the therapy of opiate addiction.
- Also useful in the therapy of opiate overdose.
- Injection is given once a month.

Chapter Review Questions

1. A patient is admitted to the emergency room with pinpoint pupils and is drowsy and incoherent. The physician administers a drug by injection, and immediately the person improves. An hour or so later, he has a relapse. The drug administered might have been:
    a. Talwin
    b. Narcan
    c. Demerol
    d. Morphine

Patient: Howard Owie				
Room 222-1	Drug	SIG	Phys	Time
	Vicodin 7.5 mg	Ť BID PRN	Smith	
	Tylenol 500 mg	ŤŤ QID	Dolt	
	Phenobarbital 50 mg	Ť TID	Scott	
	Tagamet 200 mg	Ť QD AM	Scott	

    Delmar/Cengage Learning

2. This profile is for an inpatient. Looking at the drugs, which combination should you report to the pharmacist as a possible interaction?
    a. Vicodin and Tylenol
    b. Vicodin and phenobarbital
    c. Tylenol and Tagamet
    d. Tylenol and phenobarbital

3. Which of the drugs is an overdose?
    a. Tylenol
    b. Phenobarbital
    c. Tagamet
    d. Vicodin

4. You note on the patient's chart that he has had hepatitis. You alert the pharmacist to possible contraindications with three of the drugs. Which drug might be the most appropriate to leave in his profile?
    a. Tylenol
    b. Phenobarbital
    c. Tagamet
    d. Vicodin

5. Which two drugs are a drug duplication?
    a. Tylenol and phenobarbital
    b. Tylenol and Tagamet
    c. Phenobarbital and Tagamet
    d. Vicodin and Tylenol

6. Which of the following drugs might be most likely to promote stomach ulcers?
   a. Sulindac
   b. Acetaminophen
   c. Ibuprofen
   d. Aspirin

7. Which of the following drugs has no anti-inflammatory action?
   a. Ibuprofen
   b. Ketoprofen
   c. Sulindac
   d. Acetaminophen

8. Which of the following combinations would be contraindicated?
   a. Aspirin and acetaminophen
   b. Acetaminophen and warfarin (an anticoagulant)
   c. Aspirin and warfarin
   d. Vicodin and warfarin

9. Which of the following has immediate anti-inflammatory actions?
   a. Ibuprofen
   b. Aspirin
   c. Ketoprofen
   d. Naprosyn

10. Which of the following must be absorbed through the stomach lining before it is activated?
    a. Naproxen Na
    b. Sulindac
    c. Ketoprofen
    d. Naprosyn

CHAPTER 24

Cardiovascular System Agents

Quick Study

I. General categories of cardiovascular drugs

  A. Drugs that affect the autonomic nervous system (e.g., adrenergic receptor blockers)

  B. Calcium channel blockers (e.g., verapamil, nifedipine) used in the therapy of hypertension and angina

  C. Sodium channel blockers (e.g., quinidine) used as antiarrhythmics

  D. Direct vasodilators and venodilators (e.g., hydralazine, nitroglycerin) used in the therapy of hypertension and angina

  E. ACE inhibitors

  F. Inotropic agents

  G. Diuretics

II. Uses of cardiovascular drugs

III. Mechanisms of action and adverse effects of cardiovascular drugs

IV. Physiological interactions: therapeutic and adverse effects

V. Drug interactions—due to pharmacokinetics or drug mechanism

> **NOTE**
>
> Due to the increasing difficulty of the pharmacology section of the PTCB exam, discussions in the following chapters are in-depth and technical. Before proceeding to study the following chapters, it is highly recommended that you review your physiology. For Chapter 24, it is necessary that you thoroughly understand cardiac and renal physiology, as well as the function of the autonomic nervous system, to better understand the concepts presented.

Drugs That Affect the Cardiovascular System

Recall that increased sympathetic activity functions to increase heart rate and blood pressure, and will also promote arrhythmias.

Recall that calcium influx is required for proper neurotransmission and efficient contraction of cardiac muscle.

Lower blood volume means lower pressure on the walls of the heart and blood vessels!

Drugs that directly affect the cardiovascular system are probably the most frequently prescribed group of drugs. The technician should be very familiar with them. These drugs modify heart rate, blood pressure, and cardiac conduction, as well as work to increase perfusion to organs by increasing blood flow. Drugs that modify the cardiovascular system include:

- Drugs that affect the autonomic nervous system (ANS) are useful in the therapy of hypertension, hypotension, angina, and arrhythmias. Most of the drugs prescribed are *inhibitors* of the sympathetic portion of the ANS, either directly or indirectly.

- Calcium channel blockers have a variety of actions and are useful in the therapy of hypertension, angina, arrhythmias, and congestive heart failure. Depending on the class of calcium channel blocker, these drugs may increase cardiac output and/or decrease the work of the heart.

- ACE inhibitors and angiotensin II receptor blockers decrease levels or activity of the potent vasoconstrictor angiotensin II, and are useful in congestive heart failure and hypertension.

- Vasodilators dilate *arteries* and are useful in the therapy of hypertension, congestive heart failure (CHF), and angina.

- Venodilators dilate *veins* and increase myocardial perfusion. They are useful in the therapy of angina.

- Inotropic agents increase the strength of contraction of the heart muscle and are used in congestive heart failure (CHF).

- Diuretics are agents that act at the level of the kidney to lower plasma (fluid) volume. They are useful in the therapy of hypertension, CHF, and angina.

The following discussions will list drugs by class. You should be familiar with the drug classes, what they do, and what they are used for, as well as the mechanism of action and adverse effects. Be particularly aware of the interactions of the drug with certain physiological conditions (e.g., CHF, hypertension, diabetes) and which patients should avoid taking certain drugs. Also be aware of interactions between drugs, whether by mechanism or adverse effects. Note that adverse effects are normally nothing more than an extension of the physiological effects, so a review of physiology might be helpful.

Drugs That Affect the Autonomic Nervous System (ANS)

Drugs that interfere with the ANS include:

- Beta receptor blockers
- Alpha receptor blockers
- Alpha receptor agonists
- Beta receptor agonists
- Muscarinic receptor antagonists
- Muscarinic receptor agonists

You should be familiar with these drugs and how they work, as well as their adverse effects and contraindications.

Beta Receptor Antagonists (Beta Blockers)

These drugs are targeted to block the β_1 receptor, which functions to increase heart rate and force contraction of the heart muscle. By blocking this receptor, the following occurs:

- Heart rate and cardiac output are decreased. This results in decreased blood pressure and increased tissue perfusion.
- Cardiac conduction rate is slowed, decreasing the possibility of arrhythmias.
- The production of renin is decreased, resulting in reduced production of the vasoconstrictor angiotensin II.

Adverse Effects of Beta Blockers
- The blockade of β_1 and/or β_2 receptors may interfere with the regulation of blood sugar (this is a diabetic contraindication).
- The blockade of β_2 receptors may cause bronchoconstriction (asthmatic contraindication).

Many adverse effects are caused by the blockade of β_2 receptors, so most drugs on the market are selective for the β_1 receptor. Unfortunately, none are completely without β_2 blockade (i.e., very small amounts of β_2 blockade are present, which are considered negligible).

Drugs Available

Propranolol

Brand names: Inderal, Inderal LA (sustained-release formulation)

Classification: Beta Blocker

Available as: 10 mg, 20 mg, 40 mg, 60 mg, and 80 mg tablets; solution for injection 1 mg/mL; 80 mg LA, 120 mg LA, 160 mg LA.

Special notes:

- Propranolol is a "pan beta" receptor antagonist (i.e., it blocks both β_1 and β_2 receptors equally).
- Propranolol has a membrane-stabilizing action, so it exhibits local anesthetic activity (useful in patients with arrhythmias, as it makes the membrane of the excitable cardiac cells more stable).
- Not recommended for use in diabetics or asthmatics, due to effects on blood-sugar regulation and possible bronchiolar constriction, respectively.

Atenolol

Brand name: Tenormin

Classification: "selective" β_1 adrenergic blocker

Available as: 25 mg, 50 mg, and 100 mg tablets; 5 mg/mL solution for injection.

Metoprolol succinate

Brand name: Toprol-XL

Classification: "Selective" β_1 adrenergic blocker

Available as: 50 mg, 100 mg, and 200 mg extended-release tablets.

Metoprolol tartrate

Brand name: Lopressor

Classification: "Selective" β_1 adrenergic blocker

Available as: 25 mg, 50 mg, and 100 mg tablets; 5 mg injection.

Beta Receptor Agonists

These drugs are useful in increasing the force of contraction of the heart, which raises blood pressure and cardiac output. These may be useful in cases of hypovolemia, severe hypotension, etc. These agents can also increase blood sugar. Selective β_2 receptor agonists are useful in the therapy of asthma. (These will be discussed in Chapter 25.)

Isoproterenol

Brand name: Isuprel

Available as: 0.2 mg/mL solution for injection, Inhaler.

Special notes:
- Isoproterenol stimulates both β_1 and β_2 receptors.
- Increases blood pressure, cardiac output, heart rate, blood sugar, renin, and angiotensin production.
- Is useful in patients with decreased cardiac output and decreased tissue perfusion.
- Is contraindicated in diabetics due to possible increases in blood sugar.
- May also be used in the therapy of asthma (by inhaler), as it causes bronchodilation.

Alpha Receptor Antagonists

Mechanism of action: Blockade of α_1 receptors results in a decrease in peripheral vasoconstriction, and a lowering of blood pressure and cardiac afterload.

Uses: The major therapeutic use of these drugs is in the therapy of hypertension.

Adverse effects: The major adverse effect is postural hypotension.

Doxazosin mesylate
Brand name: Cardura

Classification: α_1 adrenergic receptor antagonist

Available as: 1 mg, 2 mg, 4 mg, and 8 mg tablets.

Dosage: Must be individualized. A standard initial dose is 1 mg. Dosage is then increased stepwise to 16 mg (e.g., 1 mg, then 2 mg, 4 mg, and 8 mg, etc.).

Special notes:
- Used in the therapy of benign prostatic hypertrophy (BPH).
- May cause postural hypotension, especially in high doses.

Prazosin hydrochloride
Brand name: Minipress

Classification: α_1 adrenergic receptor antagonist

Available as: 1 mg, 2 mg, and 5 mg capsules.

Dosage: Initial dose of 1 mg, increasing gradually to a total daily dose of up to 20 mg.

Special notes:
- Used in the therapy of hypertension.
- May cause postural hypotension.
- Dosage should be reduced, in combination with a diuretic.

Terazosin
Brand name: Hytrin

Available as: 1 mg, 2 mg, 5 mg, 10 mg capsules.

Dosage: 1 mg initially, increasing up to 10 mg per day.

Special notes:

- Terazosin is of the same class as doxazosin and prazosin, and thus has similar effects.
- Has an increased potency as compared to prazosin.
- May cause significant hypotension, if used in combination with certain calcium channel blockers (e.g., verapamil).

Alpha Receptor Agonists

> Use of α_1 agonists as decongestants do not produce many adverse effects, as the drug is applied topically and very little is systemically absorbed!

In emergency situations, these drugs are used intravenously in the therapy of shock. They are also used intranasally as decongestants. Adverse effects of α_1 agonists are related to increases in blood pressure.

Norepinephrine

Brand name: Levophed

Available as: 4 mg ampoule.

Special notes:

- Norepinephrine has a very high first-pass effect through the liver and is ineffective if given orally. It is always given by injection.
- Norepinephrine stimulates α_1 receptors, so blood pressure is increased.
- Norepinephrine also stimulates β_1 receptors, so heart rate, renin, and blood sugar are affected.

Epinephrine

Brand name: Adrenalin

Available as: 1:1,000 or 1:10,000 solution for injection; 10 mg/mL solution for inhalation.

Special notes:

- Epinephrine is given by intramuscular injection or IV drip. Administration must be slow, to prevent sudden increases in blood pressure.
- Epinephrine stimulates all four adrenergic receptors. A variety of effects may be seen (most are similar to those of norepinephrine), depending on how the drug is administered.
- Epinephrine stimulates the β_2 receptor, so it dilates bronchioles. It may be used in the therapy of asthma.
- Epinephrine will increase blood sugar and renin formation.

Phenylephrine

This drug is falling out of favor due to adverse effects. However, it is still used topically.

Brand name: Neo Synephrine

Available as: Solution for injection, 1% nasal spray.

Special notes:
- Systemic use (in hypotensive crisis only).
- Useful in intranasal preparations as a decongestant. It shrinks vessels in nasal mucosa, allowing drainage.
- Phenylephrine is also useful in suppository preparations (e.g., Preparation H), as its vasoconstrictor action shrinks swelling.

Tetrahydrozyline

Brand name: Various

Available in: Ophthalmic drops (e.g., Visine) and over-the-counter cold remedies.

Special notes:
- Ophthalmic: constricts blood vessels in the conjunctiva, resulting in less redness of the eye
- Decongestant—constricts blood vessels in nasal passages, resulting in increased sinus drainage
- May aggravate hypertension or benign prostatic hypertrophy (BPH) if absorbed systemically (e.g., through nasal mucosa)

Oxymetazoline

Brand name: Various (Afrin)

Available in: Over-the-counter nasal decongestants and decongestant sprays.

Special notes:
- Decongestant—constricts blood vessels in nasal passages.
- Oxymetazoline stimulates both α_2 and β_2 receptors, decreasing the possibility that the drug will aggravate hypertension or BPH.

Alpha$_2$ Receptor Agonists

- These agents decrease the release of norepinephrine by binding to the regulatory α_2 receptor on the sympathetic neuronal ending and nucleus tractus solitarius (NTS).
- Useful in the therapy of hypertension.
- Also useful in the therapy of opiate addiction, as the α_2 receptor appears to be involved in the manifestation of opiate cravings.

Clonidine hydrochloride

Brand name: Catapres

Classification: Centrally acting sympathoplegic

Available as: 0.1 mg, 0.2 mg, and 0.3 mg tablets; transdermal patch releasing 0.1 mg, 0.2 mg, or 0.3 mg/hr; 100 mcg/mL solution for injection (for use in epidural infusion).

Primary use: Centrally acting antihypertensive agent.

Secondary uses: Clonidine is used orally in the therapy of opiate addiction, as it decreases the psychological craving for opiates. It is also used as an analgesic for severe pain, via the epidural route.

Dosage: 0.1 mg bid ac hs for blood pressure therapy, 30 mcg/hr for epidural infusion.

Special notes:

- Acts directly on α_2 receptors and stimulates them, causing an *inhibition* of norepinephrine release.

- Has a *central* action—it affects the nucleus tractus solitarius (NTS) of the hypothalamus, which regulates the activity of the ANS.

- May increase the rate of platelet aggregation.

- Proper dosage interval (i.e., patent compliance with instructions) is critical to avoid cardiovascular complications.

- Abrupt withdrawal may lead to dramatically increased blood pressure levels and hypertensive crisis. This effect is *decreased* by the administration of an α_1 antagonist and *increased* by concurrent therapy with a β_1 antagonist.

- If beta blockers are given concurrently, they must be withdrawn *before* discontinuing clonidine therapy.

- Clonidine may also be used in central inhibition of severe neuropathic pain in cancer patients who do not respond satisfactorily to opiates. In this case, the solution for injection is used in a continuous-infusion epidural device.

- Epidural clonidine is not recommended for obstetrical, postpartum, or perioperative pain management, due to the risk of hemodynamic instability (e.g., hypotension and bradycardia).

Alpha methyl dopa (a-methyl dopa)

Brand name: Aldomet

Classification: Centrally acting sympathoplegic

Available as: 125 mg, 250 mg, and 500 mg tablets; 250 mg/5 mL oral suspension; 250 mg/5 mL solution for injection.

Dosage: 250 mg bid or tid for two days, increased or decreased as needed, to a maximum of 3,000 mg/day. *Maximum dose in combination therapy:* 500 mg/day.

Adverse effects: May cause rash, liver damage, GI upset, breast enlargement, joint pain, bone marrow depression. May also aggravate angina and congestive heart failure (CHF). May cause hypotension, if the patient is put under anesthesia. May interfere with standard laboratory blood analyses (e.g., SGOT, creatinine clearance).

Special notes:

- Alpha methyl dopa is termed an indirect agonist. It is a *prodrug*. It must be taken up into the adrenergic nerve terminal and converted into alpha methyl norepinephrine, which is a potent α_2 receptor agonist.

- α-methyl dopa has no activity on its own—*it must be taken up into the neuronal ending to work*. Thus, if the reuptake pump is blocked (e.g., with tricyclic antidepressants), the drug will not work.

- Indicated for hypertension in pregnant women.

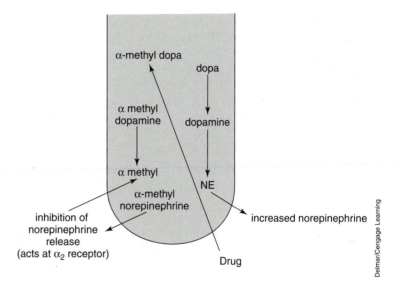

Muscarinic Antagonists

These drugs act at the level of the muscarinic receptor to block parasympathetic effects. Since the effects of the parasympathetic system are dominant over those of the sympathetic system, by blocking the parasympathetic system, *sympathetic effects are seen*.

Atropine

Brand names: Sal-Tropine, Atropisol (ophthalmic)

Available as: Single dose syringes of 5 mL and 10 mL of a 0.1 mg/mL solution (adult use); single dose syringes of 5 mL of a 0.5 mg/mL solution (pediatric use); solution for ophthalmic use; 0.4 mg/mL vial, 1 mg/mL vial.

Dosage: 0.4–0.6 mg (adult dose); 0.1–0.6 mg (neonate/pediatric dose); organophosphate insecticide poisoning: 2–3 mg IV, additional doses as needed.

Primary uses: Preanesthetic medication to reduce bronchial secretions and normalize cardiac function. Therapy of heart block, hyperactive sinus reflex. Antidote for cholinesterase inhibitor overdose (e.g., insecticides such as Malathion). Antidote for muscarine poisoning (e.g., wild mushroom poisoning). Topical ophthalmic solution for the therapy of glaucoma.

Special notes:
- Atropine crosses the blood-brain barrier and thus can cause atropine intoxication (e.g., confusion, incoordination). It decreases secretions, causing dry mouth and lack of stomach acid.

Calcium Channel Blockers

Calcium channel blockers block type "L" membrane channels for calcium, resulting in decreased calcium entry into the cells, in a dose-dependent manner. There are three basic areas that are affected. Clinically, the most important of these are:

1. Vascular smooth muscle—calcium channel blockers can relax the smooth muscle of arteries and cause vasodilation. They are therefore useful as antihypertensive and antianginal drugs.

2. Cardiac muscle—certain calcium channel blockers decrease conduction rate in cardiac tissue, resulting in a decrease in heart rate and cardiac excitability. These drugs are thus useful as antiarrhythmics and antihypertensives, as well as in the therapy of angina.

3. Calcium channel blockers can also affect neuronal tissue in high therapeutic doses. Calcium is required for the release of neurotransmitter, and calcium channel blockers can actually have a **sympatholytic** effect.

Physiology Review

Skeletal muscle obtains the calcium needed for contraction from intracellular stores, whereas cardiac muscle and smooth muscle obtain calcium from outside of the cell. Thus, skeletal muscle is not affected by calcium channel blockers, while vascular and cardiac muscle are.

NOTE

The adverse effects of calcium channel blockers include flushing, dizziness, edema, constipation, and nausea.

Classes of Calcium Channel Blockers

There are several classes of calcium channel blockers, but the majority of these drugs are of a new class: the dihydropyridines. The vast majority of calcium channel blockers prescribed belong to this class (exceptions are verapamil and diltiazem, described in this section). Drugs belonging to this class are selective for vascular smooth muscle and have little or no effect on the heart.

Nifedipine

Brand names: Adalat CC, Procardia, Procardia XL

Available as: 10 mg and 20 mg capsules; 30 mg, 60 mg, and 90 mg extended-release tablets.

Primary uses: Antianginal and antihypertensive therapy.

Dosage: 10–20 mg tid (immediate-release capsules); 30–60 mg daily (extended-release tablets); doses vary by patient. *Maximum daily dose:* 120 mg.

Storage: Sustained-release tablets should be stored below 30°C.

Special notes:

- Nifedipine has a negligible effect on cardiac tissue.
- Half-life is 2 to 5 hours.
- Extensively metabolized by the liver, so half-life and duration of action increase in the elderly or those with hepatic impairment (e.g., excessive drinkers).
- Overdose—this drug is not removed by hemodialysis.
- Therapeutic effects and patient tolerance of formulations from different manufacturers are not equal.
- Nifedipine does not affect neuronal transmission—it has essentially no sympatholytic effects.

Nicardipine

Brand name: Cardene

Available as: 20 mg and 30 mg capsules.

Primary use: Therapy of chronic stable angina.

Dosage: 20–40 mg tid. Doses are lowered in patients with renal or hepatic insufficiency (e.g., geriatric patients).

Special notes:

- Nicardipine has no effect on cardiac tissue.
- Useful in the management of congestive heart failure.

Nimodipine

Brand name: Nimotop

Available as: 30 mg capsules.

Primary use: Therapy of subarachnoid hemorrhage.

A unique use for calcium-channel blockers is the treatment of bone pain associated with cyclosporine therapy in transplant patients.

The effect of a particular calcium channel blocker on smooth muscle or cardiac muscle depends on its classification!

Dosage: 60 mg q4h, or 30 mg q4h if the patient has reduced liver function (e.g., cirrhosis). Supplied as unit dose packs of 30 mg and 100 mg.

Special notes:

- Nimodipine crosses well into the brain and is selective for *cerebral* arterioles.
- This drug is not to be taken with food or administered by parenteral injection.

Amlodipine

Brand names: Norvasc, Lotrel (amlodipine and benazepril combination), Caduet (with atrovastatin), Azor (with olmesartan), Exforge (with valsartan), Exforge HCT (with valsartan and HCTZ), Twynsta (with telmisartan)

Available as: 2.5 mg, 5 mg, and 10 mg tablets.

Primary uses: Therapy of chronic stable angina, vasospastic angina, and hypertension.

Dosage: 5 mg qd, reduced to 2.5 mg qd in geriatric patients or patients who are small or hepatically compromised.

Special notes:

- Long half-life allows for once-daily dosing.
- Dispensed as amlodipine besylate.

Calcium channel blockers with significant effects on cardiac conduction include:

Verapamil

Brand names: Calan, Isoptin, Verelan, Verelan SR, Verelan PM (chronotherapeutic), CoVera HS

Classification: Phenylalkylamine calcium channel blocker

Available as: 40 mg, 80 mg, and 120 mg tablets; 120 mg, 180 mg, and 240 mg extended-release tablets; 120 mg, 180 mg, 240 mg, and 360 mg extended-release capsules; 2.5 mg/mL solution for injection.

Proprietary formulations:

Veralan PM: This formulation of verapamil is used in the therapy of essential hypertension. This is a controlled-onset-and-release formula that is supplied as hard gelatin capsules in 100 mg, 200 mg, and 300 mg strengths.

Dosage: 200 mg hs.

Calan and Calan SR (sustained-release formulation):

Available as: 40 mg, 80 mg, and 120 mg tablets; hard gelatin sustained-release capsules of 240 mg, 180 mg, and 120 mg; sustained-release capsules of 240 mg, 180 mg, and 120 mg.

Primary uses: Therapy of hypertension, certain atrial arrhythmias, and angina.

Dosage: varies according to use.

- Angina: 80–100 mg tid (reduced in geriatric patients).
- Antiarrhythmia 240–480 mg/day (in three to four divided doses), depending on the type of arrhythmia.
- Hypertension: 80 mg tid (immediate-release tablets), 180 mg qd (sustained-release caplets), 140–240 mg qd ac (sustained-release capsules), 200 mg hs (controlled-onset capsules).

Special notes:
- Decreases excitability and the rate of cardiac conduction, making it useful as an atrial antiarrhythmic.
- Relaxes vascular smooth muscle, making it useful in the therapy of hypertension and patients with low cardiac ejection fraction.
- Has approximately equal effects on both cardiac tissue and vascular smooth muscle.
- Inhibitory effects may be produced on the sympathetic nervous system.

Diltiazem
Brand names: Cardizem, Dilacor, Tiazac, Tiamate, Cartia XT, Taztia XT, Diltiazem HCl, Cardizem SR, Cardizem CD, Dilacor XR, Cardizem mono-vial for continuous infusion (75 mg of diltiazem plus 100 mg of mannitol)

Available as: 30 mg, 60 mg, 90 mg, and 120 mg tablets; 5 mg/mL solution for injection; 60 mg, 90 mg, 120 mg (Cardizem SR); 180 mg, 240 mg, and 300 mg (Cardizem CD); and 360 mg extended-release capsules.

Special notes:
- Has a strong effect on cardiac conduction. It is therefore useful in the therapy of variant anginas, where fatal arrhythmias may occur.
- Effective in the therapy of supraventricular arrhythmias, due to its ability to slow conduction in the atrioventricular node.
- A potent vasodilator, making it useful in the therapy of hypertension.

Inhibitors of Angiotensin-Converting Enzyme (ACE Inhibitors)

Angiotensin II is a potent vasoconstrictor that is produced through a cascade of events in the plasma. Renin, released from the kidney, acts on a blood protein, *angiotensinogen*, to form *angiotensin I*, which is then acted upon by ACE to form *angiotensin II*. ACE also breaks down *bradykinin*, a potent *vasodilator*. The net result is vasoconstriction and an increase in blood pressure. This is more of a problem in females than males, as angiotensinogen levels are higher in women than in men.

ACE inhibitors are competitive antagonists of ACE—they bind to angiotensin I and compete with ACE for binding sites. The effects of the drugs are thus dose-dependent.

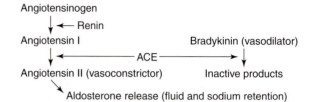

ACE inhibitors:

- Are useful in the therapy of hypertension, particularly in persons who are obese and those with existing cardiac problems.

- ACE inhibitors have been shown to be less effective in populations of African descent, due to certain genetic differences.

- The inhibition of angiotensin II formation results not only in less vasoconstriction, but less release of aldosterone, as well. This results in less fluid and sodium retention.

- ACE inhibitors may increase renal blood flow, so they are contraindicated in renal patients.

Adverse effects: Hypotension, possible rash, altered sense of taste, and dry cough. Serious adverse effects include bone marrow suppression and renal damage.

> **NOTE**
>
> *ACE inhibitors are contraindicated in pregnancy.* When used in pregnancy during the second and third trimesters, ACE inhibitors can cause injury and even death to the developing fetus.

New ACE inhibitors are being added to the market all the time. The generic names usually end in "pril" (some end in "prat"), so you can recognize them easily.

Drugs Available

Benazepril

Brand name: Lotensin

Combination drugs: Lotensin HCT (benazepril/hydrochlorothiazide combination), Lotrel (benazepril/amlodipine combination)

Available as: 5 mg, 10 mg, 20 mg, and 40 mg tablets.

Dosage: Initial dose: 10 mg/day (5 mg in patients with renal impairment). Maintenance dose: 20–40 mg/day.

Storage: Protect from moisture—dispense in a tight container.

Special notes:

- Benazepril is a prodrug—it is metabolized to the active form benazeprilat.

- Benazepril, like all ACE inhibitors, is contraindicated in pregnancy.

- Potassium supplements or salt substitute (e.g., potassium chloride) should not be used by patients taking benazepril.

- Concurrent diuretic therapy may cause hypotension, particularly with initial therapy.

Captopril

Brand name: Capoten

Combination drug: Capozide (captopril plus hydrochlorothiazide)

Available as: 12.5 mg, 25 mg, 50 mg, and 100 mg tablets.

Primary uses: Therapy of hypertension, CHF, left ventricular failure, and diabetic nephropathy.

Dosage: 25 mg bid or tid, increasing to 50 mg, if needed. Maximum dosage: 50 mg tid. Dose may be increased further, in combination with a diuretic, if the patient is nonresponsive under close supervision.

Special notes:

- Associated with a high degree of adverse effects, compared to other drugs of its class.

- Has a short half-life of 3–4 hours.

- Captopril's structure contains sulfur, so it may be contraindicated in sulfur-allergic patients.

- Contraindicated in pregnancy.

- May be used in conjunction with beta receptor blockers or diuretics.

- Hypotensive effects are additive with diuretics.

- Racial differences—the antihypertensive effects of captopril are less in African American populations than Caucasian, and a higher rate of drug-induced angioedema is also seen in these populations, with captopril administration.

- Tablets may have a slight sulfur odor.

Enalapril

Brand names: Vasotec, Vaseretic (enalapril with hydrochlorothiazide), Lexxel (enalapril with felodipine), Teczem (controlled-release tablet of 180 mg enalapril plus 5 mg diltiazem)

Available as: 2.5 mg, 5 mg, 10 mg, and 20 mg tablets; 1.25 mg/mL solution for injection.

Primary uses: Therapy of left ventricular dysfunction, heart failure, hypertension.

Dosage: 10–40 mg/day, initial dose of 5 mg/day. If administered in combination with a diuretic or to a renally impaired patient, dosage is reduced by approximately 50% (adjusted according to blood pressure response). Intravenous dose: 1.25 mg administered over a 5-minute period. The IV dose may be repeated every 6 hours.

Special notes:

- Contraindicated in pregnancy.
- Should not be administered with potassium supplements (including salt substitutes), as hyperkalemia may result.
- Enalapril is a prodrug. It is enzymatically converted into its active form, *enalaprilat* (also marketed separately under the brand name Vasotec I.V.). Conversion takes about 4 hours.
- Enalaprilat has a half-life of approximately 14 hours.
- Enalapril is associated with less adverse effects than captopril.
- Once-per-day dosage.

Fosinopril sodium

Brand name: Monopril

Available as: 10 mg, 20 mg, and 40 mg tablets.

Primary uses: Antihypertensive therapy.

Dosage: Initial dose of 20 mg. Maintenance dose range is normally 20–40 mg/day, but dosages as high as 80 mg can also be prescribed. Normal dosages may be used in patients with diminished.

Special notes:

- Prodrug—metabolized to fosinoprilat.
- Positive adverse-effect profile. Adverse effects are mild (nausea, cough).
- May be used in combination with thiazide diuretics.

Ramipril

Brand name: Altace

Available as: 1.25 mg, 2.5 mg, 5 mg, and 10 mg capsules.

Lisinopril

Brand names: Prinivil, Zestril

Available as: 2.5 mg, 5 mg, 10 mg, 20 mg, and 40 mg tablets.

Combination Drugs

Brand names: Prinzide, Zestoretic (lisinopril with hydrochlorothiazide) (HCTZ)

Primary uses: Adjunct in the therapy of hypertension, heart failure, myocardial infarction.

Dosage: 10 mg/day. Dosage range: 20–40 mg/day, increasing to 80 mg, if warranted.

Storage: The drug should not be frozen or exposed to temperatures above 80°F.

Special notes:
- Lisinopril is the active metabolite of enalaprat.
- The half-life is approximately 14 hours.
- Once-per-day dosage.
- Transient hypotension may occur following the initial dose of lisinopril.
- Should not be administered in conjunction with increased potassium intake.

Angiotensin II Receptor Blockers

The use of angiotensin II receptor blockers during the second and third trimesters of pregnancy can cause death to the developing fetus. Therapy should be discontinued as soon as the pregnancy is detected.

These agents are simply competitive antagonists of angiotensin II at its receptor. Effects are dose-dependent. Less adverse effects are seen with these drugs than with the ACE inhibitors, due to less bradykinin available, but the total blood-pressure–lowering effect is also less. Angiotensin II receptor blockers reduce the effects (not levels) of angiotensin II (e.g., vasoconstriction and increased secretion of aldosterone, a hormone that retains sodium and water from the renal tubules). Unlike the ACE inhibitors, angiotensin II receptor blockers do not have an effect on the levels of bradykinin (a blood factor that promotes vasodilation), so the effects may be more predictable.

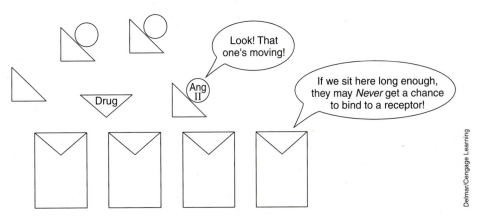

Drugs Available

Candesartan cilexetil
Brand name: Atacand

Combination drugs: Atacand HCT (candesartan with hydrochlorothiazide)

Available as: 4 mg, 8 mg, 16 mg, or 32 mg tablets.

Dosage: Initial recommended dosage is 16 mg, administered as a daily dose. Typical daily dosages range from 8 mg to 32 mg, administered once or twice

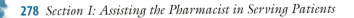

daily, with or without food. No dosage adjustment is necessary for geriatric patients.

Special notes:

- Candesartan cilexetil is converted to candesartan during absorption through the intestinal wall.
- Major adverse effects are headache and dizziness.
- No drug interactions have been identified.

Irbesartan

Brand name: Avapro

Available as: 75 mg, 150 mg, and 300 mg tablets.

Combination Drugs

Brand name: Avalide (irbesartan and HCTZ)

Dosage: 150 mg qd. Dosage for patients who are volume- or salt-depleted: 75 mg. No dosage adjustment is necessary for geriatric patients.

Special notes:

- No significant drug interactions have been reported.
- Adverse effects are mild and infrequent.

Telmisartan

Brand name: Micardis

Available as: 40 mg and 80 mg tablets.

Dosage: Starting dose of 40 mg once per day. Normal dosage range is between 20-80 mg/day.

Special notes:

- Telmisartan may cause severe hypotension in volume-depleted patients.
- Tablets should not be removed from the protective blister until immediately before administration.

Valsartan

Brand name: Diovan

Available as: 80 mg and 160 mg capsules; Diovan HCT: 12.5 mg of valsartan with either 80 mg or 160 mg of HCTZ.

Dosage: 80–320 mg once a day, as monotherapy. No dosage adjustment is necessary for geriatric patients, but dose must be lowered by 50% if the patient is volume-depleted.

Storage: Store below 86°F (30°C), in a tight container.

Losartan potassium

Brand names: Cozaar, Hyzaar (with HCTZ)

Available as: 25 mg and 50 mg tablets.

Dosage: 50 mg qd. Dosage reduction of 50% is required in volume-depleted patients. No adjustment is needed for geriatric or renally compromised patients (e.g., dialysis patients).

Special notes:
- The oldest drug of the class.
- Extensively metabolized and has a high first-pass effect ($T_{1/2}$ = 2 hours).
- Metabolism of losartan produces an active metabolite ($T_{1/2}$ = 6 to 9 hours).
- Extensively bound to plasma albumin, so it may have drug-binding interactions.
- Dosage should be reduced in patients with reduced hepatic function.
- Cozaar tablets contain potassium in the following amounts: 2 mg in the 25 mg tablet, and 4 mg in the 50 mg tablet.

Direct Vasodilators

Direct vasodilators act at the level of arteriolar smooth muscle to relax it, resulting in dilation of the arteriole. The following drugs are useful in the therapy of congestive heart failure, hypertension, and angina.

Drugs Available

Hydralazine
Brand names: Apresoline, Apresazide (hydralazine and HCTZ)
Available as: 10 mg, 25 mg, 50 mg, or 100 mg tablets.

Special notes:
- Causes postural hypotension.
- Increases renin-angiotensin activity.

Diazoxide
Brand name: Hyperstat IV
Available as: Solution for injection.

Special notes:
- Used in the therapy of hypoglycemia (by oral administration) and hypertension (vintravenous administration).
- Causes dilation of peripheral arterioles by inhibiting potassium outflow.
- Most useful in acute situations (e.g., patients with malignant hypertension).
- Causes increased retention of fluid and sodium, decreased renal filtration.

- Enhances loss of uric acid and retention of potassium.
- Increases blood glucose through inhibition of insulin release.
- Half-life 21 to 36 hours, increased to 53 hours in renally compromised patients.

Venodilators (Nitrates)

These drugs act at the level of the vein to relax venous smooth muscle and increase capacitance. They work through increasing levels of nitric oxide, which in turn increases cellular levels of *cyclic GMP*, a smooth-muscle relaxant. The effects of these drugs are dose-dependent—the more nitric oxide that is produced, the more dilation is seen. These drugs primarily cause dilation of veins, and so have the following general effects:

1. A decrease in the filling of the heart (preload), leading to increased cardiac efficiency.
2. An increase in tissue perfusion, leading to increased oxygen delivery to the tissues.
3. Pooling of blood in the lower extremities (i.e., legs).

Venodilators are not useful in the therapy of hypertension, as they do not significantly affect arteriolar smooth muscle. Adverse effects include:

- Nausea and vomiting
- Fainting (syncope)
- Postural hypotension, leading to dizziness
- Palpitations, increased heart rate
- Headache, due to arteriolar dilation
- Occasionally methemoglobinemia, due to oxidation of hemoglobin

Drugs Prescribed

Nitroglycerin
Brand names: Nitrol (ointment), Nitro-BID, Nitrostat, Nitroquick (sublingual preparations), Nitro-Dur, Nitro Trans, Nitro Disc, Minitran TDS (patch formulations)

Available as: 0.3 mg, 0.4 mg, and 0.6 mg SL tablets; sublingual spray; 5 mg/mL injection; 2% ointment; 2.5 mg, 6.5 mg, and 9 mg capsules; 0.1 mg/hr, 0.2 mg/hr, 0.3 mg/hr, 0.4 mg/hr, and 0.6 mg/hr patches.

Special notes:
- Has a very rapid onset.
- Very short-acting (15–30 minutes), so not suitable for maintenance therapy.

- Very unstable—degrades quickly.
- Should be packaged in glass, as it reacts with most forms of plastic (this includes preparation of IVs).
- Must be stored away from light in a cool, dry place.
- Used for acute attacks (except skin patch, which is used as short-term prophylaxis).
- Dosage limit for sublingual administration: one dose every 15 minutes and no more than four doses per hour (limit of five doses).
- Tolerance to effects can occur with repeated, frequent dosage. This tolerance extends to other nitrate drugs (e.g., isosorbide nitrates) as well—other nitrates will produce less of an effect after repeated administration of nitroglycerin.
- Intermittent dosage is recommended to reduce tolerance and dependence.
- 24-hour prophylaxis cannot be achieved, even with the patch, as tolerance is produced.

Isosorbide mononitrate

Brand names: Ismo, Monoket, Imdur

Available as: 20 mg tablets (Ismo, Monoket); Imdur tablets contain 30 mg, 60 mg, or 120 mg of isosorbide mononitrate in an extended-release formulation.

Special notes:
- The nitrate group is cleaved off of the molecule and reacts intracellularly to cause relaxation of venous smooth muscle.
- Orally administered.
- Less first-pass effect than nitroglycerin.
- Longer duration of action than nitroglycerin.
- Effects are more predictable than those of isosorbide dinitrate.

Isosorbide dinitrate

Brand name: Isordil

Available as: 5 mg, 10 mg, 20 mg, 30 mg, or 40 mg tablets.

Special notes:
- Isosorbide dinitrate is converted to isosorbide mononitrate, releasing a nitrate group. This nitrate group is converted to nitric oxide in the lining of the blood vessel (vascular endothelium) and causes dilation of the vessel.
- Behaves much like isosorbide mononitrate, except that two nitrates are produced instead of one.
- The production of two nitrates, instead of only one, makes the effects of the drug slightly less predictable than that of isosorbide mononitrate. There is no way to tell how quickly the second nitrate will be taken off in relation to the first (i.e., how steady of an effect will be produced).

Sodium nitroprusside

Brand names: Nitropress, Nitroprussin

Available as: 50 mg flip-top vial containing 25 mg/mL solution for injection.

Dosage: Nitroprusside should be infused at a rate of 0.5–10 pg/kg/min or less (0.5–10 pg/kg/min 0.0005–0.001 mcg/kg/min).

Special notes:

- Must be diluted in large amounts of D_5W before infusion.
- Can cause a precipitous drop in blood pressure, resulting in decreased perfusion and oxygen deprivation in tissues (ischemia).
- Rapidly degraded by any trace contaminants that may be present in the solution or packaging. In this event color changes may occur.
- Very sensitive to light and should be stored and dispensed in a light-proof container or IV bottle.
- Dilates both arterioles and veins.
- Used in the therapy of malignant hypertension.
- Administered intravenously protected from light, in a supervised setting.
- Produces cyanide as a by-product, which is buffered by hemoglobin. Excessive doses may cause toxicity.

Inotropic Agents

Physiology Review

Cardiac muscle is composed of contractile filaments made of actin and myosin, which overlap. The end (head) of the myosin molecule is an enzyme, which cleaves a phosphate group off of the body's energy source: ATP. This results in the release of energy and cyclic AMP (cAMP), which regulates the contractile process. The contractile process starts with the binding of calcium to proteins surrounding the actin and ends with the degradation of cAMP by *phosphodiesterase*. By increasing the amount of calcium present or inhibiting phosphodiesterase (which allows the cAMP to stay around longer), we increase the number of active contractile filaments and increase the force of contraction.

Inotropic agents increase the strength of contraction of cardiac muscle. There are three classes of drugs presently used to increase contractile force:

- The cardiac glycosides, which increase the amount of calcium available and thus increase the force of contraction.
- The bipyridines, which decrease the activity of phosphodiesterase and therefore increase levels of cAMP.
- The methylxanthines, which inhibit phosphodiesterase and increase levels of cAMP.

Cardiac Glycosides

> Cardiac glycosides have a very narrow therapeutic window—there is not much difference between the effective plasma level and the toxic plasma level. Thus, patients need to be made aware that the dosage regimen must be followed very accurately, and that if they miss a dose, they should not double the next dose.

Cardiac glycosides inhibit the actions of the cellular pump that pumps sodium out of the cell and potassium back in, after the action potential has occurred. The result is a buildup of sodium in the cell that can then exchange for calcium. As heart cells depend on calcium from the outside, the trapping of calcium in the cell and the additional pumping of calcium in from outside causes a large amount of calcium to be available for contraction and increases the number of contracting muscle fibers.

At the same time that sodium levels are building up within the cell and activating the sodium/calcium exchange, the potassium is building up outside of the cell. This can cause abnormalities in heart conduction. *Potassium levels are thus critical in a patient on cardiac glycosides and must be monitored closely.*

The adverse effects of cardiac glycosides include CNS effects such as fatigue, drowsiness, mental confusion, and yellow/blurring vision, and gastrointestinal effects such as gastrointestinal irritation, resulting in nausea and vomiting. In addition, increased urinary output may be seen.

The toxicity of cardiac glycosides is manifested in two stages:

> Cardiac glycosides are useful in a regimen for congestive heart failure and may also be useful in the therapy of supraventricular arrhythmias, as they slow conduction in the AV node.

1. Early effects are seen as a slowing of heart rate (*bradycardia*). Patients should be advised to monitor their heart rate at regular intervals, particularly after a dose. If the heart rate falls below 60 beats per minute, this may signify the beginning of toxicity.

2. Later effects—rapid heart rate (tachycardia) is seen. Sympathetic effects (e.g., mydriasis, diaphoresis) may also be seen. Fatal arrhythmias may develop, if left untreated.

There are two cardiac glycosides presently in use. The choice of drug to use depends on the individual patient, age, and state of health. These drugs are usually combined with a diuretic, such as torsemide or furosemide, to decrease fluid volume.

Drugs Prescribed

Digoxin
Brand names: Lanoxicaps, Lanoxin

Available as: 0.05 mg, 0.1 mg, and 0.2 mg capsules; 0.125 mg, 0.25 mg, and 0.5 mg tablets; 0.05 mg/mL elixir; 0.1 mg/mL and 0.25 mg/mL injection.

Special notes:
- Eliminated by the kidney, so it is not suitable for patients with decreased renal function.

Digitoxin
Brand name: Crystodigin

Available as: 0.1% oral solution; 0.1 mg tablets; 0.2 mg/mL solution for injection.

Dosage: 600 mcg as the initial (digitalizing) dose, then 200 mcg every 6 hours thereafter.

Special notes:
- May be taken with food, but not fiber.
- Should not be taken within 6 hours of antacids or binding polymers (e.g., sucralfate, cholestyramine, Kaopectate).
- Should be taken at the same time every day.
- Has a narrow therapeutic window.
- Has synergistic effects with other antiarrhythmic agents (e.g., quinidine, which also has potassium interactions).
- Serum potassium levels are critical with this drug—diuretics (e.g., thiazides) or potassium supplementation may have detrimental effects. Potassium levels should be evaluated regularly.
- *Signs of toxicity:*
  - lightheaded feeling
  - nausea
  - palpitations
  - wheezing
  - itching
  - swelling of extremities, face, or neck
- Metabolized by the liver. These metabolites are active. They are dumped into the bile, secreted into the intestine, and reabsorbed (**enterohepatic recycling**).
- *Very long half-life* due to active metabolites.
- Used in the therapy of atrial and supraventricular arrhythmias.
- Not suitable for patients with decreased hepatic function.
- This drug is falling out of favor—digoxin is more frequently prescribed.

Dopamine
Available as: 40 mg/mL solution and 80 mg/mL solution for injection.

Special notes:
- Stimulates dopaminergic receptors in the heart and increases its force of contraction. It also stimulates cardiac beta receptors to further increase contractile force.
- Short duration of action.
- Dopamine therapy maintains renal blood flow, which is of concern in heart failure.

Dobutamine

Brand name: Dobutrex

Available as: 12.5 mg/mL solution for injection.

Special notes:
- Ultra-short half-life (on the order of 5–10 minutes), so it is only given intravenously.
- Increases renal blood flow—helps to avoid renal shutdown.
- Dispensed as a mixture of isomers to maximize beneficial effects and minimize adverse effects
- Unlike dopamine, dobutamine has no direct stimulation of cardiac tissue.

Phosphodiesterase Inhibitors

Phosphodiesterase inhibitors presently consist of two classes of drugs: the methylxanthines (e.g., caffeine, theophylline) and the newest class of drugs, the bipyridines (e.g., amrinone and milrinone). These drugs increase levels of cAMP, resulting in longer and stronger contraction of cardiac muscle. Caffeine is not used clinically.

Bipyridines

> **NOTE**
>
> Bipyridines are newly established drugs on the market, so limited data is currently available.

Amrinone

Brand name: Inocor IV

Available as: Solution for intravenous infusion.

Dosage: 0.75 mg/kg, infused over 10–15 minutes. Maximum dose: 1 mg/kg. Maintenance dose: 2–15 mcg/kg.

Special notes:
- Used only in acute situations. Short-term parenteral use only under supervision.
- Used in the therapy of CHF that does not respond to first line drugs (e.g., digoxin).
- 4–6 hour half-life.
- Should not be diluted directly into dextrose solutions—dilution in saline or administration through a piggyback IV is required.
- Patients with an allergy to sulfur should not receive amrinone.
- May cause myocardial ischemia (lack of oxygen to the heart).

Milrinone

Brand name: Primacor

Available as: 1 mg/10 mL or 20 mL single-dose vial; 200 mcg in 100 or 200 mL D$_5$W.

Dosage: 50 mcg/kg over 10 minutes. Infused Dose: 0.375 mcg-0.75 mcg/kg/min to a daily dose of up to 1.1 mg/kg.

Special notes:
- Intravenous furosemide may not be administered in the same IV line as milrinone. A chemical reaction will occur and a precipitate will form in the solution.
- Short-term parenteral use only.
- Administered by IV drip only.

Sodium Channel Blockers

Sodium channel blockers are used as local anesthetics. They decrease excitation of conductive tissue. As agents used to block pain, they decrease the firing of pain neurons. These drugs also decrease conduction in nodal tissue and are useful as antiarrhythmics.

Useful drugs include:

Lidocaine

Brand name: Xylocaine

Available as: 10 mg/mL, 20 mg/mL, 40 mg/mL, 100 mg/mL, and 200 mg/mL solution for injection; premixed IV solution.

Special notes:
- Not taken orally, as it is degraded on the first pass through the liver. It is administered by intravenous drip.

Quinidine

Brand names: Quinaglute Dura, Quinidex

Available as: 324 mg extended-release tablets.

Special notes:
- Highly protein bound, so it has the potential for drug interactions.
- Blocks potassium channels as well as sodium channels. Thus, the amount of time needed to repolarize the heart is lengthened.
- Because of the changes in cardiac conduction, this drug may cause a potentially fatal arrhythmia called *torsades des points,* which can lead into ventricular fibrillation.
- The hallmark of quinidine toxicity is *cinchonism,* which is characterized by headache, dizziness, and ringing in the ears.

Disopyramide

Brand name: Norpace

Available as: 100 mg and 150 mg capsules.

Special notes:
- Long half-life.
- Strong negative inotropic actions.
- Anticholinergic effects.

Drugs Used to Decrease Fluid Volume (Diuretics)

Diuretics act on the nephron to increase retention of sodium in the urine, decrease the concentrating ability of the renal medulla, or increase the excretion of water and salts. Four types of diuretics will be discussed.

Loop Diuretics

> Newer drugs are increased in potency:
> torsemide
> bumetanide
> furosemide

These drugs act by disrupting the concentration mechanism in the kidney. As a result, the urine is very dilute, which means that more water is eliminated. As water is eliminated, the plasma becomes more concentrated, drawing water out of tissues and decreasing edema.

Adverse Effects
- Toxicity to the ear (ototoxicity), as they decrease the amount of fluid in the inner ear.
- Loop diuretics should be supplemented with potassium tablets because they cause significant potassium loss.

Thiazide Diuretics

Thiazide diuretics act at the distal end of the nephron and impair the ability of the kidney to reabsorb chloride (and thus sodium) into the body. As sodium attracts water (i.e., has a "layer of hydration"), this means that water is also retained in the urine, along with the sodium. These drugs also inhibit carbonic anhydrase.

Adverse Effects
- Potassium loss, to a lesser extent than loop diuretics.
- These drugs will cause alterations in glomerular filtration rate (GFR), including a slowing of GFR and a decreased rate of urine formation.
- Caution should be taken in patients with a sulfa allergy due to the potential for cross-sensitivity allergy.

Carbonic Anhydrase Inhibitors

> Carbonic anhydrase inhibitors are not very effective diuretics! Their major clinical use is in the therapy of glaucoma.

These drugs inhibit the conversion of carbon dioxide to carbonic acid, a process that utilizes water and brings it back into the body. The result is a slight loss of water and a large loss of bicarbonate, producing alkaline urine.

Special notes:

- Carbonic anhydrase inhibitors cause excretion of bicarbonate. Thus, they produce alkaline urine and may cause systemic acidosis. They may, however, be useful in correcting systemic alkalosis.
- The inhibition of the conversion of carbonic acid to carbon dioxide and water results in decreased formation of aqueous humor and decreased intraocular pressure. These drugs are thus useful as opthalmic preparations in the therapy of glaucoma.

Potassium-Sparing Diuretics

These drugs are very poor diuretics. They are used in combination with a potassium-wasting diuretic (e.g., thiazides), or they may be used as monotherapy if fluid retention is not severe. They may also be used if concurrent medical conditions prohibit the use of a more potent diuretic.

There are two major groups of potassium-sparing diuretics:

- The *aldosterone antagonists* (e.g., spironolactone), which compete with aldosterone for binding sites on its receptor. These drugs are only effective in patients with elevated levels of aldosterone.
- The *membrane-stabilizing agents* (e.g., triamterene, amiloride), which decrease the excitability of renal tubular cells and prevent sodium and potassium transport.

Osmotic Diuretics

Osmotic diuretics are used **intravenously**, under supervised conditions (e.g., in a hospital). They are sugar polymers that bind to water and are filtered into the urine. As a result, they prevent the reabsorption of water and cause diuresis. There is no selective loss of one ion with these drugs—salt loss is more uniform.

Adverse Effects

- Dehydration (fluid replacement may be necessary).
- Diarrhea if taken orally (osmotic laxative effect).
- Headache, nausea, and vomiting. The major use of osmotic diuretics is reduction of increased intracranial pressure. These drugs rapidly decrease intracranial pressure due to injury, hematoma, and swelling of the brain.

Frequently Prescribed Diuretics

Acetazolamide

Brand name: Diamox

Classification: Carbonic anhydrase inhibitor.

Available as: 125 mg and 250 mg tablets; 500 mg sustained-release tablet; 500 mg powder for injection; ophthalmic solution.

Amiloride hydrochloride

Brand name: Midamor

Classification: Potassium-sparing diuretic.

Available as: 5 mg tablet.

Spironolactone

Brand name: Aldactone

Classification: Aldosterone inhibitor, potassium-sparing diuretic.

Available as: 25 mg, 50 mg, and 100 mg tablets.

Bumetanide

Brand name: Bumex

Classification: Loop diuretic.

Available as: 0.5 mg, 1 mg, and 2 mg tablets; 0.5 mg/2 mL solution for injection.

Furosemide

Brand name: Lasix

Classification: Loop diuretic.

Available as: 20 mg, 40 mg, and 80 mg tablets; 10 mg/mL solution for injection; 40 mg/5 mL oral solution.

Torsemide

Brand name: Demedex

Classification: Loop diuretic.

Available as: 5 mg, 10 mg, 20 mg, and 100 mg tablets; 10 mL ampules containing 2 mg/mL or 5 mg/mL solutions for injection; multidose vial containing 10 mg/mL solution for injection.

Storage: 15–30°C (9–86°F). Do not freeze.

Chlorothiazide

Brand name: Diuril

Classification: Thiazide diuretic.

Available as: 250 mg and 500 mg tablets.

Special notes:
- Less bioavailable than hydrochlorothiazide, so less frequently prescribed.

Hydrochlorothiazide

Brand names: Esidrex, Ezide, Oretic

Classification: Thiazide diuretic.

Available as: 12.5 mg capsules; 25 mg, 50 mg, and 100 mg tablets; 50 mg/5 mL oral solution.

Special notes:
- More bioavailable than chlorothiazide.

Triamterene and hydrochlorothiazide

Brand names: Dyazide, Maxzide

Classification: Combination drug (potassium-sparing diuretic with HCTZ).

Available as: 25 mg thiazide/50 mg triamterene and 50 mg thiazide/100 mg triamterene capsules; 25 mg thiazide/37.5 mg triamterene and 50 mg thiazide/75 mg triamterene tablets.

Drugs Used in the Therapy of Inappropriate ADH Secretion (SIADH) Syndrome

Demeclocycline

Brand name: Declomycin

Classification: Antidiuretic hormone (ADH) antagonist

Available as: 150 mg and 300 mg tablets; 300 mg capsule

Special notes:
- Demeclocycline is a low-potency tetracycline antibiotic but is not used as an antibiotic. Among the drug's adverse effects is the ability to suppress ADH. It is this effect that makes it a useful drug in the therapy of SIADH. The drug exhibits the characteristic effects of the tetracyclines such as promoting photosensitivity, and binding divalent ions such as calcium and magnesium.

Drugs Used to Reduce Blood Cholesterol

Bile Binding Resins

Bile binding resins, as the name implies, bind bile salts in the intestine. This prevents them from being absorbed and reused. Since bile salts are necessary for the digestion of fats, the body must then use cholesterol stores to make new bile salts. This lowers cholesterol stores (particularly LDL) and thus total cholesterol. These drugs are not useful for lowering triglyceride levels, only cholesterol (specifically the LDL form).

Recall that the body uses cholesterol to make bile salts, which are made in the liver, stored in the gallbladder, and released into the duodenum when fatty foods are being digested. Once they emulsify the fats, the bile salts are reabsorbed into the body for reuse.

Types of hypercholesterolemia:

- Elevated LDL level, or in its more virulent form, familial hypercholesterolemia
- Familial combined dyslipidemia (elevated dense LDL, elevated triglyceride-rich lipoprotein remnants, and elevated VLDL)
- Type IV dyslipidemia, the so-called atherogenic lipoprotein profile (low HDL, high LDL, and moderately elevated VLDL)
- Elevated triglycerides— the chylomicronemia syndrome (triglycerides 1,000 mg/dL)
- Type III dyslipidemia (markedly elevated levels of remnant triglyceride-rich lipoproteins)

Adverse effects: These drugs are not palatable and therefore have low patient compliance. They can cause constipation and may cause liver toxicity.

Cholestyramine

Brand names: Prevalite, Questran

Available as: 4 g/9 g suspension or 378 g cans with calibrated scoop.

Dosage: One pouch (9 g), which contains 4 g of cholestyramine once or twice a day, with periodic increases in dose up to four pouches per day. The maximum daily dose is six pouches. Doses should be taken with meals.

Drugs That Interfere with Triglyceride Synthesis (Fibrates)

The enzyme *lipoprotein lipase* breaks down VLDL. Fibrates increase the synthesis of this enzyme, resulting in decreased levels of VLDL. These drugs are useful in hypertriglyceridemia, as they decrease blood levels of triglycerides.

Adverse effects: Anemia, myositis (inflammation of muscle).

Interactions:

1. Anticoagulants. These drugs will increase anticoagulant effects.
2. Fibrates and statins synergize and will produce significantly more myositis if used together. Use with caution.

Gemfibrozil

Brand name: Lopida

Available as: 600 mg tablet.

Dosage: 1,200 mg, administered in two divided doses (600 mg bid), 30 minutes before the morning and evening meal.

Clofibrate

Brand name: Atromid-S

Available as: 500 mg capsules.

Dosage: 2 g per day, in divided doses.

Storage: Protect from light, do not freeze. Avoid excessive heat.

Inhibitors of HMG CoA Reductase

These drugs inhibit the first step in cholesterol biosynthesis. Thus, cholesterol synthesis is inhibited in a *dose-dependent* manner. These drugs are extremely efficacious, but have recently come under fire for the production of muscle dysfunctions. A large amount of recent evidence indicates that these drugs are extremely useful in coronary heart disease. They change not only the character of atherosclerotic plaques but also the character of vessel walls, increasing coronary perfusion.

Contraindications may potentiate the effects of anticoagulants such as warfarin. *Grapefruit juice* decreases the rate of breakdown of the drug and may lead to toxic levels, and/or an increase in adverse effects.

Fluvastatin
Brand names: Lescol, Lescol XL
Available as: 20 mg and 40 mg capsules, 80 mg (XL).

Lovastatin
Brand name: Mevacor
Available as: 10 mg, 20 mg, and 40 mg tablets.

Simvastatin
Brand name: Zocor
Available as: 5 mg, 10 mg, 20 mg, and 40 mg tablets.

Rosuvastatin
Brand name: Crestor
Available as: 5 mg, 10 mg, 20 mg, and 40 mg tablets.

Ezetimibe
Brand name: Zetia
Available as: 10 mg tablet.
Dosage: 10 mg daily.

Special notes:
- Inhibits the absorption of cholesterol.
- Often given with *statin* drugs.
- Can take up to two weeks for full benefits to take effect.

Omega-3-acid ethyl ester
Brand name: Lovaza
Available as: 1 gram capsule.
Dosage: 4 g daily in two divided doses or once daily.

Special notes:
- An omega-3 fatty acid derived from fish oil.
- Works by decreasing the production of triglycerides.
- Side effects include back pain, unpleasant taste, and belching.
- Adverse effects include fever, chills, and chest pain.

Drugs That Affect the Blood and Blood Clotting

Drugs that affect the blood include **anticoagulants**, which interfere with the clotting cascade; **antithrombolytic agents**, which interfere with platelet aggregation; and **thrombolytic agents**, which can break down an existing clot.

Anticoagulants

Anticoagulants interfere with various stages of the clotting cascade in blood plasma. They do not have a major effect on platelets. There are two main anticoagulant drugs in widespread use. These are *heparin*, which is used intravenously, and *warfarin*, which is taken orally.

Heparin

Heparin is a carbohydrate polymer that *potentiates* a natural anticoagulant called antithrombin III. This substance interferes with the formation of thrombin, which is required for clot formation. Because heparin is essentially a sugar, it would be digested if given orally. Thus, heparin is only administered subcutaneously and by IV drip.

Heparin (Heparin sulfate proteoglycan)
Brand names: Heparin, Hep-Pak

Available as: 10 units/mL, 100 units/mL, 1,000 units/mL, 5,000 units/mL, 10,000 units/mL, 20,000 units/mL.

Enoxaparin
Brand name: Lovenox

Available as: 30 mg, 40 mg, 60 mg, 80 mg, and 100 mg prefilled syringes.

Special notes:
- Used for prophylaxis or treatment of deep vein thrombosis.
- Considered a low molecular weight heparin.
- Administered subcutaneously.

Warfarin

Warfarin is an oral anticoagulant that inhibits the recycling of vitamin K. Since vitamin K is required for the action of several clotting factors that are necessary for the clotting cascade, and warfarin effectively decreases liver stores of vitamin K, these clotting factors no longer function and clotting decreases in a dose-dependent manner.

Warfarin sodium
Brand name: Coumadin

Available as: 1 mg, 2 mg, 2.5 mg, 3 mg, 4 mg, 5 mg, 6 mg, 7.5 mg, and 10 mg tablets; 5 mg powder for injection.

Special notes:

- Warfarin is highly protein bound, so drug interactions due to plasma protein binding may occur.
- Because liver stores of vitamin K must be used up before the clotting factors become inactive, this drug has a delayed clinical onset.
- Recovery from the drug is also delayed, as vitamin K stores must be replenished before clotting can resume.
- Warfarin should be discontinued seven days prior to surgery.
- Food interactions exist—foods that contain vitamin K, such as green, leafy vegetables, should be avoided.
- Antibiotics decrease the number of vitamin K–producing bacteria in the intestine and can amplify the effects of warfarin.

Antithrombotic Agents

These drugs interfere with the actions of the platelet plug and decrease platelet aggregation. This may result in a decrease in the number of small clots (thrombi) that routinely form in the course of normal blood flow, due to random platelet activation.

Aspirin (low dose–80 mg)

- Aspirin inhibits the formation of platelet thromboxanes, resulting in decreased platelet aggregation.
- Aspirin taken at doses therapeutic for pain (e.g., 300 mg) will not have the beneficial effects of the lower dose, as vascular prostacyclin synthesis is also inhibited.
- It should be discontinued seven days prior to surgery.

Clopidrogrel

Brand name: Plavix

Available as: 75 mg tablet.

Special notes:

- Blocks ADP receptors, preventing fibrinogen binding.
- Reduces platelet adhesion and aggregation.
- Should be discontinued seven days prior to surgery.

Ticlopidine

Brand name: Ticlid

Available as: 250 mg tablet.

Special notes:

- Interferes with binding of the clotting protein fibrinogen to the platelet membrane, resulting in decreased platelet aggregation.
- Long duration, as the drug binds to platelets.
- May increase bleeding, as it interferes with clotting proteins as well.

Thrombolytic Drugs

Thrombolytic drugs break up formed clots. They act from within the clot to lyse (break up) the clot. The dangers of thrombolytic drugs lie in the formation of smaller clot pieces that can block small vessels and cause myocardial infarction or stroke.

These drugs are administered intravenously. They are extremely expensive (they can cost more than $1,000 per dose), so they are not used routinely. Their use is limited to life-threatening situations or potential loss of limb or organ.

> Thrombolytic drugs break up formed clots. They act from within the clot to lyse (break up) the clot.

Streptokinase

Brand name: Streptase

Available as: 250,000 units, 1.5 mil units, and 750,000 units powder for injection.

Special notes:
- IV or intracardiac (IC) administration.
- Derived from bacterial sources and is a natural product. Contamination may arise, if bacteria used to make the drug become infected with a bacterial virus, etc.

Urokinase

Brand name: Abbokinase

Available as: 250,000 unit solution for injection.

Special notes:
- Urokinase is derived from urine and is a natural product. Its potency is decreased as compared to streptokinase.

Tissue plasminogen activator (TPA)—alteplase

Brand names: Activase, Cathflo

Available as: 2 mg, 50 mg, 100 mg (Activase); 2 mg (Cathflo) solution for injection.

Special notes:
- TPA is a naturally occurring substance that activates plasminogen, which in turn causes the dissolution of fibrin in the clot. This results in clot lysis. It is a natural product and is extremely costly.

Chapter Review Questions

1. Which of the following drugs might be contraindicated in a diabetic patient?
   a. Nifedipine
   b. Isoproterenol
   c. Enalapril
   d. Lidocaine

2. Digoxin is a member of which class of drug?
   a. calcium channel blocker
   b. sodium channel blocker
   c. beta blocker
   d. cardiac glycoside

3. Calcium channel blockers such as nifedipine would affect:
   a. heart rate
   b. blood sugar level
   c. vessel diameter
   d. renin levels

4. A direct vasodilator:
   a. affects both arteries and veins
   b. would be a drug such as isosorbide mononitrate
   c. would affect arterial diameter
   d. would cause postural hypotension

5. A patient presents with severe bradycardia. He confesses that he missed a dose of his medication and doubled the next one. The drug in question is probably:
   a. Isuprel
   b. Lanoxin
   c. Adalat
   d. Bumex

6. Which of the following drugs would cause postural hypotension?
   a. Minipress
   b. Cardura
   c. Nitrostat
   d. all of the above drugs would cause postural hypotension

John Q. Patient

Drug	Date dispensed	Refills
Catapres 0.2 mg	2/11/10	2
Captopril 12.5 mg	2/11/10	3
Lasix 40 mg	2/11/10	3

7. The drug profile above shows that John Q. Patient:
   a. is overmedicated
   b. has high blood pressure
   c. has congestive heart failure
   d. has an arrhythmia

8. Which of the following drugs will have synergistic effects?
   a. Atropine and Isoproterenol
   b. Adalat and Prazosin
   c. Verapamil and Doxazosin
   d. Atropine and Clonidine

9. Procardia has its major effects on:
   a. the heart
   b. veins
   c. arterioles
   d. the brain

10. Which of the following drugs has a delayed onset of action?
    a. Enalapril
    b. Coumadin
    c. Heparin
    d. both a and b

11. Which of the following drugs might have similar effects?
    a. Prazosin and Adalat
    b. Candesartan and Capoten
    c. Isuprel and Tenormin
    d. Enalapril and Isoproterenol

12. Which of the following may be given orally?
    a. Heparin
    b. Diazoxide
    c. Mannitol
    d. Warfarin

13. Mr. Hoad has a clot in his leg. If the following drugs were to be considered, which carries the risk of small-vessel occlusion, resulting in a stroke, or MI?
    a. Streptokinase
    b. TPA
    c. Heparin
    d. Warfarin

14. Mrs. Jones complains that she gets dizzy when she stands suddenly. This could be due to the effects of which drug?
    a. Captopril
    b. Isosorbide mononitrate
    c. Verapamil
    d. Isuprel

15. Which of the following is not useful for maintenance therapy, due to its short half-life?
    a. TPA
    b. Lasix
    c. Nitroglycerin sublingual tablets
    d. Nimotop

Pulmonary Agents

Asthma

The most common lung disorder treated pharmacologically is asthma. The objective in the treatment of asthma is to increase bronchiolar diameter. This may be done with the following drug classes:

- **Sympathetic agonists:** Drugs that stimulate the β_2 receptor will cause bronchodilation, due to an increase in cyclic AMP. Those that block the receptor will inhibit this bronchodilation, and may cause bronchoconstriction (depending on what other factors are present).

- **Muscarinic antagonists:** Since acetylcholine can cause bronchoconstriction, blocking receptors for acetylcholine may cause bronchodilation. These drugs are less effective in the therapy of asthma, as the parasympathetic system has less of an effect in the lung than the sympathetic system.

- **Methylxanthines:** These are phosphodiesterase inhibitors and raise the level of cAMP, resulting in dilation of bronchioles. This class of drugs includes caffeine and theophylline.

- **Steroids and other anti-inflammatory drugs:** These drugs will decrease the inflammatory response in the lung, which may be initiated by airborne pollutants, stress responses, or similar factors. These drugs decrease the inflammatory response by stabilizing *mast cells*, which secrete histamine, as well as stabilizing intracellular lysosomes, which release toxic substances.

- **Leukotriene antagonists:** This is the newest class of therapy for asthma. Leukotrienes are prostanoid derivatives that may be released in response to irritation, and which cause constriction of smooth muscle—in this case bronchiolar smooth muscle. The production of these agents is not affected by cyclooxygenase inhibitors or steroids. By antagonizing these inflammatory agents, bronchioles remain dilated.

Drugs Prescribed

Sympathetic Agonists

Drugs that are useful in asthma are selective agonists at the β_2 adrenergic receptor. Those that are nonselective will also be useful but will have more adverse effects (e.g., tachycardia, changes in blood sugar regulation, changes in blood pressure, etc.).

Albuterol

Brand names: Proventil HFA, Ventolin HFA, Ventolin Diskus, ProAir, Accuneb, VoSpire

Classification: Beta adrenergic agonist

Available as: 90 mcg/dose metered-dose inhaler; 0.021%, 0.042%, 0.083%, and 0.5% solution; 2 mg/5 mL syrup; 200 mcg capsule; 2 mg and 4 mg tablets; 4 mg and 8 mg extended-release tablets.

Special notes:
- Albuterol is very selective for the β_2 receptor. It has negligible β_1 activity, so there is a decreased incidence of adverse cardiac effects.
- Inhaled forms of albuterol have increased efficacy compared to oral forms.

Levalbuterol

Brand name: Xoprenex

Available as: Solution for nebulization; 0.31 mg/3 mL, 0.63 mg/mL, 1.25 mg/3 mL.

Special notes:
- An isomer of albuterol.
- Has fewer side effects.

Metaproterenol

Brand name: Alupent

Available as: 10 mg, 20 mg tablets; dosed inhaler; 10 mg/5 mL oral solution; 0.4%, 0.6%, and 5% nebulizing solution.

Special notes:
- Has a rapid onset—within minutes.
- Primarily a β_2 receptor.
- Used as a bronchodilator.

Pirbuterol

Brand name: Maxair

Available as: Metered-dose inhaler.

Special notes:
- A short acting bronchodilator.
- Used as a selective β_2 agonist.
- Preferred agent in pregnant women.

Terbutaline

Brand names: Brethine, Bricanyl

Available as: Metered-dose inhaler; 1 mg/mL injection; 2.5 mg and 5 mg tablets.

Special notes:
- Long acting.
- Considered a β_2 agonist.
- Can also be used to stop premature labor.

Salmeterol

Brand name: Serevent

Classification: β_2 adrenergic agonist

Available as: 21 mcg/dose inhaler.

Special notes:
- Highly selective, inhaled β_2-agonist indicated for the long-term treatment of asthma and for prevention of bronchospasm in adults with reversible obstructive airway disease.
- Long duration of action allows twice per day dosing.
- The onset of therapeutic action is delayed, so use is prophylactic only.

- May be combined with a fast-acting corticosteroid (e.g., fluticasone) to provide rapid onset and long duration.
- May be useful in obstructive pulmonary disease.
- Not useful in acute asthma attacks, as onset is too slow.

Salmeterol/Fluticasone
Brand name: Advair

Available as: 100 mcg, 250 mcg, or 500 mcg of fluticasone with 50 mcg salmeterol in a Diskus inhalant device.

Special notes:
- A synergistic combination.
- Used as a maintenance medication for asthma or COPD.
- Comes in an inhaled powder form.

Formoterol fumarate
Brand name: Foradil

Available as: 12 mcg capsules for inhalation.

Primary Uses: Prophylactic use only. Not indicated for acute use. Used in conjunction with corticosteroid therapy—not used alone.

Dosage: Twice daily administration—one capsule (12 mcg) by Aerolizer inhalation

Storage: 15–25°C.

Special notes:
- Parenteral use for treatment of status asthmaticus.
- May produce changes in sleep and behavior.

Formoterol/Budesonide
Brand name: Symbicort

Available as: Powder for inhalation.

Special notes:
- Used for maintenance therapy.
- Also an anti-inflammatory.
- Considered a beta$_2$ adrenergic agonist.

Muscarinic Antagonists

Ipratropium bromide
Brand name: Atrovent

Classification: Cholinergic antagonist, bronchodilator

Available as: 0.018 mg/dose metered-dose inhaler; 0.03% nasal spray; 0.02% solution for inhalation.

Special notes:
- Still prescribed, but used less often, as compared with newer drugs—the selective role of acetylcholine in asthma is relatively small.
- Works well for COPD patients.

Ipratropium/Albuterol
Brand names: Combivent, DuoNeb
Available as: Metered inhaler (Combivent); 0.5 mg/2.5 mg per 3 mL nebulizing solution (DuoNeb).

Methylxanthines

Theophylline
Brand names: TheoDur, SlowBid, SlowPhyllin, Respbid, Quibron, Theolair, Uni-Dur
Available as: 100 mg, 200 mg tablets; 80 mg/15 mL syrup.

Special notes:
- Pharmacological mechanisms other than increased cAMP are involved in the actions of theophylline in the therapy of asthma.
- Theophylline works mainly in the periphery and has no central effects. Thus, adverse effects are decreased. Cardiac effects may be seen with high doses, or if taken orally.
- Some adverse effects are insomnia, tremors, seizures, and diarrhea.
- Less useful for acute attacks of asthma, as onset is slower than that of other drugs.
- Rarely prescribed anymore.

Dyphylline
Brand names: Lufyllin, Lufyllin GG (dyphylline with guaifenesin)
Available as: 200 mg and 400 mg tablets.
Dosage: 15 mg/kg q6h.

Special notes:
- Used in the therapy of asthma, and to relieve spasm of the bronchi associated with chronic bronchitis and emphysema.
- Has greater potency than theophylline.
- For oral use.

Oxytriphylline
Brand name: Choledyl SA.
Available as: 400 mg and 600 mg tablets.

Corticosteroids

These drugs are glucocorticoids. They decrease inflammation, resulting in decreased swelling of bronchiolar tissue and increased airway space. Taken systemically, steroids cause inhibitory effects on the adrenal gland, and require gradual withdrawal, in order to allow the adrenal gland to resume normal functioning. Inhaled steroids present less of a problem in this regard, but abrupt withdrawal is still not recommended.

Corticosteroids also inhibit the immune system and may decrease production of certain hormones, if used chronically in a systemic formulation. They can stunt growth and cause osteoporosis, to name just a few effects caused by decreased immunity and hormone production. They are metabolized by the liver and may affect liver function. Depending on the amount of mineralocorticoid activity present in the drug, edema of the face and extremities may also be seen. Dosage of corticosteroids is individualized to the particular patient and his or her condition.

Corticosteroids used in the therapy of asthma include:

> Taken systemically, steroids cause inhibitory effects on the adrenal gland, and require gradual withdrawal, in order to allow the adrenal gland to resume normal function.

Beclomethasone
Brand names: Vanceril DS, Vancenase AQ, Beconase AQ, Qvar

Available as: 40mcg/dose, 80 mcg/dose metered-dose inhalers (Qvar); 0.42 mg/dose and 0.84 mg/dose nasal spray (Beconase/Vancenase).

Special note:
- Substantially more potent than other corticosteroids.

Fluticasone
Brand names: Flonase, Flovent HFA, Flovent Diskus

Available as: 110 mcg/dose, 220 mcg/dose, and 440 mcg/dose metered-dose inhaler; 50, 100, 250 mcg/dose diskus, 0.05 mg/dose nasal spray.

Special notes:
- Most potent of the aerosol corticosteroids.
- May cause edema if taken orally, as it has mineralocorticoid activity.

Mometasone furoate
Brand names: Nasonex, Elocon

Available as: Nasal suspension; lotion, cream, ointment (Elocon).

Triamcinolone acetonide
Brand names: Nasocort AQ, Azmacort

Available as: Nasal inhaler, oral inhaler.

Budesonide
Brand names: Rhinocort AQ, Pulmicort

Available as: Nasal inhaler, powder of oral inhalation.

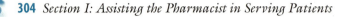

Methylprednisolone

Brand names: Medrol, Depo Medrol, Solu Medrol

Available as: 2 mg, 4 mg, 8 mg, 16 mg, 24 mg, and 32 mg tablets (Medrol); 12 mg/mL, 40 mg/mL, and 80 mg/mL solution for injection (Depo Medrol—acetate form); 40 mg, 125 mg, 500 mg, 1 g, and 2 g powder for injection (Solu Medrol—sodium succinate form).

Special notes:
- A relatively low potency corticosteroid.
- Intended for short-term treatment.

Prednisone

Brand names: Deltasone, Meticorten, Orasone

Available as: 1 mg, 2.5 mg, 5 mg, 10 mg, 20 mg, and 50 mg tablets; 5 mg/ 5 mL syrup.

Special notes:
- The least potent of the corticosteroids, resulting in a greater incidence of adverse effects.
- Used for short-term treatment only.

Leukotriene Receptor Antagonists

These drugs inhibit the inflammatory action of leukotrienes.

Montelukast

Brand name: Singulair

Available as: 10 mg tablet (adult), 4 mg, and 5 mg chewable tablet (pediatric), granules.

Special notes:
- Administered in the fasting state.
- Highly plasma protein bound.
- Doses above 10 mg/day do not show additional therapeutic effect.
- Dose is a single dose of 10 mg to be taken in the evening.

Zafirlukast

Brand name: Accolate

Available as: 10 and 20 mg tablets.

Special notes:
- Dose reduction may be required in the elderly and hepatically impaired.
- Long half-life—10 hours.

- Inhibits several leukotrienes—broader spectrum of action.
- Food reduces bioavailability by 40%, so drug should be administered in the fasting state.
- Inhibits P_{450} isoenzymes CYP2C9 and CYP3A4, so drug interactions are possible.
- Dosage: 20 mg twice daily, one hour before or at least two hours after meals.

Chapter Review Questions

1. Which of the following is given orally?
   a. Medrol
   b. Flovent
   c. Beclovent
   d. Depo-Medrol

2. Which of the following would be most useful in an acute asthma attack?
   a. Albuterol
   b. Singulair
   c. Theolair
   d. Prednisone

3. Serevent belongs to which class of drugs?
   a. methylxanthines
   b. β_2 agonist
   c. muscarinic blocker
   d. steroid

4. Which of the following is related to caffeine?
   a. Atrovent
   b. Theo-Dur
   c. Albuterol
   d. Zafirlukast

5. Which of the following drugs is an inhaled steroid?
   a. Orasone
   b. Beclomethasone
   c. Flovent
   d. both b and c

6. Singulair is a:
   a. beta receptor blocker
   b. oral steroid
   c. inhaled steroid
   d. leukotriene receptor antagonist

7. Corticosteroids:
   a. decrease the immune system
   b. are metabolized in the kidneys
   c. increase hormone production
   d. none of the above

8. The most potent aerosol corticosteroid is:
   a. Advair
   b. Qvar
   c. Flovent
   d. Nasocort

9. Albuterol is a
   a. ß adrenergic agonist
   b. ß$_2$ adrenergic receptor
   c. Cholinergic agonist
   d. Leukotriene receptor antagonist

10. Mast cells are affected by
    a. muscarinic antagonists
    b. methylxanthines
    c. leukotrienes
    d. steroids

CHAPTER **26**

Antibiotics and Anti-Infectives

Quick Study

I. General mechanisms of action and adverse effects of antibiotics

    A. Bacteriostatic vs. bacteriocidal antibiotics

    B. General adverse effects
- Production of superinfections
- Hypersensitivity reactions

II. Mechanism of action, cross-sensitivities, uses, adverse effects, and contraindications of the various antibiotics:

    A. Penicillins and cephalosporins

    B. Aminoglycosides

    C. Tetracyclines

    D. Macrolides

    E. Fluoroquinalones

    F. Sulfa drugs

III. Combination drugs: Using two antibiotics with synergistic effects

IV. Interactions of antibiotics with other drugs

V. Antiviral drugs

VI. Antifungal drugs

VII. Antitubercular drugs

Antibiotics and Anti-infectives

> Bacteria are classified as either gram negative or gram positive, depending on whether or not they absorb a particular kind of dye. Gram-positive organisms have a less developed cell wall than gram-negative organisms and are thus easier to target.

Antibiotics are a group of drugs that target bacteria. Bacteria are single-celled organisms that have a cell wall and cellular machinery, and are capable of cell division—unlike viruses, which are not cells and must use a human cell as a "host" in order to replicate. Because of this, many antibiotics target this cellular machinery within the bacterium, which is required for cellular replication, and inhibit its function. Because viruses are not real cells and do not have this cellular machinery, antibiotics are not effective in the treatment of viral infections.

Bacteria have a substantial cell wall surrounding the cell. This cell wall protects the organism from outside influences, and keeps water and salts from passing in and out of the cell. Some types of bacteria have a less substantial cell wall than others. These can be identified by placing a dye called a "Gram stain" on the bacteria, and watching to see if the dye enters the cell. If it does, the bacteria are classified as "gram positive" (abbreviated "g^+"). If the dye is not allowed into the cell, the bacteria are classified as "gram negative" ("g^-").

Because gram-positive (g^+) organisms have a less developed cell wall than gram-negative (g^-) organisms, they are easier to target pharmaceutically. There are currently more antibiotics that are effective against gram-positive organisms than gram-negative organisms. Only certain drugs will target gram-negative organisms, but new therapies are being developed. A drug that is effective against both gram-positive and gram-negative organisms is called a **broad spectrum** antibiotic.

Bacteriostatic vs. Bacteriocidal Drugs

> Bacteriostatic drugs inactivate bacteria and prevent them from replicating. Thus, the patient may feel better, due to the temporary inactivation of the organisms, and stop taking the drug. If this happens, the organism will once again be able to replicate when it is released from the effects of the drug. This is why patients must be advised to take the full course of medication, regardless of how they "feel."

Antibiotics may either kill immediately, or may take a bacterial generation to have an effect. Those that kill immediately are called **bacteriocidal** drugs. Those that simply prevent the cell from replicating, and therefore take one bacterial generation to have an effect, are called **bacteriostatic** drugs.

> **NOTE**
>
> Antibiotics are not specifically targeted to one organism. Thus, they may promote yeast infections, by decreasing certain bacterial populations and allowing the yeast to grow unchecked.

Superinfections

The intestine is normally populated with a large number of bacteria, called "flora" (since they are supposed to be there, we call them "normal flora"). These organisms assist in digestion, manufacture vitamins and lipid compounds, and also assist in the activation of certain drugs. Many of these organisms, by themselves, are deadly, virulent bacteria (for example, *e. coli* is present in large numbers in the intestine and can cause severe diarrhea and even death). Since there are so many species of bacteria that must survive on food and water coming through the digestive tract, they compete for food. This keeps the growth rate of the organisms in check.

Most antibiotics target certain strains of bacteria, so, when they are taken orally, and hit the digestive tract at full strength, they selectively target and kill a certain population of bacteria. This leaves the other strains of intestinal flora with more nutrients, and can initiate an increase in growth of these potentially lethal organisms. This may cause a severe bacterial infection, on top of the infection that the antibiotic is supposed to cure. This second infection, caused by the antibiotic, is called a **superinfection** and can be life-threatening.

> Taking an antibiotic when it is not warranted may be very dangerous, as it may cause a virulent bacterial infection!

> **NOTE**
>
> It is especially important that patients be advised as to the dangers of superinfections, and that antibiotics not be taken unless prescribed (e.g., a specific bacterial infection has been diagnosed). Taking antibiotics without regard to the underlying infection may not only be ineffective against the condition, but will promote bacterial resistance to the antibiotic, and may cause a superinfection, as well.

General Adverse Effects of Antibiotics

In addition to possible superinfections, adverse effects of the various antibiotics may vary somewhat. In general, adverse effects of antibiotics are as follows:

- Antibiotics that are taken orally may also cause *gastrointestinal distress*, due to the actions of the drug on the intestine itself.
- An increase in the frequency of yeast infections may be seen.
- Many antibiotics (e.g., penicillins and sulfa drugs) cause **hypersensitivity reactions**, which can be life-threatening.
- They can potentially decrease the effectiveness of birth control.
- Antibiotics can increase INR in patients taking warfarin.

Hypersensitivity Reactions

Hypersensitivity reactions are instigated by the release of histamine, and may begin with a rash (hives), and progress to wheezing and shortness of breath. The patient may eventually go into anaphylactic shock. Mild hypersensitivity reactions, such as a rash, may be an indication of a possible serious reaction with the next dose of drug, and should be taken seriously.

Hypersensitivity reactions can be life-threatening. The severity of a hypersensitivity reaction may be decreased by premedication with corticosteroids (e.g., prednisone, beclomethasone), and a combination of corticosteroids and intravenous epinephrine may be used to minimize a reaction, once it has begun. It is, of course, best to avoid such a reaction entirely, using your knowledge of pharmacology and the information contained in the patient profile.

Drugs Prescribed

Penicillins

> The *beta lactam ring portion* of the penicillin structure is largely responsible for hypersensitivity (allergic) reactions. Therefore, drugs with similar structures, such as cephalosporins and monolactams, may cause allergic reactions in penicillin-sensitive patients.

Penicillins act by binding to specific "penicillin binding proteins" (PBPs) in the bacterial cell wall and inhibiting cell wall synthesis. Thus, the cell wall is incompletely formed, and holes or "fenestrations" are present that allow molecules to pass in and out of the cell. The result is *cell lysis*—the cell breaks apart.

Penicillins are called beta lactam antibiotics, due to a certain part of the molecular structure, called the beta lactam ring. There are many penicillins, which are grouped together according to when they were discovered. We call the oldest drugs "first generation"; the newest to date are "fifth-generation" drugs. The efficacy of the drugs and their duration of action vary with each generation, as does the resistance of the drugs to substances made by certain bacteria. This designation is still noted in the cephalosporins, a derivative of penicillins, discussed later in the chapter.

Most penicillins are acid-labile—they are rapidly broken down by stomach acid. Many of the newer penicillin drugs are more resistant to acid hydrolysis, and may be taken orally. *In general, the older penicillins may not be effective orally depending on the bacteria present.*

> Oral antibiotics may reduce the efficacy of contraceptives, resulting in pregnancy.

Consequences of Antibiotic Therapy—Important Points to Consider

1. *Decreased activity of oral contraceptives*—oral contraceptives are activated in the gut by microorganisms present. Thus, the use of antibiotics, which may kill these organisms, can interfere with the activity of the contraceptive, resulting in unexpected pregnancy.

2. *Increased bleeding and bruising*—microorganisms in the gut manufacture a large portion of the body's stores of vitamin K. Use of oral antibiotics may eliminate these organisms, thus decreasing vitamin K stores. This may result in increased prothrombin time (PTT), and decreased ability of the blood to clot, so the patient may be prone to excessive bruising and bleeding, with injury. Because of this, the use of antibiotics will also potentiate the actions of warfarin.

Penicillin Allergy

Many patients are allergic to penicillin. With the first dose, the patient may experience a generalized rash (**urticaria**, or hives). With subsequent doses,

anaphylaxis may be seen. The patient experiences wheezing, cannot breathe, and goes into shock. This reaction can be life-threatening. If a patient has experienced a rash with a penicillin drug, it is not wise to expose him or her a second time.

Treatment of an anaphylactic reaction may include antihistamines (e.g., diphenhydramine), and steroids (e.g., beclomethasone), usually in combination with epinephrine.

Penicillin Resistance

> The most common form of bacterial resistance is the production by the bacteria of an enzyme that degrades penicillin, called penicillinase.

Certain bacteria have developed a *resistance* to penicillin, simply because it has been used so much. There are many forms of bacterial resistance. The most common form of resistance is when the bacteria make an enzyme that degrades the penicillin, called penicillinase. We have now developed drugs to inactivate the penicillinase, as well, which are given along with the penicillin. These include clavulanic acid, sulbactam, and tazobactam.

- These drugs (penicillinase inhibitors) act as competitive antagonists (i.e., false substrates) of penicillinase. They are similar in structure to penicillin, so the enzyme will not know the difference and may act on the drug, as well as the penicillin. Since these drugs have no pharmacological activity of their own, they will not cause toxic effects, but increase the amount of penicillin available to act on the bacteria. They are normally included in certain penicillin formulations along with the penicillin, but may also be sold separately.

Modified Penicillin Derivatives

Penicillins have been chemically modified to be more effective in the therapy of disease. Some have been modified to be effective against penicillinase-resistant organisms, for example, and some are "extended spectrum" antibiotics and have an effect on a broader range of organisms. Examples of these drugs are listed in Table 26-1 and Table 26-2.

Table 26-1	Extended spectrum penicillins
amoxicillin	mezlocillin
ampicillin	piperacillin
carbenicillin	ticarcillin

Table 26-2	Penicillinase resistant penicillins
cloxacillin	nafcillin
dicloxacillin	oxacillin

Penicillins available for prescription include:

Penicillin G

This drug was the first penicillin and is the oldest on the market. *It is not effective orally.* It is still marketed as an oral formulation, but very large doses must be taken to compensate for the acid degradation, so this formulation is infrequently prescribed. It is most effective in the injectable form.

Brand names: Pencil G, Pfizerpen, PenG SOD (Na form)

Available as: Powder for reconstitution—1 million units/vial, 5 million units/vial, 20 million units/vial.

Special notes:

- Penicillin G is bacteriocidal.
- It is normally measured in millions of units.
- It is administered parenterally—intravenous drip or intramuscularly, for a slow administration. *Rapid administration may cause hypersensitivity reactions.*
- It is primarily marketed as the sodium or potassium salt of penicillin G (Penicillin G-Na or Penicillin G-K, respectively).
- It is normally dispensed as powder for injection, which must be reconstituted according to label directions.

Sodium and Potassium Salts of Penicillin

The problem with the sodium and potassium formulations of penicillin in the body is that the salt may accumulate and can shift electrolyte balance, with long-term therapy. Penicillin G-Na in particular may cause edema, due to the influx of sodium.

Extended-Release Penicillins

Extended-release formulations contain procaine or epinephrine and are administered IM. These agents cause local vasoconstriction at the site of injection, which slows systemic absorption. This allows higher doses to be administered for a long-lasting effect. An example of this is procaine penicillin.

Penicillin V Potassium

Brand names: Pen-Vee, Beepen VK

Available as: 250 mg and 500 mg tablets; 125 mg/mL and 250 mg/5 mL powder for reconstitution as an oral suspension.

Special notes:

- This formulation is taken orally.
- Penicillin V is bacteriocidal.
- Dosage is measured in milligrams, rather than international units.

Amoxicillin

Brand names: Amoxil, Polymox, Trimox, Augmentin

Available as: 250 mg and 500 mg capsules; 125 mg and 250 mg chewable tablets; 50 mg/mL, 125 mg/5 mL, and 250 mg/5 mL powder for reconstitution (oral suspension), Augmentin: 250 mg, 500 mg, 875 mg, and 1,000 mg; 125 mg/5 mL, 200 mg/5 mL, 250 mg/5 mL, and 400 mg/5 mL oral suspension; 600 mg/5 mL ES suspension.

Extended spectrum penicillins include ticarcillin and carbenicillin.

Special notes:

- Has a broader spectrum of action than either penicillin V or penicillin G, and is more effective against gram-negative organisms.
- Acid stable, so is taken orally.
- Is bacterio*cidal.*
- Causes less diarrhea than other orally administered penicillins.

Ticarcillin

Brand names: Ticar, Timentin (with clavulinic acid)

Available as: Timentin: 3.1 g vials, 3.1 g IV piggyback.

Dosage: Adult: 3.1 g every four to six hours. Pediatric (patients three months): 200–300 mg/kg/day in divided doses (patients 60 kg); 3.1 g every four to six hours (patients 60 kg).

Storage: Concentrated solutions may be stored at room temperature for up to six hours. Diluted solutions may be frozen for up to thirty days (freezer storage is limited to seven days, if the drug is diluted in D_5W). Once thawed, solutions may not be refrozen.

Penicillinase resistant penicillins include nafcillin, oxacillin, and dicloxacillin.

Special notes:

- An extended spectrum penicillin.
- Incompatible with sodium bicarbonate.

Nafcillin

Brand name: Nafcil

Available as: Powder for injection: 500 mg, 1 g, 2 g, 10 g vials; 1 g and 2 g piggyback vials.

Dosage: 500 mg–2 g IV q 4h. Pediatric dosage: 25 mg/kg bid. Neonatal dosage: 10 mg/kg bid.

Special notes:

- Penicillinase resistant.
- Used in soft tissue infections and upper respiratory infections.
- Effective against staphylococcus.

Cephalosporin Antibiotics

Cephalosporin antibiotics are a newer class of antibiotics that have a structure and action similar to the penicillins. Like the penicillins, these drugs also bind to penicillin-binding proteins, and since there are so many of these proteins and each controls a different function in the bacterial cell, the actions of these drugs vary. As with the penicillins, the cephalosporins are grouped in "generations," according to when they were developed and their general characteristics.

First-Generation Cephalosporins

The first-generation cephalosporins have mainly a gram-positive action, with limited spectrum, and are bacteriocidal.

Cephalexin

Brand names: Keflex, Keftab, Biocef

Available as: 250 mg and 500 mg capsules/tablets; 125 mg/5 mL and 250 mg/5 mL oral suspension.

Special notes:
- Used in lower respiratory infections.
- Used for UTI infections.
- Used for prophylaxis in endocarditis and oral surgery.

Cephradine

Brand name: Velosef

Available as: 250 mg and 500 mg capsules; 250 mg/5 mL oral suspension.

Special notes:
- Used for respiratory infections.
- Can also be used in genitourinary infections.
- Used for GI infections.

Cefadroxil

Brand name: Duricef

Available as: 500 mg and 1,000 mg capsules; 250 mg/5 mL or 500 mg/ 5 mL oral suspension.

Special notes:
- Used in skin and soft tissue infections.

Cefazolin

Brand names: Kefzol, Ancef

Available as: 500 mg and 1 g vials; 1 g and 2 g PB bags.

Important Points to Note:

Cephalosporins are similar in structure to penicillins, and thus can trigger hypersensitivity reactions in penicillin-allergic patients (1 – 4%)! Patients who have had an anaphylactic reaction to penicillin are not advised to take cephalosporins. Hypersensitivity reactions may occur at any time, even after years of taking the drug without a problem.

Special notes:
- Used in gram-positive infections.
- Commonly used for surgical prophylaxis.

Second-Generation Cephalosporins

Second-generation cephalosporins have more gram-negative action, but are fairly mixed in their actions.

Cefaclor
Brand name: Ceclor

Available as: 250 mg and 500 mg capsules; 125 mg/5 mL and 250 mg/5 mL oral suspension; 187 mg/5 mL and 375 mg/5 mL extended-release oral suspension.

Special notes:
- Used for otitis media, and sinusitis.
- Can be used in UTI, and respiratory infections.
- Very expensive.

Cefuroxime
Brand names: Ceftin, Zinacef, Cefurox

Available as: Ceftin: 250 mg and 500 mg tablets, 125 mg/5 mL and 250 mg/5 mL oral suspension. Zinacef/Cefurox: 750 mg or 1.5 g vials for injection.

Special notes:
- Used to treat lower respiratory infections.
- Used for otitis media.
- Also used in skin and soft tissue infections.

Cefamandole
Brand name: Generics available only

Available as: 1 g and 2 g vials.

Special notes:
- Used for respiratory infections.
- Used to treat septicemia.
- Often used for gynecological infections.

Cefoxitin
Brand name: Mefoxin

Available as: 1 g and 2 g vials for injection.

Special notes:
- Used for gynecological infections.
- Used in respiratory infections.

Cefotetan
Brand name: Cefotan

Available as: 1 g and 2 g vials for injection.

Special notes:
- Used to treat wound infections.
- Can be used for sepsis.
- Used in skin and bone infections.

Third-Generation Cephalosporins

Third-generation cephalosporins are very efficacious drugs, with a broader spectrum of action and more efficacy against gram negative organisms. They are bacteriocidal.

Cefpodoxime
Brand name: Vantin

Available as: 100 mg and 200 mg tablets; 50 mg/5 mL and 100 mg/5 mL oral suspension.

Special notes:
- Used to treat community acquired pneumonia.
- Also used in otitis media.
- Used to treat UTI.

Cefixime
Brand name: Suprax

Available as: 400 mg tablets; 100 mg/5 mL and 200 mg/5 mL oral suspension.

Special notes:
- Used to treat UTI.
- Used for otitis media.
- Used in respiratory infections.

Cefdinir
Brand name: Omnicef

Available as: 300 mg capsules; 125 mg/5 mL and 250 mg /5 mL oral suspension.

Special notes:
- Used for pneumonia.
- Used to treat bronchitis.
- Can be used in otitis media.
- Used for sinusitis.

Ceftriaxone
Brand name: Rocephin

Available as: 250 mg, 500 mg, 1 g, and 2 g vials for injection.

Special notes:
- Used for sepsis.
- Also used for lower respiratory infections.
- Can be used for intra-abdominal infections.
- Treats meningitis.

Ceftazidime
Brand names: Fortaz, Tazidime

Available as: 500 mg, 1 g, and 2 g vials for injection.

Special notes:
- Treats pseudomonas aeruginosa infections.

Newer Generations

Fourth- and fifth-generation drugs have broader spectrum and more activity against resistant organisms.

Cefepime
Brand name: Maxipime

Available as: 500 mg, 1 g, and 2 g vials for injection.

Special notes:
- Used for community acquired pneumonia in adults.
- Can be used in UTI.
- Used in pyelonephritis.
- Used for febrile neutropenia.

Macrolide Antibiotics

Macrolide antibiotics are a class of drugs that has expanded greatly over recent years. They are bacteriostatic, and work by inhibiting bacterial protein synthesis, at the level of the ribosome. *It should be noted that, since the ribosomes of bacteria and humans are different, these drugs do not affect human cells.* These drugs may promote diarrhea, and also may affect cytochrome P_{450}, causing drug interactions.

Macrolide antibiotics presently marketed include:

Erythromycin

Erythromycin is marketed in several forms, according to its use and method of administration. For example, erythromycin base and erythromycin stearate are oral formulations, and erythromycin lactobionate is the intravenous form. Erythromycin is the drug of choice in Legionnaires' disease.

Adverse effects: Diarrhea. Extreme nausea and vomiting. Ototoxicity (seen mainly with high dose or intravenous administration). Irritation and inflammation of the veins with intravenous administration. Inhibition of cytochrome P_{450}, resulting in drug interactions. May cause hepatic dysfunction. Patients taking antibiotics containing erythromycin should be monitored for proper hepatic function. May cause pseudomembranous colitis (a potentially serious inflammation of the colon). May promote theophylline toxicity if concurrently administered with theophylline.

Erythromycin Base

This form is used for oral and topical administration.

Brand names: E-Mycin, Ery-Tab, T-Stat.

Available as: 250 mg enteric-coated capsule; 250 mg and 500 mg tablets; 333 mg and 500 mg tablets/coated particles; 250 mg, 333 mg, and 500 mg enteric-coated tablets; 2% gel/jelly; 2% ointment; 5 mg/g ophthalmic ointment; 2% pad; 1.5% and 2% solution; 2% swab.

Erythromycin Ethylsuccinate (with Sulfasoxazole)

Brand names: E.E.S., Eryped, Pediazole (with sulfasoxazole)

Available as: 400 mg tablets, 200 mg/5 mL and 400 mg/5 mL suspension (EES); flavored syrup—200 mg of erythromycin, 600 mg sulfasoxazole per 5 mL (Pediazole).

Erythromycin Stearate

Brand names: Eramycin, Erythrocin

Available as: 250 mg and 500 mg tablets.

Dosage: 250 mg q 6h, or 500 mg q 12h.

Storage: Store below 86°F.

Erythromycin Lactobionate

Brand names: Erythrocin, Erythrocin LA, Erythrocin Lactobionate IV

Available as: 500 mg and 1 g vials for injection.

Dosage: 500 mg every six hours for three days, depending on the condition treated. Doses can range from 250 mg up to 1–4 g per day.

Special notes:

- Used in conjunction with erythromycin stearate.
- May be used to treat rickettsial infections in patients that do not tolerate tetracyclines.
- Must be diluted with sterile water (no preservatives) to prevent formation of a gel-like precipitant.
- Further dilution should be in normal saline for stability; if D_5W is required, then sodium bicarb must be added.

Azithromycin

Brand name: Zithromax

Available as: 250 mg, 500 mg, and 600 mg tablet; 100 mg/5 mL, 200 mg/5 mL, and 1 g/packet oral powder for reconstitution; 15 mg/3mL injection.

Special notes:

- Long half-life allows for once-a-day dosing.
- Given over three to five days instead of seven to ten days.
- Can be given orally or by intravenous administration.
- Not significantly metabolized.
- Has poor CNS penetration, so it is not useful in the treatment of meningitis.
- Useful in the therapy of Lyme disease.
- Can be used for respiratory infections and otitis media.

Clarithromycin

Brand names: Biaxin, Biaxin XL

Available as: 250 mg and 500 mg tablets; 125 mg/5 mL and 250 mg/5 mL granules for reconstitution.

Special notes:

- Available in immediate-release or extended-release formulations.
- Extensively metabolized by the liver, producing an active metabolite.
- Bacterio*static* in low doses, bacterio*cidal* in higher doses.
- Leaves a metallic taste in the mouth.
- Should not be refrigerated once reconstituted.

Aminoglycoside Antibiotics

Aminoglycoside antibiotics inhibit protein synthesis. Aminoglycosides are unique in that they bind to the bacterial ribosome *irreversibly* and thus are bacteriocidal. Aminoglycosides are not first-line drugs, as they have a variety of serious adverse effects. Aminoglycosides can cause:

- Ototoxicity—there is a direct action on the auditory nerve (eighth cranial nerve). This may cause permanent deafness, particularly in children.

- Nephrotoxicity—the amount of nephrotoxicity produced varies with the individual drug, and is dose related. It is reversible if the drug is withdrawn quickly enough.

- Nephrotoxicity is most prominent with gentamycin, amikacin, and tobramycin.

- Skeletal muscle blockade—skeletal muscle contraction can be inhibited by these drugs, and respiratory paralysis may result.

- Deafness in the developing child; hence, aminoglycosides are contraindicated in pregnancy.

- Ototoxic effects synergize with loop diuretics; hence, aminoglycosides are contraindicated with loop diuretics.

> **NOTE**
>
> Aminoglycosides should not be used in the elderly, or in a patient who is dehydrated, as serum levels will increase and severe toxicity may result.

Drugs of the aminoglycoside class that are frequently prescribed include:

Streptomycin Sulfate
Brand name: Streptomycin
Available as: 400 mg/mL solution for intramuscular injection.

Special notes:
- May produce severe neurotoxicity and should not be used in combination with other agents that may also cause neurotoxicity.
- Renal function must be monitored during therapy (e.g., creatinine clearance). Serum drug levels should also be monitored in patients with reduced renal clearance.
- Streptomycin may cause synergistic reactions with skeletal muscle blockers or general anesthetics. The drug should not be given during, before, or immediately after inhalation anesthesia.

- Adverse effects are increased with intravenous therapy. Therapy should not be administered without adequate facilities for monitoring renal and neurological function.

Gentamicin

Brand names: Garamycin; Ophthalmic preparations: Genoptic, Gentacidin

Available as: 40 mg/mL for injection, 10 mg/mL solution for injection (pediatric); 3 mg/mL ophthalmic solution.

Special notes:

- Broad spectrum antibiotic.
- May be used concurrently with penicillins.
- May cause ototoxicity if taken for five days or more. Gentamycin is particularly ototoxic in children.
- Narrow therapeutic window—8 g/dL is therapeutic; 12 g/dL enters the toxic range.
- Use is limited to severe infections.

Tobramycin

Brand names: Nebcin (tobramycin sulfate), Tobrex

Available as: 40 mg/mL, 10 mg/mL (pediatric); 0.3% ophthalmic solution and ointment (Tobrex).

Special notes:

- Similar to gentamycin, but has more activity against aminoglycoside-resistant organisms.

Vancomycin

Brand name: Vancocin

Available as: 125 mg and 250 mg capsules, 250 mg/5 mL oral solution, 500 mg and 1 g vials for injection.

Special notes:

- A glycopeptide antibiotic
- Used for staphylococcal infections.
- Covers streptococcal infections.
- Used in infections that are resistant to traditional antibiotics.
- The dose should be decreased for renal-impaired patients.
- Can cause red-man syndrome in 1–10% of patients.

Tetracycline Antibiotics

Tetracyclines are a very old but still useful class of antibiotics used to treat atypical bacteria. They are bacteriostatic, and work by inhibiting protein synthesis within the bacterial cell. Tetracyclines have the unique property of

Tetracyclines have a unique property of being able to enter mammalian cells to affect organisms growing within cells. They are thus drugs of choice for intracellular (e.g., rickettsial) infections, such as Rocky Mountain Spotted Fever.

Tetracyclines produce a toxic by-product as they break down. Patients must be warned not to use the product after the expiration date! The drug must be discarded!

being able to enter mammalian cells to affect organisms growing within cells. They are thus *drugs of choice for intracellular (e.g., rickettsial, mycoplasmic) infections,* such as Rocky Mountain Spotted Fever and psittacosis. They are *ineffective against viruses or fungi.*

Adverse effects: Digestive upset. Photosensitivity—patients should be advised to stay out of the sun. Contraindicated with other drugs that cause photosensitivity (e.g., carbamazepine).

Tetracyclines bind to complex divalent ions, such as iron, magnesium, and calcium. Because the drugs form insoluble complexes with these ions, the drug cannot pass into the blood, but remains in the intestine. It will not be absorbed, and will have no therapeutic effect. A patient taking oral tetracyclines should be aware that:

- the drugs cannot be taken with food or with milk, as they will not be absorbed.
- the drugs cannot be used in conjunction with antacids that contain calcium, magnesium, or aluminum, nor can they be taken with mineral supplements (e.g., iron, calcium, magnesium).
- the drugs will enter developing bone and form complexes with the calcium in the bone, weakening the bone structure. This is a problem with children and will cause staining of teeth and brittle bones. The only exception to this problem is with doxycycline, which does not complex calcium but prefers to complex iron.
- tetracyclines are contraindicated in pregnancy, as the drug will enter fetal bone and disrupt bone formation.
- tetracyclines are contraindicated in nursing and in children under eight years.

Tetracycline Hydrochloride ("Tetracycline")
Brand names: Achromycin V, Sumycin

Available as: 250 mg, and 500 mg capsules; 3% ointment; 1% ophthalmic solution.

Special notes:
- Eliminated by the kidney, so it is not the drug of choice in a patient with poor renal function.
- Has a relatively short half-life (eight to nine hours), but can be dosed twice daily, although four times a day is preferred.
- Has a strong "post-antibiotic effect" (PAE)—the killing effect continues for six to eight hours after the drug has been cleared from the body.
- Has a broad spectrum of action—both gram-positive and gram-negative organisms are affected.

- Most useful in gram-negative infections, as resistance has developed in most gram-positive organisms.
- Very inexpensive.

Doxycycline

Brand names: Periostat, Doryx, Monodox, VIBRA-TABS, Atridox, doxycycline

Available as: 50 mg/5 mL syrup, 25 mg/5 mL oral suspension, coated tablets, powder for reconstitution (parenteral)—100 mg or 200 mg vials. Periostat (doxycycline hyclate): 20 mg tablets. Doryx (doxycycline hyclate): 75 mg and 100 mg enteric-coated capsules. Monodox (doxycycline monohydrate): 50 mg or 100 mg capsules.

Storage: Reconstituted solutions should be refrigerated.

Atridox (Doxycycline Hyclate)

Atridox is a controlled-release formulation of doxycycline hyclate used in the therapy of periodontitis ("trenchmouth"). The dosage form is designed to be placed at the base of the gum.

This formulation consists of a two-syringe system—one syringe contains doxycycline, the other contains the delivery system. When mixed together, and applied to the base of the gum, the mixture solidifies and becomes a controlled-release system, which releases the drug locally for up to seven days.

Dosage: Variable. The finished product contains 42.5 mg of doxycycline in 500 mg of polymer.

Storage: The unmixed syringes should be stored refrigerated (2–8°C). They may be stored at room temperature for up to three days. They should then be discarded.

Special notes:

- Doxycycline is very lipid soluble, so it is very useful in CNS infections.
- Has a lower degree of calcium binding, so less interactions.
- No food interactions—may be taken with meals.
- Post-antibiotic effect: 28 hours.
- Once-daily dosing.
- Limited renal elimination, so it is a preferred drug for renal patients.

Minocycline

Brand names: Minocin, Dynacin

Available as: 50 mg, 75 mg, 100 mg capsules; 100 mg vial.

Special notes:

- Considered the most active tetracycline.
- Is long-acting.
- Most lipid soluble of the tetracyclines.
- Useful in meningitis.
- Recently shown to be useful in the treatment of rheumatoid arthritis.
- Administered orally or intravenously.

Sulfa Drugs

Sulfa drugs are another older class of drugs. They are most frequently prescribed in combination with other drugs (e.g., trimethoprim) for the therapy of kidney infections. They are also used as ophthalmics.

The Mechanism of Action of Sulfa Drugs

Sulfa drugs act by inhibiting the uptake of para-amino-benzoic-acid (PABA) by bacteria. The PABA is used by the bacteria to make folic acid, which is necessary for DNA synthesis. Without it, the bacteria cannot reproduce, and die (bacteriostatic).

> Sulfa drugs may cause damage to kidney tubules if the patient does not drink sufficient water! The drug will precipitate out in concentrated urine, forming crystals that will damage the kidney!

Adverse effects: Rash: This is a symptom of hypersensitivity, and may lead to more serious complications if the drug is not discontinued. Kidney damage: Sulfa drugs are eliminated through the urine. These drugs are only soluble in water at low concentrations (e.g., a little drug and a lot of water). Therefore, if the patient does not drink enough water, the urine becomes concentrated, and the drug will crystallize in the urine. When this happens, the sharp crystals of drug can damage the renal tubules and cause kidney failure. Photosensitivity. Discoloration of urine.

Sulfasalazine

Brand names: Azulfadine, Azulfidine EN (Sulfasalazine EC—delayed-release tablet)

Available as: 500 mg tablets.

Primary Uses: Used in the therapy of rheumatoid arthritis and ulcerative colitis.

Dosage: Loading dose of 4 g for the first day, then maintenance dosage of 2 g daily; pediatric dose (>2 years): 40–60 mg/kg/day in divided doses.

Sulfamethoxazole

Brand name: Gantanol

Available as: 0.5 g tablets (green, scored).

Dosage: Adult dose: 2 g loading dose, 1 g bid thereafter; pediatric: 40–60 mg/kg loading dose, 25–30 mg/kg thereafter. Maximum dose: 75 mg/kg in 24 hours.

Special note:

* Should not be administered to children under two years of age, due to renal clearance and renal toxicity.

Trimethoprim/sulfamethoxazole

Brand names: Bactrim, Bactrim IV, Bactrim DS (double strength–160 mg trimethoprim and 800 mg sulfamethoxazole), Bactrim PED (pediatric formulation), Bethaprim PED; Cotrim, Cotrim Pediatric, Cotrim DS; Septra, Septra IV, Sulfameth-Tri, Sulfatrim

Available as: 80 mg trimethoprim/400 sulfamethoxazole tablets; 160 mg trimethoprim/800 mg sulfamethoxazole double-strength tablets; 40 mg trimethoprim and 200 mg sulfamethoxazole/5 mL oral suspension; 16 mg trimethoprim and 80 mg sulfamethoxazole/mL concentrate for injection; suspension needs to be shaken–stored at room temperature.

Special notes:

* Trimethoprim is an antibiotic that interferes with the utilization of folic acid by bacteria (recall that folic acid is necessary to make DNA). Recall that sulfa drugs interfere with the **synthesis** of folic acid. The drugs thus act synergistically.

Erythromycin-sulfisoxazole

Brand name: Pediazole

Available as: Flavored suspension; granules for reconstitution.

Dosage: 200 mg erythromycin/600 mg sulfisoxazole/5 mL (teaspoon).

Fluoroquinolone Antibiotics

Fluoroquinolone antibiotics inhibit the enzyme that supercoils DNA. This enzyme is called *topoisomerase I* or *DNA gyrase* and regulates the coiling of DNA. If the enzyme is not present (and active), the DNA cannot be copied, and the cell cannot replicate or make proteins that are necessary for it to survive.

Fluoroquinolone antibiotics:

* Are effective against gram negative rods.
* Have a significant post-antibiotic effect—cell death continues after the drug is withdrawn.
* May cause nausea and vomiting.
* Causes photosensitivity.

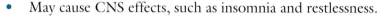
- May cause CNS effects, such as insomnia and restlessness.
- Should be used with caution in patients prone to seizures.
- Interact with divalent ions (absorption is reduced) and so must not be given within 2 hours of administering antacids.
- *Have interactions with theophylline*—these drugs interfere with the metabolism of theophylline and will cause increased plasma levels.

Ciprofloxacin

Brand names: Cipro, Ciloxan (opthalmic)

Classification: DNA topoisomerase (Types II and IV) inhibitor

Available as: 100 mg, 250 mg, 500 mg, and 750 mg, and 1,000 mg tablets; 250 mg/5 mL and 500 mg/5 mL oral suspension, 3% ophthalmic solution. Intravenous solutions: 10 mg/mL (20 mL, 40 mL, and 120 mL per vial), 20 mg/mL (100 mL per vial), and 40 mg/mL (200 mL vial), 0.2% premixed solution in D_5W, available in containers of 100 mL or 200 mL

Dosage: 250 mg–500 mg every 12 hours, orally. Intravenous administration: 200–400 mg every 12 hours, to be administered in a 60-minute infusion.

Storage: Oral dosage forms are stored at controlled room temperature. Intravenous solutions are stored below room temperature, between 5°C and 25°C.

Special notes:
- Should not be administered orally in conjunction with antacids or supplements of iron, magnesium, or calcium, as these ions will delay absorption.
- Intravenous administration must be very slow and in dilute solution, as the drug is irritating to the veins.
- Ready-to-use solutions for infusion. These solutions can leach out contaminants from plastic packaging during shelf storage.
- Food delays absorption of the drug.
- Renal excretion, so dosage must be reduced in renally compromised patients.
- Should not be used in individuals under the age of 18 (as with all the fluoroquinolones).

Ofloxacin

Brand names: Floxin, Ocuflox

Classification: DNA topoisomerase (Types II and IV) inhibitor

Available as: 200 mg, 300 mg, and 400 mg tablets; 0.3% ophthalmic solution; 4 mg/mL, 20 mg/mL, and 40 mg/mL solution for injection.

Special notes:
- Useful in systemic infections.
- Excreted through the urine.

Levofloxacin

Brand names: Levaquin, Quixin

Available as: 250 mg, 500 mg, and 750 mg tablets, 0.5% ophthalmic solution, 25 mg/mL and 5 mg/mL injection.

Special note:
- Ophthalmic formulation used in bacterial conjunctivitis.

Norfloxacin

Brand name: Noroxin

Available as: 400 mg tablet.

Special notes:
- Treats urinary tract infections and cystitis.

Urinary Antiseptics

Nitrofurantoin

Brand names: Macrodantin, Macrobid

Available as: 25 mg, 50 mg, and 100 mg capsules; 100 mg extended release capsules; 25 mg/5 mL suspension.

Drugs That Are Effective against Viruses and Fungi

Viruses and fungi function quite differently from bacteria. Fungi are plant-based and replicate from spores. Viruses are very simple organisms that consist of a strand of DNA or RNA, inside of a protein shell or "coat."

Viruses

Viruses have no means of generating energy or of self-replication. They must use a cellular host in order to replicate. Basically, the virus comes in contact with a suitable host cell, attaches to it, and "injects" its DNA or RNA into the cell. It then uses the organelles of the host cell to make new protein coats and DNA or RNA strands and, as more and more of these small viruses (called "virions") are formed, the cell eventually bursts (lyses), releasing the viruses to the circulation. The newly formed viruses repeat the process, and a viral infection is begun.

Viruses, in general, tend to be rather short lived, but mutate very quickly, evading the human immune system. This is why a patient may contract a viral infection several times (e.g., a cold, or the "flu"). Some viruses remain dormant for long periods of time and suddenly become active.

Antiviral Agents

Acyclovir

Brand name: Zovirax

Available as: 200 mg capsule; 400 mg and 800 mg tablets; 500 mg and 1,000 mg powder for injection; 200 mg/5 mL suspension; 5% ointment.

Special notes:
- Useful in the therapy of herpes infections.
- Prevents viral replication by inhibiting viral thymidine kinase.
- Only accumulates in virally infected cells, so host cell toxicity is minimal.

Valicyclovir

Brand name: Valtrex

Available as: 500 mg and 1,000 mg caplets.

Special note:
- This drug is a prodrug. It is converted to acyclovir after absorption.

Vidarabine

Brand name: Vira-A ophthalmic ointment

Available as: 30 mg/g topical ointment.

Special notes:
- Produces chemicals toxic to host cells.
- Teratogenic—causes birth defects, so it is used topically.
- Used topically in the therapy of keratitis due to herpes zoster infections.

Antiretroviral Drugs (Used in the Therapy of AIDS)

These drugs are derivatives of nucleosides, and disrupt the transcription of DNA and RNA.

The Human Immunodeficiency Virus (HIV)

The AIDS virus is a very different kind of virus, called a *retrovirus*. This virus attaches to specific receptors on its host cell, the T-lymphocyte. Like an ordinary virus, it attaches and injects its RNA into the cell. The cell then makes viral DNA from the RNA, which then becomes incorporated into the DNA of the host cell. When the host cell replicates, the gene for the AIDS virus is replicated along with it. This gene may be dormant for a long period of time, but eventually it becomes active and HIV particles are produced and released, inhibiting the function of the immune system and beginning the progression of the disease.

Drugs Used in the Therapy of AIDS

Mechanism of Action

Drugs used in the therapy of AIDS act to inhibit the transcription of the viral RNA into DNA, by mimicking the structures of DNA nucleosides, and inserting themselves into the viral DNA molecule as it is formed. The newly formed DNA is thus unstable and the strands break. Unfortunately, the constant rate of mutation of the viruses limits the effectiveness of these drugs.

Drugs available include:

Azidothymidine (AZT)

Generic name: Zidovudine

Brand name: Retrovir

Available as: 300 mg tablets; 100 mg capsules; 50 mg/5 mL syrup; 10 mg/mL solution for IV injection.

Special notes:

- Deoxythymidine analog.
- Affects rapidly dividing host cells (e.g., bone marrow), so produces anemia.
- Produces CNS effects, such as insomnia and headaches.

Didanosine

Brand name: Videx

Available as: 25 mg, 50 mg, 100 mg, 150 mg, and 200 mg chewable tablets; powder packets for oral solution in 100 mg, 167 mg, or 250 mg, 10 mg/mL pediatric solution, sustained-release capsules: 125 mg, 200 mg, 250 mg, and 400 mg.

Adverse effects: May cause inflammation of the pancreas (pancreatitis), which may be fatal. May cause enlargement of the liver and lactic acidosis.

Special note:

- This drug is degraded by acid (acid labile), so must be administered on an empty stomach.

Antifungal Drugs

These drugs are used in the therapy of systemic or topical yeast infections, and superficial fungal infections (e.g. ringworm, nail fungus).

Fluconazole

Brand name: Diflucan

Available as: 50 mg, 100 mg, 150 mg, and 200 mg tablets; 50 mg/5 mL and 200 mg/5 mL powder for reconstitution; 2 mg/mL vials for injection, 200 mg/100 mL, and 400 mg/200 mL IVPB vials for injection.

Special notes:
- Acts as an enzyme inhibitor. It inhibits fungal cytochrome P_{450}, resulting in a nonfunctional cell.
- May be used systemically or topically.
- Useful in vaginal yeast infections (topical, orally) and the therapy of nail fungus (systemic administration).

Ketoconazole

Brand name: Nizoral

Available as: 2% cream; 1% shampoo; 200 mg tablet.

Special notes:
- Acts to inhibit the synthesis of fungal cell membranes.
- Oral and topical use only; not used parenterally.
- May cause nausea and vomiting.
- Decreases cholesterol synthesis with prolonged therapy; may affect steroid hormone production.

Antitubercular Drugs

These drugs affect the organism *mycobacterium tuberculii*. This particular strain of bacteria is difficult to eradicate, as it has a thick, waxy coating that makes penetration by conventional antibiotics difficult. Thus, antibiotics in general are not effective in the therapy of tuberculosis.

Drugs available:

Isoniazid (INH)

Brand name: Nydrazid

Available as: 100 mg and 300 mg tablets; 50 mg/5 mL oral syrup.

Special notes:
- Age-related hepatitis. Risk of hepatitis is increased by age and alcohol consumption.
- Regular liver function tests should be performed, including SGOT (now called AST), and SGPT (now called ALT).

Rifampin
Brand names: Rifadin, Rimactane
Available as: 150 mg and 300 mg tablets; 600 mg solution for injection.

Rifampin Isoniazid Combination
Brand name: Rifamate
Available as: Capsules containing 300 mg rifampin and 150 mg isoniazid.

Chapter Review Questions

1. An antibiotic that will kill both gram-negative and gram-positive organisms is called a(n):
   a. efficacious antibiotic
   b. antistatic antibiotic
   c. broad spectrum antibiotic
   d. totally awesome antibiotic

2. A drug that kills bacteria directly is called:
   a. bacteriostatic
   b. bacteriocidal
   c. an antifungal
   d. efficacious

3. A patient comes into the pharmacy, complaining of a severe yeast infection that just started after beginning her new drug therapy. The drug responsible might be:
   a. her contraceptive medication
   b. Amoxil
   c. Aspirin
   d. the contraceptive in combination with the Amoxil

4. A patient takes large doses of oral cefamandole without consulting a physician. He really has a viral infection, not a bacterial infection. Which of the following is most likely to happen?
   a. he will experience cardiovascular complications
   b. he will develop a rash
   c. he will develop a superinfection
   d. the viral infection will get worse

5. A patient is allergic to penicillin. The following drugs appear on the hospital order for her therapy. You would call the attention of the pharmacist to which drug?
   a. Tobramax
   b. Ceclor
   c. Zithromax
   d. Isoniazid

6. A patient is taking oral contraceptives. She takes amoxicillin for an infection. Which of the following could happen?
   a. she could be miraculously cured
   b. she could develop a superinfection
   c. she could become pregnant, in spite of the contraceptives
   d. she could develop hearing loss

7. Tazobactam may be given with penicillin for what reason?
   a. it stabilizes the penicillin
   b. it inhibits penicillinase
   c. it is a defense against penicillin resistance
   d. both b and c are correct

8. Which of the following is orally active?
   a. Penicillin G
   b. Penicillin G potassium
   c. Polymox
   d. Nafcil

9. A local anesthetic, such as procaine, may be added to a penicillin bolus because:
   a. the penicillin is more effective
   b. the penicillin effects last longer
   c. it allows a larger dose to be administered, for a longer lasting effect
   d. it stabilizes the penicillin

10. Which of the following has a high degree of activity against gram-negative organisms?
    a. Penicillin G
    b. Amoxicillin
    c. Penicillin V
    d. Nydrazid

11. Which of the following is a macrolide antibiotic?
    a. Ocuflox
    b. Doxycycline
    c. Ceclor
    d. Zithromax

12. Erythromycin and gentamicin:
    a. are both aminoglycoside antibiotics
    b. can cause ototoxicity
    c. can cause renal failure
    d. have nothing in common

13. A patient is dehydrated and has a bacterial infection. Which of the following would be contraindicated?
    a. Bactrim
    b. Erythromycin
    c. Biaxin
    d. Zithromax

14. Which of the following is an ophthalmic antibiotic solution?
    a. Doryx
    b. Nebcin
    c. Ocuflox
    d. Biaxin

15. Which of the following requires routine liver function tests?
    a. Isoniazid
    b. Floxin
    c. Bactrim
    d. Pen-Vee-K

16. Which of the following may produce toxic products after its expiration date?
    a. Macrodantin
    b. Tetracycline
    c. Cipro
    d. both b and c

17. Which of the following causes sun sensitivity?
    a. Gentamicin
    b. Tetracycline
    c. Minocycline
    d. all of the above

18. A drug useful in herpes infections is:
    a. Myconazole
    b. Isoniazid
    c. Videx
    d. Zovirax

19. Miconazole and ketoconazole are used in the therapy of:
    a. pneumonia
    b. viral infections
    c. fungal infections
    d. tuberculosis

20. Which class of drugs are structurally similar to penicillin?
    a. Cephalosporins
    b. Macrolides
    c. Aminoglycosides
    d. Antivirals

CHAPTER 27

Cancer Chemotherapeutic Agents

Quick Study

I. General types of cancer chemotherapeutics

  A. Cell cycle–specific agents—act at a specific point in the cellular replication cycle, and must be administered by continuous infusion
  B. Non-cell cycle–specific agents—act at any place in the cell cycle, and may be dosed at intervals

II. General mechanisms of cancer chemotherapeutic drugs

  A. Alkylating agents:
    1. Drugs that alkylate DNA, preventing accurate copying of DNA, and thus inhibit cell replication
    2. DNA crosslinkers—drugs that crosslink DNA strands
  B. Antimetabolite antineoplastic drugs:
    1. Drugs that interfere with the utilization of folic acid, thus interfering with DNA synthesis (e.g., methotrexate)
    2. Drugs that interfere with the synthesis of DNA nucleotides (e.g., 5-FU)
    3. Use of leukovorin with the various types of antimetabolite drugs
  C. Drugs that affect spindle formation in mitosis
    1. Taxanes—interfere with the attachment of mitotic spindles
    2. Vinca alkaloids (e.g., vincristine, vinblastine)—interfere with microtubule formation
  D. Drugs that affect the coiling of DNA and thus inhibit DNA replication
    1. Topoisomerase inhibitors (etoposide, teniposide)
    2. Campothectins (topotecan, irinotecan)

E. Antibiotic chemotherapeutic agents
   1. Anthracyclines—severe cardiac toxicity
   2. Bleomycin—can cause severe pulmonary toxicity
F. Adverse effects of the various cancer chemotherapeutic agents—Adverse effects vary with each drug class and are normally an extension of the effects of the drugs on normal cells, which are rapidly dividing (e.g., hair follicles, blood and immune cells). These include:
   1. Nausea and vomiting
   2. Alopecia (loss of hair)
   3. Bone marrow suppression
   4. Immunosuppression
G. Drugs used in combination with cancer chemotherapeutics (to decrease the adverse effects)
   1. Erythropoietin (for bone marrow suppression)
   2. Antiemetic therapy

Introduction

Cancer chemotherapeutics are rapidly becoming a large part of pharmacy practice. There are pharmacists who devote themselves entirely to the therapy of cancer patients, and new drugs for cancer therapy are being developed and marketed constantly. It is wise for the pharmacy technician to be familiar with these drugs.

Drugs used for cancer chemotherapy differ widely in their mechanism of action, duration, and how they affect the cell cycle. Other areas to be considered when determining a therapy are adverse effects, effects of the drugs on existing physiological conditions of a patient, and interactions with other prescribed and over-the-counter drugs.

Choice of Therapy

Physiology Review

When cells divide, the process occurs in cyclic stages (the cell cycle), designated by letters: The "S" phase is the preparatory phase, where the building blocks of DNA synthesis and RNA synthesis are formed. G0 and G1 are the initial phases of the cell cycle, where DNA and proteins are made, which are necessary for cell division. DNA is then copied, and chromosomes are formed. The "M" phase is where the chromosomes line up on protein spindles in the cell and break apart, forming the DNA for two cells, which then break apart. Interruption of this cell cycle at any stage prevents cellular replication and tumor growth.

Cell Cycle–Specific Agents

The choice of therapy depends on the growth rate of the tumor, and the characteristics of the tumor, as well as potential toxicity as compared with patient age and state of health. Many chemotherapeutic agents are **cell cycle specific**—meaning that the activity of these agents occurs only in one specific phase of the cell cycle (e.g., prophase, if the drug interferes with the formation of DNA; or metaphase, if a drug inhibits the formation of mitotic spindles). In therapeutic terms, this means that the drug is effective at only one stage of cell division and therefore targets a single group of cells at a time. Because cells within a tumor may be in different phases of the cell cycle at any given time, cell cycle–specific agents must be given by continuous infusion, and possibly over a long period of time, as the drug must be in the blood when each cell enters the specific phase in which the drug is effective. The increased time of exposure to the drug in continuous therapy may result in increased toxic effects.

Agents That Are Not Cell Cycle Specific

Drugs that are not cell cycle specific may act at any place in the cell cycle. This results in increased efficacy, as the drug can act on more cells—instead of just cells in a particular stage of division, these drugs can act on tumor cells that are in any stage of division. Because of this, these drugs do not need to be given by continuous infusion, as the drug will affect cells in various stages of the replication cycle as soon as therapeutic levels are attained. Drugs that are not cell cycle specific are also more likely to be administered on an outpatient basis, as the drug can be administered by bolus injection every few days, or taken orally.

Central-Line Infusion

Cancer chemotherapeutics may often be administered through a catheter inserted into a large vein, such as the jugular vein, which results in central infusion (in the chest area), rather than infusion through a peripheral vein in the arm or hand. Central infusion tends to minimize adverse effects, as the drug is diluted by the blood right away, and does not come in contact with as much of the body, in its concentrated form.

Adverse Effects of Cancer Chemotherapeutics

With cancer chemotherapeutics, adverse effects are often an extension of the therapeutic action of the drug.

> **EXAMPLE**
>
> Drugs that are effective in lymphocytic metastases (e.g., acute or chronic lymphoblastic leukemia) inhibit immune function as part of their therapeutic effect. Thus, a major adverse effect may be susceptibility to infection.

> **EXAMPLE**
>
> Drugs that inhibit cellular replication at the level of DNA (e.g., cisplatin, methotrexate) may also affect rapidly dividing normal cells, such as blood cells and hair cells. Thus, they cause suppression of the bone marrow (*myelosuppression*), whereas those that inhibit other areas of the cell cycle may not. These drugs are also more likely to cause hair loss.

Minimizing Adverse Effects

- **Central-line infusion** produces the same therapeutic effects as continuous infusion, but produces less adverse effects.
- Drugs that are synergistic in therapeutic mechanism (but have different adverse effects) may be used in **combination therapy**. Lower doses of each drug may be used to decrease the probability of adverse effects.
- *Radiation sensitizers*—some drugs sensitize tumor tissue to the effects of radiation, which increases the effects of radiation therapy. Since low doses of drug are often all that is necessary for maximum efficacy, adverse effects are dramatically decreased.

Major Chemotherapeutic Drugs, by Class

Alkylating Agents

Recall that DNA must uncoil and come apart to be copied—the presence of these foreign bulky chemical groups on the DNA prevents this. Thus, accurate copying of the DNA strand is prevented.

The alkylating agents are an older class of drugs. This class of drugs contains several subclasses, many of which are still widely used today. Alkylating agents act by chemically reacting with DNA—adding a chemical group called an *alkyl group* to certain parts of DNA. (RNA may also be affected at high doses.) These drugs may have active sites at one or both ends of the molecule.

Depending on where the active sites are, the drugs may crosslink DNA strands (leading to lack of DNA replication), or simply cause errors in DNA replication and fragmentation of DNA strands. The ultimate result in either case is an inability of the tumor cells to replicate.

> Adverse effects of alkylating agents are due to the effects of the drug on rapidly dividing normal cells, and may include bone marrow suppression, pulmonary toxicity, and gonadal toxicity.

Therapeutic Effects of Alkylating Agents

Most alkylating agents are non-cell cycle specific and will affect cells at any stage of division. Thus, cell division, particularly in a tumor with rapidly dividing cells, is halted in a manner that is dose-dependent (the larger the dose, the more cells that are affected). Those cells that divide *less* rapidly (e.g., normal tissue) have the opportunity to repair the damaged DNA and are less affected by the drug.

Use of Alkylating Agents

Due to their ability to obstruct cell division, alkylating agents are most useful in the treatment of smaller tumors, which have more dividing cells, but they may also be useful in some slower-growing tumors.

Alkylating agents basically are categorized into three groups, each with slightly different characteristics:

1. Nitrogen-containing drugs (e.g., nitrogen mustards and nitrosoureas)
2. Platinum-containing compounds (e.g., cisplatin and carboplatin)
3. Non-classical alkylating agents (e.g., procarbazine)

Nitrogen Mustards and Their Derivatives

Nitrogen mustards and their derivatives are the oldest alkylating agents presently marketed and are declining in use. They are derived from sulfur mustard gas used in World War II. Most are used infrequently, due to strong toxicity, and for specific applications. These drugs may cause alopecia (hair loss), particularly in high or intravenous doses, as well as bone marrow depression and vomiting (emesis).

Nitrogen mustards cause a decrease in the rate of growth of lymphoid tissue and are thus useful in the treatment of lymphomas. Mechlorethamine is the only pure nitrogen mustard still in use, but its use is restricted to the treatment of Hodgkin's disease. Cyclophosphamide, ifosfamide chlorambucil, and melphalan are derivatives of nitrogen mustard, and exhibit less toxicity. These drugs also have limited use.

The most frequently prescribed drugs include:

Cyclophosphamide

Brand name: Cytoxan

Available as: 25 mg and 50 mg tablets; powder for injection in single-use vials of 100 mg, 200 mg, 500 mg, 1 g, and 2 g (vials contain 75 mg of mannitol per 100 mg of drug).

Special notes:
- Used in the therapy of multiple myeloma, lymphomas, and lymphoid leukemias.

- Cyclophosphamide is useful in the treatment of lymphomas. It is also useful in treatment of autoimmune disease and in transplantation, due to its immunosuppressant effect.

Ifosfamide

Ifosfamide is a newer drug, derived from cyclophosphamide. It is useful in the therapy of sarcomas and testicular carcinomas. Both cyclophosphamide and ifosfamide can cause inflammation of the bladder with bleeding (hemorrhagic cystitis).

Brand name: Ifex

Available as: 1 g and 3 g vials, to be diluted to 50 mg/mL with sterile water.

Dosage: 1.2 g/m^2/day for five days.

Special notes:
- Used as third-line chemotherapy in germ cell testicular cancer.
- Ifosfamide is only available in combination packages with Mesnex, a protective agent for the renal system.
- Severe bone marrow toxicity.

Nitrosoureas

The nitrosoureas and related drugs are also derived from nitrogen mustards. These drugs have limited use, and include carmustine, lomustine, and streptozocin.

- Carmustine may be used as adjunct therapy for brain tumors, as it crosses the blood-brain barrier.
- Lomustine may be used as a last-resort therapy in lung cancer.
- Streptozocin is directly toxic to pancreatic cells and thus is used strictly as an agent to combat islet cell carcinoma.

Carmustine and lomustine are notable for the production of a delayed bone marrow suppression, which may manifest several weeks after discontinuation of therapy. Streptozocin, however, exhibits no myelosuppression.

Carmustine

Brand names: BiCNU, Gliadel (wafer)

Available as: 100 mg vials, packaged with a 3 mL vial of diluents (BICNU), 7.7 mg wafer (Gliadel).

Dosage: 150–200 mg/m^2 every six weeks

Storage: Refrigerated

Special notes:
- Used in combination therapy for the treatment of lymphomas, multiple myeloma, and brain tumors.
- Causes severe bone marrow depression.

Lomustine
Brand name: CeeNU

Available as: dose pack of capsules, containing two 100 mg capsules, two 40 mg capsules, and two 10 mg capsules.

Special notes:
- Used in the therapy of Hodgkin's disease and brain tumors.

Unclassified Agents

Thiotepa
Thiotepa may be used in the therapy of breast and bladder cancer; however, it is rarely used as a cancer chemotherapeutic agent at the present time. The major use of this drug is as a preparative agent in bone marrow transplantation in the therapy of breast cancer.

Brand name: Thioplex

Available as: 15 mg lyophilized powder for injection.

Dosage: Rapid IV administration at 0.3–0.4 mg/kg. Doses are given at one to four-week intervals

Storage: Refrigeration; must be protected from light at all times

Special notes:
- Used (rarely) in the therapy of adenocarcinoma of the breast and ovary.
- Must be filtered through a 0.22 micron sterile filter before administration.

Busulfan
Brand names: Busulfex, Myleran

Available as: 10 mL single dose ampules containing 60 mg of drug (Busulfex), 2 mg tablet (Myleran).

Storage: Refrigeration

Special notes:
- Used in the preparation of bone marrow/stem cell transplants.
- Once used in the therapy of myelogenous leukemia; now used to destroy the myeloid cell line prior to an allergenic bone marrow transplant for leukemia.
- High doses can lead to lung problems and/or seizures.

Platinum-Containing Compounds

These drugs are DNA crosslinking agents—they form crosslinks between DNA strands, effectively binding the strands together so that they cannot separate and be copied. Thus, cellular replication is halted. These drugs are highly toxic. The three drugs of this class are cisplatin, carboplatin, and the newest drug oxaliplatin.

Carboplatin is unique in that it must first enter the cell before it is activated. Once inside the cell, the ring structure of the drug reacts with water to form the active form of the drug, which effectively crosslinks the strands of DNA and RNA. Because the drug is activated *inside* of the tumor cell, adverse effects are reduced. Crosslinks formed by carboplatin are also more stable than those formed by cisplatin, so the effects are longer lasting; however, cisplatin crosslinks are formed more quickly (six to eight hours post administration) than those of carboplatin (eighteen hours post administration).

Cisplatin

Brand names: Platinol, Platinol AQ (aqueous formulation)

Available as: 50 mL and 100 mL amber glass vials of 1 mg/mL solution for injection.

Dosage: 50–100 mg/m^2

Special notes:

- Hypersensitivity reactions (allergic reactions) may occur.
- Bone marrow suppression, alopecia, and nausea are likely to occur.
- Patients should be adequately hydrated, during and after administration.
- Contraindicated in pregnancy, as in all chemotherapeutic agents.
- Chemically reacts with aluminum—any portion of the intravenous infusion set containing aluminum may cause a black precipitate to be formed.
- Toxic to the kidney, ear, and bone marrow.

Carboplatin

Brand name: Paraplatin

Available as: 50 mg, 150 mg, and 450 mg vials of powder for injection.

Dosage: 360 mg/m^2 every four weeks

Storage: Diluted solutions should be discarded after eight hours.

Special notes:

- Used in the therapy of advanced ovarian carcinoma (second-line therapy).
- Carboplatin has a much more favorable adverse effect profile than cisplatin; however, it does suppress bone marrow more than cisplatin. Carboplatin is also a *radiation sensitizer*—concurrent use with radiation therapy potentiates the effects of radiation.

Antitumor Antibiotics

Some antibiotics have antitumor activity. These include dactinomycin, bleomycin, mitomycin, and doxorubicin.

Alkylating Agents That Are Antibiotics

The only antibiotic in use that acts as an alkylating agent is mitomycin. Mitomycin is activated inside the cell and is concentrated in tumor tissue. The active metabolite binds to guanine residues and may form crosslinks with DNA, resulting in inhibition of DNA synthesis.

Mitomycin

Brand name: Mutamycin

Available as: 20 mg powder for injection, 5 mg vial, 40 mg vial. To be diluted to 0.5 mg/mL.

Storage: 0.5 mg/mL solution is stable for 14 days if refrigerated, or seven days at room temperature.

Special notes:

- Mitomycin is used in combination therapy.
- Mitomycin is light sensitive.
- Severe bone marrow toxicity may occur.
- Mitomycin acts as a radiation sensitizer. It is thus used in combination with radiation therapy. Mitomycin may also cause breakage of DNA strands, and is therefore a potent carcinogen and teratogen.

Table 27-1	Unique Adverse Effects of Selected Alkylating Agents
Drug	**Adverse Effect**
Cisplatin	nephrotoxicity, ototoxicity, peripheral neuropathy
Cyclophosphamide	hemorrhagic cystitis, cardiotoxicity
Ifosfamide	hemorrhagic cystitis, confusion leading to coma
Mitomycin	carcinogenic agent—may promote tumor formation; potent teratogen—may cause severe birth defects
Procarbazine	potential for hypertensive crisis due to inhibition of MAO; disulfiram-like reactions may occur

Antimetabolite Antineoplastic Drugs

This class of drugs interferes with cellular metabolism and the production of DNA by mimicking vital nutrients, or blocking reactions that synthesize a nutrient. Again, several subclasses exist, which have different actions. These drugs interfere with the utilization of folic acid, which is normally used to make thymidine, a component of DNA. Adverse effects for this group of drugs include suppression of the immune system (immunosuppression), rash, hair loss (alopecia), and vomiting (emesis).

Inhibitors of Folic Acid Utilization

The prototype for this class of drugs is methotrexate. Also included in the class is 5-fluorouracil, or 5-FU (because it has a slightly different mechanism, it is actually classified as a purine antagonist).

Methotrexate

Methotrexate is an inhibitor of the enzyme dihydrofolate reductase (DHFR), which is involved in the cellular cascade that results in the production of thymidine, a building block for the synthesis of DNA. The lack of thymidine results in DNA strand breakage and decreased cellular reproduction. RNA is not affected, as thymidine is not used in RNA.

Brand names: Trexall, Methotrex, Rheumatrex DP

Available as:
- Powder for injection: 20 mg and 1 g vials.
- Solution for injection: single-use vials: 50 mg, 100 mg, 200 mg, and 250 mg.
- Multi-use vials: 50 mg in 2 mL, 250 mg in 10 mL.
- Tablets: 2.5 mg tablets (Rheumatrex).
- Tablets: 5 mg, 7.5 mg, 10 mg, 15 mg (Trexall).

Adverse effects: Rash, immunosuppression, bone marrow suppression, and liver fibrosis (rare)

Special notes:
- Used in the treatment of choriocarcinoma, acute lymphocytic leukemia, breast cancer, and other cancer types.
- Used in the therapy of rheumatoid arthritis (due to its immunosuppressant properties).
- Methotrexate exhibits cell selectivity—the drug is selectively concentrated in lymph tissue, making it useful in the therapy of acute lymphoblastic leukemia, as well as treatment of choriocarcinoma and moderate grade lymphomas (grades 3 and 4). Methotrexate is also useful in treatment

of cancers of the breast and bladder, and is used intrathecally to treat malignant disease that has spread to the meninges. Intrathecal preparations should always be compounded with preservative-free diluents.

- Tumor cell resistance to this drug is not uncommon. Cells may produce altered DHFR or increased levels of DHFR. Entrance of the drug into the tumor cell may also be inhibited.

Leucovorin Rescue

Normal cells exposed to methotrexate can be "rescued" from the effects of the drug by the administration of leucovorin (reduced folic acid). The leucovorin allows for normal activity of DHFR, and allows production of thymidine. High doses of methotrexate can therefore be administered therapeutically, and the normal cells "rescued" with leucovorin. This provides for a significant effect on the rapidly dividing tumor cells, while minimizing effects on normal tissue.

Leucovorin calcium
Brand names: Leucovorin CA, Wellcovorin

Available as: 5 mg, 10 mg, 15 mg, and 25 mg tablets.

Injection: 50 mg, 100 mg, 250 mg, and 350 mg powder; 50 mL solution (10 mg/mL)

Storage: 15–30°C; protect from light

Pyrimidine Antagonists

5-FU can be useful in both rapidly growing tumors and more slow-growing tumors. In rapidly proliferating tumors, the major mechanism is inhibition of thymidylate synthase. In slow-growing tumors, the major mechanism is intercalation into nucleic acids. The drug inserts itself into the DNA structure, preventing the DNA from being copied.

This class of drugs inhibits the synthesis of DNA by inhibiting the synthesis of nucleotides.

5-Fluorouracil (5-FU)
5-Fluorouracil is a prodrug that is converted to an altered building block of DNA. Fluorouracil interferes in nucleic acid function, by inactivating a key enzyme required for the synthesis of DNA.

Brand names: Aducil, Efudex

Available as: 50 mg/mL solution for injection (10 mL multi-use vials); Efudex: topical preparation.

Dosage: Should not exceed 800 mg/day. Normal dosage is 12 mg/kg IV/day for four days, then 6 mg/kg/day every other day for an additional six days, beginning on day 6.

Administration: 5-FU may be administered orally, but administration by central line substantially reduces adverse effects. Survival rate appears to be independent of method of administration.

Adverse effects: include bone marrow suppression, thrombocytopenia, and hand-and-foot syndrome (in hand-and-foot syndrome, the patient experiences reddening of the palms and the soles of the feet—this is thought to be due to blood vessel damage caused by the drug).

Special notes:
- Solution may discolor slightly during storage—potency and safety are not affected.
- 5-FU is useful in the therapy of a variety of tumor types, alone or in combination with other drugs.

Use of Leucovorin with 5-FU

When used in conjunction with 5-FU, leucovorin produces the opposite effect of its use with methotrexate. Instead of rescuing cells, it *potentiates* the actions of the drug, by allowing more cofactor to be made and thus increasing the number of stabilized enzyme-cofactor complexes. This reduces the amount of enzyme available, and decreases the synthesis of thymidine. Thus, the use of leucovorin allows lower doses of 5-FU to be administered, decreasing the severity of adverse effects.

Capecitabine

Capecitabine is converted intracellularly to 5-FU. It thus has decreased adverse effects as compared with intravenous 5-FU—the adverse effect profile mimics the actions of 5-FU administered by central line.

Brand name: Xeloda

Dosage: 2,500 mg/m² per day in two doses, with food, for two weeks, followed by a one-week rest period.

Adverse effects: diarrhea, mucositis, and hand-and-foot syndrome.

Special notes:
- Used in the therapy of breast cancer, which is resistant to anthracycline antibiotics and paclitaxel.

Cytarabine

Cytarabine is a prodrug. It is metabolized intracellularly to an agent that competitively inhibits DNA polymerase, resulting in decreased DNA synthesis. The drug is also directly incorporated into both RNA and DNA, resulting in altered DNA and RNA synthesis.

Brand names: Cytosar U, DepoCyt (liposomal formulation)

Available as: 100 mg, 500 mg, 1 g, and 2 g vials of powder for injection (Cytosar); 50 mg/mL injectable suspension (DepoCyt).

Storage: Solutions made with bacteriostatic water for injection must be used immediately.

> Administration of 5-FU by rapid infusion, or in high doses, produces the highest level of myelosuppression. Administration of the drug by slow infusion reduces the incidence of myelosuppression to less than 15%.

Special notes:

- Cytarabine is not active orally.
- Powder for injection is reconstituted with bacteriostatic water USP.
- Solutions preserved with benzyl alcohol should not be used for dilution, if the drug is to be used for intrathecal injection (as well as any other type of preservative).
- Cytarabine must be administered by continuous infusion.
- Used in the therapy of acute myeloid and lymphoid leukemias. Also used in combination with anthracyclines (e.g., idarubicin) for induction therapy of acute myelogenous leukemia (AML). Used intrathecally to treat malignant disease that has spread to the meninges.

6-Mercaptopurine and Thioguanine

These agents have a narrow spectrum of activity. They are normally used only for maintenance therapy in patients with acute lymphocytic leukemia (ALL). They are metabolized to the nucleotide form of the nucleic acid (e.g., guanine) via hypoxanthine-guanine phosphoribosyl transferase (HGPRT). The nucleotide form is recognized by synthetic enzymes, and acts as a false substrate in the purine synthesis pathway.

6-Mercaptopurine

Brand name: Purinethol

Available as: 50 mg tablets.

Storage: Cool (15–25°C), dry place

Special notes:

- Only available orally.
- Used in the therapy of acute lymphocytic, lymphoblastic, or myelogenous leukemia.

6-Thioguanine

Brand name: Lanvis

Available as: 40 mg tablets, 75 mg injection (investigational).

Storage: Cool (15–25°C), dry place

Toxicity: These drugs cause rapid tumor cell lysis, which may precipitate gout.

Special notes:

- Only available for oral administration.
- Used in the therapy of acute, non-lymphocytic leukemia only.

Fludarabine

Fludarabine is a relatively new antimetabolite agent. It has significant activity against slow-growing lymphoid tumors and is indicated for the treatment of CLL. It is not effective against hairy cell leukemia.

Fludarabine phosphate

Brand name: Fludara

Available as: 50 mg single-dose glass vials, containing 50 mg of mannitol.

Dosage: 25 mg/m² for five consecutive days. Therapy may repeat in 28 days.

Storage: Refrigerated

Toxicity: Myelosuppression

Special notes:

- Fludarabine is a cell cycle–specific agent. It acts to inhibit DNA polymerase and interfere with cellular replication.

- Fludara should be diluted in 2 mL of sterile water for injection. The drug should fully dissolve in 15 seconds or less. The solution should be used within eight hours.

- Used in the therapy of B-cell chronic lymphocytic leukemia (CLL).

- Used as second-line therapy, if standard therapy with an alkylating agent is ineffective.

Pentostatin

Pentostatin is an antimetabolite agent. It has significant activity against slow-growing lymphoid tumors. Pentostatin is useful in the treatment of patients with active hairy cell leukemia who have not received previous treatment, or who have not responded to treatment with alpha interferons. Its use in the therapy of hairy cell leukemia has declined in favor of cladribine, which has a very high efficacy against hairy cell leukemia.

Pentostatin is structurally similar to a component of DNA that is necessary for DNA synthesis. Thus, it interferes with DNA synthesis. It is cell cycle specific. Pentostatin has the greatest effect in lymphocytes, particularly T-lymphocytes. Thus, this drug has an immunosuppressant effect. Reductions in T-cell numbers persist for long periods of time (months or years) posttreatment. It may take as much as four to five months to achieve a therapeutic response.

Brand name: Nipent

Available as: Powder for reconstitution—10 mg vial (with 50 mg mannitol—dilute with saline).

Storage: Refrigerated; dilute solution is stable at room temperature for eight hours

Contraindications: Pentostatin should not be used in combination with fludarabine, as extreme pulmonary toxicity may occur. Concurrent administration of allopurinol, colchicine, or probenecid for preexisting gout: Pentostatin may increase serum uric acid, due to rapid cell lysis. Concurrent administration of agents that suppress bone marrow (e.g., carbamazepine, felbamate, alkylating chemotherapeutic agents). Concurrent radiation therapy—bone marrow suppression may occur. Pentostatin is cleared by the kidney, so dosage should be reduced in patients without adequate renal function.

Special notes:
- Pentostatin is an antimetabolite drug.
- Not recommended for combination therapy with other drugs.
- Given as a bolus or intermittent infusion. Continuous infusion is not recommended.
- May worsen gout.
- Not approved for pediatric use.
- May promote viral skin infections (e.g., herpes, rash).
- Pentostatin does cross the blood-brain barrier, and may have CNS effects.
- Intravenous fluids must be administered before and after treatment.
- The major adverse effect is myelosuppression. Pentostatin may also cause severe allergic reactions (ranging from severe rash/hives to anaphylaxis).
- Due to its immunosuppressant effects, pentostatin may cause secondary malignancies (e.g., lymphoid tumors). Infertility may also occur.

Taxanes

Taxanes are plant alkaloids. They affect the arrangement of spindles in metaphase, interfering with cell replication. They are cell cycle specific.

Docetaxel
Brand name: Taxotere

Available as: 80 mg and 20 mg vials of concentrate for infusion, "premix" solution—10 mg/mL.

Storage: Refrigerated

Special notes:
- Docetaxel affects the formation of the cellular spindle "anchors" (centrosomes) in S phase, resulting in lack of mitotic spindle integrity.
- The drug also has limited effects on cells in the M phase (metaphase).
- Used in the therapy of breast and lung cancers.
- Should not be administered to patients with insufficient liver function.
- Not approved for pediatric use.
- It can cause edema and neurotoxicity.

Paclitaxel

Brand names: Taxol, Paxtene, Onxol, Abraxane

Available as: Multi-dose vials containing 30 mg/5 mL, 100 mg/16.7 mL, 300 mg/50 mL.

Dosage: 175 mg/m² over three hours, every three weeks. Dosage for Kaposi's sarcoma: 100–135 mg/m² q two to three weeks based on dose chosen

Adverse effects: Hematologic toxicity—bone marrow suppression, thrombocytopenia, hypersensitivity reactions (small fraction of patients), increased susceptibility to infection, fever, edema, skin toxicity—rash/hives on feet and hands, change in pigmentation of nails, inflammation of the mouth, cardiovascular effects, particularly hypotension and arrhythmias, febrile neutropenia, confusion, seizures, pulmonary edema, respiratory distress, interstitial pneumonia, neurotoxicity.

Drug interactions: Drug interactions may occur with medications metabolized by the cytochrome P_{450} system—specifically cytochrome. These include major macrolide antibiotics, certain antifungal drugs, and others.

Administration: Administration of paclitaxel as a second course of therapy after a regimen of cisplatin may result in severe bone marrow suppression. If paclitaxel therapy is instituted after therapy with an anthracycline antibiotic, an P_{450CA} increased incidence of congestive heart failure is seen. If paclitaxel is given concurrently with an anthracycline (e.g., doxorubicin), an increase in plasma levels of the anthracycline may be seen, leading to severe cardiac complications.

Contraindications: Severe hypersensitivity reactions occur in about 2% of patients and may be fatal. Patients who experience hypersensitivity reactions should be taken off of the drug and not be reinstituted. Patients with neutrophil counts 1,500 cells/mm³ should not have taxane therapy, due to myelosuppressant effects. For patients with AIDS, this limitation drops to 1,000 cells/mm³.

Resistance:
- "Multidrug resistance"—due to alterations in cellular drug efflux pump.
- Alterations in the alpha- and beta-tubulin subunits which decrease the rate of polymerization into microtubules.

Special notes:
- Paclitaxel affects the formation of mitotic spindles, resulting in inhibition of mitosis. It stabilizes microtubules, so that the normal assembly/disassembly procedure required for cellular transportation and mitosis cannot take place. In addition, it promotes aggregation of microtubules into bundles, rendering them nonfunctional.
- Used in the treatment of breast cancer; may also be used for non-small cell lung cancer.
- Second-line agent for the treatment of AIDS-related Kaposi's sarcoma.

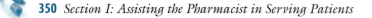

- Should not be stored in containers made of polyvinylchloride (PVC).
- Premedication with dexamethasone, diphenhydramine, or cimetidine is required to prevent possible hypersensitivity reactions.
- Cytotoxicity of the drug correlates with total dosage, rather than prolonged exposure, making the drug virtually schedule-independent. It has greatest effect on rapidly proliferating cells.

Topoisomerase Inhibitors

Etoposide and Teniposide

Etoposide and teniposide are plant alkaloids and inhibitors of topoisomerase II. Unlike the anthracyclines, these drugs do not bind directly to the enzyme, but stabilize the complex formed by the enzyme and DNA. When DNA and topoisomerase II are bound together, and can no longer dissociate, both are inactivated and further progression in the cell cycle is halted. DNA strand breaks develop, and the cell dies. These drugs are cell cycle specific.

Etoposide

Brand names: Vepesid, Toposar, VP-16

Available as: 50 mg capsules; 100 mg, 150 mg, 500 mg, and 1 g vials of powder for injection. Etoposide phosphate: 100 mg single-dose vials.

Dosage: Testicular cancer: Used in combination therapy, doses are 50–100 mg/m^2/day IV on a five-day regimen, *or* 100 mg/m^2/day given only on days 1, 3, and 5 of a five-day regimen. Lung cancer: Used in combination therapy, 35 mg/m^2/day for five days or 50 mg/m^2 for four days, IV. Therapy may be repeated at three- to four-week intervals.

Storage: Store under refrigeration (2–8° C); protect from light.

Forms: Etoposide and etoposide phosphate. Etoposide phosphate is more water soluble than etoposide. This form may have fewer adverse effects.

Adverse effects: Bone marrow suppression. White cell count is lowest around two weeks into therapy. Recovery from suppression may occur as early as three weeks post therapy. Nausea and vomiting. Changes in blood pressure (hypertensive or hypotensive episodes). Allergic reactions, including anaphylaxis, particularly during initial infusion. Alopecia. Infrequent adverse effects, such as GI distress, abdominal pain, Stevens-Johnson syndrome, cortical blindness, and hepatotoxicity.

Contraindications: Concurrent use of levimasole, cyclosporine.

Special note:
- Used in refractory testicular tumors and small cell lung cancer.

Teniposide

Teniposide is a phase-specific cytotoxic drug, acting in the late S or early G_2 phase of the cell cycle.

It causes dose-dependent single- and double-stranded breaks in DNA and RNA; protein crosslinking of DNA strands also occurs.

Brand name: Vumon

Available as: 10 mg/mL, 5 mL vials.

Dosage: 250 mg/m² weekly for four to eight weeks, in combination with vincristine and prednisone. Teniposide is administered intravenously, and should be dispensed from a nonreactive glass IV bottle or polyolefin bag to prevent extraction of plastic components. The central line administration apparatus must be thoroughly cleaned before using it with teniposide, as any residual polymer chemicals (e.g., heparin) may cause precipitation of the drug and occlusion of the line.

Storage: Refrigeration; drug may be frozen; protect from light.

Adverse effects: Severe myelosuppression with delayed recovery. Nausea and vomiting. Alopecia. Hypersensitivity reactions. CNS depression, particularly with prior administration of phenothiazine-type antiemetics (e.g., Compazine). Hypotension.

Contraindications: Hepatic insufficiency. Concurrent therapy with drugs that depress the central nervous system (e.g., antihistamines, sedative-hypnotic drugs, anticonvulsant drugs, narcotics, etc.). Concurrent therapy with drugs that are highly plasma protein bound (e.g., warfarin, carbamazepine, benzodiazepines, etc.).

Special notes:
- Used as initial (induction) therapy of acute lymphoblastic leukemia in children.
- Useful in the therapy of refractory childhood ALL.
- Severe hypotension may result if given by rapid injection—intravenous infusion is used.
- Teniposide should not be administered by bolus injection.

Camptothectins

The camptothectins, topotecan and irinotecan, are inhibitors of the enzyme topoisomerase I, which regulate the uncoiling of DNA prior to replication. They are highly cell-cycle phase specific, and cause defects in DNA repair, resulting in strand breakage. RNA is also affected.

These drugs are used in the therapy of refractive ovarian cancer, and in the therapy of small cell lung cancer.

Topotecan

Brand name: Hycamtin

Available as: 4 mg single-dose vials of lyophilized powder; package of 1 or 5; 0.25 mg and 1 mg capsules.

Dosage: Dosage of topotecan is 1.5 mg/m² IV in a 30-minute infusion per day, for five days. A subsequent period of 16 days drug-free completes a 21-day course. Cervical cancer is dosed at 0.75mg/m² for 3 days. Dosage adjustment does not appear to be necessary in patients with mild renal impairment or hepatic dysfunction. In the same way, dosage adjustment is not required in the elderly, unless renal clearance is impaired.

Storage: Solution is stable for 24 hours at room temperature and normal lighting.

Adverse effects: Nausea and vomiting are most frequent. Total alopecia, including body hair. Mild hepatotoxicity. Thrombocytopenia (rare). Dermatitis (rare).

Contraindications: Bone marrow depression may be severe, if given in conjunction with cisplatin. Interactions with other medications have not fully been elucidated.

Special note:
- Used as second-line therapy for carcinoma of the ovary and small cell lung cancer.

Antibiotic Chemotherapeutic Agents

Bleomycin

Bleomycin is an older drug that is relatively cell cycle specific (G_2 and M phases).

Bleomycin exerts its effects on DNA through a multistep process. Initially, the DNA forms a complex with iron and oxygen, in the presence of DNA. This stabilizes the molecule by complexing it. This complex then binds to DNA.

The binding of the bleomycin complex to DNA occurs at certain nucleotide sequences via electrostatic interactions and partial intercalation of bleomycin into the DNA molecule. In addition to stabilizing the molecule, the bleomycin complex causes single- and double-strand breaks.

Brand names: Bleocin, Blenoxane

Available as: Vials of powder for injection containing 15 units or 30 units.

Dosage: Given weekly or biweekly, parenterally (IV, IM, SC). After a 50% response, in the treatment of Hodgkin's lymphoma, a maintenance dose is given of 1 unit (0.025 mg) daily or 5 units weekly IV or IM.

Storage: Refrigeration; drug should be discarded after the expiration date.

Adverse effects: Bleomycin causes pulmonary toxicity. This presents initially as pneumonitis, which progresses to pulmonary fibrosis. Post-therapy, bleomycin can make the adverse pulmonary effects due to oxygen administration worse. Rash and occasional vascular toxicities may be seen.

Special notes:
- Used in the therapy of squamous cell carcinoma, testicular carcinoma, and lymphomas.
- Considered palliative treatment for Hodgkin's and non-Hodgkin's lymphoma, testicular carcinoma, and squamous cell carcinomas of the head and neck.
- Bone marrow suppression is not seen, as bone marrow tissue contains a high level of bleomycin hydrolase, which inactivates the drug.
- Therapy should be initiated with a very low dose (0.2 units) because of the possibility of anaphylactic reactions.
- Given by IM, IV, and SC routes.
- A dose-related pulmonary toxicity is seen.
- Loss of potency may result if the drug is reconstituted in D_5W or other sugar solutions.

Anthracycline Antibiotics

Anthracycline antibiotics are a group of highly toxic drugs with specific efficacies. Anthracyclines intercalate between base pairs in DNA, causing the helix to change shape, which interferes with strand elongation. They are cell cycle nonspecific.

Doxorubicin HCl (liposomal injection)
Brand name: Doxil

Available as: Vial of 2 mg/mL, 10 mL or 25 mL.

Dosage: 20 mg/m² over 30 minutes, once every three weeks for Kaposi's syndrome

Storage: Refrigerated; short-term freezing permitted

Special notes:
- Used in the therapy of metastatic carcinoma of the ovary and Kaposi's sarcoma.
- Bolus injection is not recommended.

Doxorubicin
Brand names: Adriamycin, Adriamycin PF, Rubex

Available as: 10 mg, 20 mg, 50 mg, (2 mg/mL); 10 mg, 20 mg, 50 mg single-dose polypropylene vials (2 mg/mL); 150 mg multidose glass vial.

Dosage: For treatment of ovarian carcinoma: 50 mg/m² infused at a rate of 1 mg/minute repeated every four weeks for as long as tumor progression continues to be inhibited, and cardiotoxicity is not manifested. Four courses of therapy may be necessary before tumor regression is seen.

Storage: Diluted solution is stable for 15 days under refrigeration, 7 days at room temperature and ambient lighting.

Adverse effects: The dose-limiting adverse effect of doxorubicin is cardiotoxicity, including congestive heart failure. Other adverse effects include: bone marrow depression, hand-and-foot syndrome, dry mouth, nausea, and vomiting.

Contraindications: Doxorubicin should be used with caution in the elderly, and patients with compromised heart function.

Special notes:
- This drug is *cardiotoxic* and *may cause congestive heart failure.*
- Doxorubicin should not be given as a bolus dose, as the risk of cardio-toxicity is greatly increased.

Dactinomycin

Dactinomycin is an anthracycline antibiotic, similar to doxorubicin.

Brand name: Cosmegen, (Actinomycin-D)

Available as: Powder for injection—0.5 mg vials with 20 mg mannitol added.

Dosage: Drug dosage depends on the type of tumor and the needs of the patient

Adverse effects: Adverse effects are delayed. Emesis may occur during therapy, but other adverse effects do not generally occur for several weeks after cessation of therapy. Adverse effects are serious and include: bone marrow depression, liver toxicity (including hepatomegaly, hepatitis, and ascites), corrosion of soft tissue with extravasation at the injection site, GI and mouth ulceration, alopecia, skin rashes, and emesis.

Contraindications: Previous courses with daunorubicin or doxorubicin can potentially cause cardiotoxicity.

Special note:
- Useful as part of a combination drug regimen in the treatment of Wilm's tumor, childhood rhabdomyosarcoma, Ewing's sarcoma, gestational trophoblastic neoplasia, and nonseminiferous metastatic testicular cancer (in a combination regimen with cyclophosphamide, bleomycin, vinblastine, and cisplatin).

Daunorubicin HCl

Brand names: Cerubidine, Daunoxome (daunorubicin citrate—liposomal formulation)

Available as: Single-dose vials containing 20 mg of doxorubicin and 100 mg mannitol.

Dosage: Adult dosage—45 mg/m² for three days. Pediatric dose: 75 mg/m² weekly in combination with prednisone and vincristine

Storage: Reconstituted solution is stable for 24 hours at room temperature, 48 hours under refrigeration; protect from light.

Adverse effects: Dose-limiting toxicity includes myelosuppression and cardiotoxicity (the cardiotoxicity of daunorubicin is decreased as compared with doxorubicin). Other adverse effects include: thrombophlebitis and/or tissue necrosis at the injection site, alopecia, nausea and vomiting, hyperuricemia (especially in patients with leukemia), fever and chills, anaphylaxis (rare).

Special notes:

- Used in the therapy of non-lymphocytic leukemia, in combination with cytosine arabinoside.

- Daunorubicin *must be administered by continuous infusion* and not by any other parenteral route, as tissue necrosis will occur.

- Indicated for treatment of remission in leukemic disorders—AML (adults) and ALL (children and adults).

Idarubicin

Idarubicin is similar to (is an *analog* of) doxorubicin, and has similar uses and properties. Idarubicin is less lipophilic, and therefore has less cardiotoxicity than doxorubicin or daunorubicin. It has a greater affinity for DNA and increased DNA binding, as compared with doxorubicin, and is more readily taken up into target cells. In addition, idarubicin inhibits the uptake of thymidine into cancer cells at lower concentrations, and may thus be considered more potent.

Idarubicin has orphan drug designation for acute myelogenous leukemia, acute lymphoblastic leukemia in pediatrics, chronic myelogenous leukemia, and myelodysplastic syndrome.

Brand name: Idamycin

Available as: Single-use vials of 1 mg/mL solution in 5 mL, 10 mL, and 20 mL strengths.

Dosage: 12 mg/m²/day for three days, in combination with cytarabine (100 mg/m² for seven days)

Storage: Refrigeration; protect from light

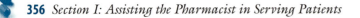

Special notes:
- Used in the therapy of acute myeloid leukemia in adults.
- Must be given slowly, in a dilute intravenous solution (IV drip), as tissue necrosis may occur.
- Cardiotoxic.
- Should not be mixed directly with other drugs or exposed to alkaline pH.

Drugs Used in Combination with Cancer Chemotherapy

The major uncomfortable and/or potentially debilitating adverse effects of cancer chemotherapy are bone marrow depression and nausea/vomiting. There are drugs that are used in combination with cancer chemotherapeutics to combat these effects and improve the well-being of the patient.

Drugs Used in the Therapy of Bone Marrow Suppression

The major drug effective against red blood cell loss is actually a hormone—erythropoietin.

Epoetin alfa

Brand names: Epogen, Procrit

Available as: 10 mL vials containing 2,000 units/mL, 3,000 units/mL, 4,000 units/mL, and 10,000 units/mL in trays of 6 or 25 vials; 1 mL and 2 mL multidose 20,000 unit vials of preserved solution.

Dosage: 50–100 units/kg three times weekly; administered intravenously or SC

Storage: 2–8°C; do not freeze or shake

Special notes:
- For use in cancer patients receiving continuous chemotherapy for at least two months.
- Is intended for patients with bone marrow depression. It is not indicated for use in patients with simple anemia, due to lack of vitamins or iron.
- Hemoglobin should be 10–13 g/dL for appropriate treatment with erythropoetin.

Filgrastim

Brand name: Neupogen

Available as: 300 mcg and 480 mcg vials or prefilled syringes.

Storage: Must be refrigerated; no shaking. It can be warmed to room temperature for administration. Can remain out of the refrigerator no longer than 24 hours.

Special notes:
- A white blood cell stimulator.
- Neupogen is produced by recombinant DNA technology.
- Also reduces the time to neutrophil recovery.

Pegfilgrastim
Brand name: Neulasta

Available as: 0.6 mL syringe (6 mg dose).

Storage: Must be refrigerated; no shaking. It can be warmed to room temperature for administration. Can remain out of the refrigerator no longer than 48 hours.

Special notes:
- Decreases the incidence of infection from febrile neutropenia.
- Neulasta is a covalent conjugate of Neupogen.

Drugs Used in the Therapy of Emesis

There are several drugs used in the therapy of nausea and vomiting in the hospital setting for chemotherapy treatment. In addition, certain antihistamines may alleviate nausea as well (e.g., meclizine). The following drugs are used:

Metoclopramide HCl
Brand name: Reglan

Available as: 5 mg and 10 mg tablets, 5 mg/5 mL syrup for oral administration; parenteral formulations: 5 mg/mL single dose vials of 2, 10, or 30 mL single-dose ampules of 2 mL.

Special note:
- Reglan antagonizes dopamine, but does not cross into the brain. Thus, there are fewer adverse effects than with Compazine.

Prochlorperazine maleate
Brand name: Compazine

Available as: 5 mg and 10 mg tablets; 15 mg and 10 mg sustained-release spansules; 2 mL and 10 mL vials of 5 mg/mL injectable solution; 2.5 mg, 5 mg/5 mL syrup; 2.5 mg, 5 mg, or 25 mg suppositories.

Special note:

- Prochlorperazine is a phenothiazine class of antipsychotic. It has strong antiemetic effects, but can produce the same adverse effects as other drugs of the class (e.g., Parkinson's-like effects). It may also affect the heart, as it has peripheral effects on dopamine.

Prochlorperazine edisylate

Brand name: Compazine

Available as: 5 mg/mL solution for parenteral use; 2 mL cartridges for injection.

Special notes:

- Total parenteral dosage should not exceed 40 mg/day.
- May cause Parkinson's-like symptoms, especially in children.

Ondansetron

Brand name: Zofran

Available as: 2 mg/mL injection; 4 mg/5 mL oral solution; 4 mg, 8 mg, and 24 mg tablets, also orally disintegrating tablets.

- It is a Selective 5-HT$_3$ receptor agonist.
- It should be administered 30 minutes prior to chemotherapy.
- It is used in chemo-induced emesis.

Chapter Review Questions

1. Which of the following drugs is cardiotoxic?
   a. Methotrexate
   b. Doxorubicin
   c. Topotecan
   d. Reglan

2. Which of the following may be taken orally?
   a. Reglan
   b. Idamycin
   c. Cytoxan
   d. both a and c

3. Which of the following is used in the therapy of nausea caused by cancer chemotherapy?
   a. Reglan
   b. Compazine
   c. Epoetin
   d. both a and c

4. Which of the following can be given by subcutaneous injection?
   a. Taxol
   b. Reglan
   c. Bleocin
   d. Adriamycin

5. A patient is on methotrexate chemotherapy. Which of the following would be contraindicated?
   a. Amoxil
   b. A B-vitamin supplement containing folinic acid
   c. Cardioquin
   d. Calan

6. Which of the following should be administered by central line infusion?
   a. Bleocin
   b. 5-FU
   c. Methotrexate
   d. Topotecan

7. Procrit is available in:
   a. tablet form.
   b. 10 mL multidose vials.
   c. 1 mL single use vials.
   d. frozen solution.

8. Which of the following cancer chemotherapeutics is used in the therapy of arthritis, due to over-activity of the immune system?
   a. Topotecan
   b. Adriamycin
   c. Methotrexate
   d. 5-FU

9. Which drug is considered a "rescue drug"?
   a. leucovorin
   b. Reglan
   c. Taxol
   d. INH

10. Which drug is a nitrogen mustard derivative?
    a. Cisplatin
    b. Methotrexate
    c. Taxotere
    d. Cyclophosphamide

CHAPTER 28

Gastrointestinal System Agents

Quick Study

I. Drugs that inhibit the secretion of gastric acid

    A. Histamine antagonists
    B. Muscarinic antagonists

II. Drugs that inhibit the formation of gastric acid

    A. Proton pump inhibitors—mechanism of action
    B. The therapy of ulcers—different drugs with varying properties and uses

III. Drugs that neutralize gastric acid—onset, duration, efficacy, and potential adverse effects

    A. Sodium bicarbonate–based drugs—rapid onset, short duration, may cause systemic alkalosis
    B. Calcium carbonate–based drugs—intermediate onset and duration. These drugs cause calcium rebound
    C. Magnesium carbonate–based drugs—intermediate onset and duration; these drugs also have laxative properties
    D. Aluminum-containing drugs—slow onset, long duration; these drugs may contribute to the etiology of Alzheimer's disease

IV. Cytoprotective agents

    A. Prostanoids—effects and adverse effects
    B. Coating agents—sucralfate and bismuth subsalicylate (Pepto-Bismol)

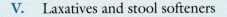

V. Laxatives and stool softeners

    A. Irritant laxatives
    B. Bulk laxatives
    C. Stool softeners (e.g., docusate, glycerin)

VI. Antidiarrheals

    A. Binding agents (e.g., Kaopectate)
    B. Opiates (e.g., loperamide, propoxyphene)

VII. Drugs used in the therapy of parasitic infections (anthelmintics)

Histamine (H2) Receptor Antagonists

Physiology Review

Gastric acid is made by separating carbonic acid into bicarbonate (base) and acid (H^+) and adding sodium chloride, forming hydrochloric acid (HCl) and sodium bicarbonate ($NaHCO_3$). This separation is done by the **proton pumps** in the parietal cells of the stomach lining. In order for the acid to be released, we also need calcium, histamine, and/or acetylcholine. Blocking receptors for histamine or acetylcholine will decrease the amount of acid secreted into the stomach, as will blockade of the proton pump. In the same way, increased amounts of acetylcholine or calcium will *increase* the secretion of stomach acid.

Gastric acid is made in the parietal cells of the stomach lining. The release of gastric acid is dependent on certain hormones, as well as acetylcholine and histamine. If the actions of either acetylcholine or histamine are blocked, the secretion of gastric acid will correspondingly decrease.

Drugs that block histamine receptors in the stomach lining must first be absorbed into the body and enter the parietal cells of the stomach from the blood. They then act to inhibit the release of acid into the lumen of the stomach. Because they must first be absorbed, rather than acting directly on the stomach lining, they do not have immediate effects. H_2 receptor antagonists:

- have a delayed onset, but a long duration of action (up to nine hours).
- have major drug interactions, as they will change the clearance rate of other drugs—H_2 antagonists are also extensively metabolized, and affect the cytochrome P_{450} system. They thus will alter the rate of metabolism of drugs using the same enzyme system.
- interfere with the absorption of drugs that are normally absorbed through the stomach (e.g., aspirin), because they decrease acidity.

Drugs

Cimetidine

Brand names: Tagamet, Tagamet HB (OTC)

Available as: 200 mg, 300 mg, 400 mg, and 800 mg tablets; 150 mg/mL and 300 mg/50 mL solution for injection, 300 mg/5 mL liquid; also available OTC in 200 mg tablets.

Special notes:
- Cimetidine is the oldest of the drugs in the class and the least potent.
- This drug has a potent effect on cytochrome P_{450} and may produce a variety of drug interactions.
- Cimetidine has weak anti-androgenic activity and may cause male infertility with frequent or prolonged use.

Ranitidine

Brand names: Zantac, Zantac OTC

Available as: 150 mg and 300 mg tablets; 25 mg effervescent tablet; 150 mg granules for reconstitution; 15 mg/mL syrup; 25 mg/mL injection. Zantac OTC: 75 mg tablets.

Special notes:
- Ranitidine is more potent than cimetidine—approximately 10 to 15 times as potent.
- Useful in the therapy of peptic ulcers.
- Less effect on cytochrome P_{450} than cimetidine.

Famotidine

Brand names: Pepcid, Pepcid AC

Available as: 20 mg and 40 mg tablets; 10 mg/mL solution for injection; 40 mg/5 mL powder for reconstitution. Pepcid AC (OTC): 10 mg tablets, 10 mg chew tab.

Special notes:
- 1,000 times as potent as cimetidine.
- Famotidine has no effect on cytochrome P_{450} and thus produces no enzyme-related drug interactions.
- The injectable form must be refrigerated.

Nizatidine

Brand names: Axid, Axid AR (OTC)

Available as: 150 mg and 300 mg capsules; Axid AR (OTC): 75 mg tablets; 15 mg/1 mL oral solution.

Special note:
- Newest of the H_2 antagonists—increased potency, with decreased drug interactions.

Drugs That Neutralize Gastric Acid: Antacids

Antacids are weakly basic drugs that chemically react with stomach acid, forming a salt and water. They have an immediate onset and relatively short duration of action. For the most part, they are sold over the counter. Antacids can interfere with drug absorption, and can increase the elimination of certain drugs (e.g., drugs that are weak acids and are eliminated by the kidney). It may decrease the rate of elimination of drugs that are weak bases. Binding to other medications may also occur; therefore, it is suggested to administer 2 hours apart from other medications.

Drugs That Are Commonly Sold Over the Counter

> Sodium bicarbonate will increase the rate of elimination of drugs that are weak acids and are eliminated through the urine, and decrease the elimination of those that are weak bases.

Sodium bicarbonate (Alka-Seltzer)
Sodium bicarbonate acts very rapidly to neutralize acid. It is also rapidly absorbed, so it can produce systemic alkalosis with frequent or excessive dosing.

Calcium carbonate (Tums, Rolaids)
Calcium carbonate has a longer duration of action than sodium bicarbonate and is more potent. The problem with calcium-containing antacids is that calcium stimulates acid secretion, so, once the acid is neutralized by the carbonate, more is released, due to the actions of the calcium. This is called *calcium rebound*.

Magnesium hydroxide (Rolaids, Milk of Magnesia)
Magnesium hydroxide is not well absorbed, and thus has fewer systemic actions than calcium carbonate or sodium bicarbonate, and has a longer duration of action. It will also act as a laxative, so overuse can cause diarrhea.

Aluminum hydroxide (Mylanta)
Aluminum hydroxide is a potent acid neutralizer and has a very long duration of action. Aluminum has, however, been linked to the etiology of Alzheimer's disease. It can also lead to constipation.

Proton Pump Inhibitors

Proton pump inhibitors inhibit the cellular pump that is responsible for making gastric acid (see Figure 28-1). These drugs are unique in that they require activation by an acid environment before they will have an effect. Thus, *if*

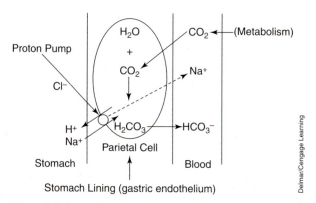

Figure 28-1: A Schematic Representation of Gastric Acid Production

these drugs are taken when they are not needed (e.g., if increased production of gastric acid is not present), they will not work. These drugs:

- are absorbed in the duodenum.
- are highly plasma protein bound (97%).
- have a fast onset (about an hour) and long duration (up to three days).
- are most effective when given 30 minutes prior to a meal.

Additionally, these drugs:

- enter the stomach lining from the blood, and must be activated before they will work.
- inhibit the actions of cytochrome P_{450}, so drug interactions may be seen.
- are effective against the stomach bacteria (*H. pylorii*) that causes ulcers when given in combination with an antibiotic. This makes them very useful in the therapy of gastric ulcers.

Drugs Prescribed

Omeprazole

Brand name: Prilosec

Available as: 10 mg and 20 mg delayed-release tablets; 10 mg and 20 mg OTC formula; 2.5 mg/5 mL and 10 mg/15 mL oral suspension (powder packets to be diluted).

Special note:
- This drug is the oldest and least potent of the class.

Esomeprazole

Brand name: Nexium

Available as: 20 mg and 40 mg delayed-release tablets.

Special note:
- Esomeprazole is similar to omeprazole (it is the S-isomer of omeprazole). It has a very high degree of activity against *H. pylorii* when used in combination with an antibiotic.

Lansoprazole

Brand name: Prevacid

Available as: 15 mg and 30 mg delayed-release tablets; 15 mg disintegrating tablet; 15 mg and 30 mg granule packets; 15 mg and 24 mg OTC tablets.

Special note:
- This drug has an extremely long duration of action—acid suppression lasts 24 hours.

Pantoprazole

Brand name: Protonix

Available as: 20 mg and 40 mg tablets; 40 mg injection; 40 mg granule packet.

Special notes:
- It suppresses gastric acid secretion by inhibition of parietal cells (H^+/K^+ ATP pump).
- The unlabeled use is for peptic ulcer disease.
- It can cause diarrhea and abdominal pain.
- The injection form must be stored in the refrigerator.
- It has a very short half-life (approx. 1 hour).

Cytoprotective Agents

These agents coat and protect the stomach lining. They form a protective barrier to stomach acid and promote healing of ulcers.

Misoprostol

Brand name: Cytotec

Classification: Synthetic prostaglandin, anti-ulcer drug

Available as: 100 mcg and 200 mcg tablets.

Special notes:
- Misoprostol increases mucous production from the stomach lining.
- May decrease acid secretion.
- May be used as a prophylactic, and also forms a protective barrier around an existing ulcer.
- Has a rapid onset—inhibition of gastric acid secretion occurs within 30 minutes.

- Misoprostol has a high first-pass effect through the liver, producing an active metabolite.
- Is contraindicated in pregnancy, as it may cause contraction of uterine smooth muscle.
- It is also used to ripen the cervix in preparation for delivery.

Sucralfate
Brand name: Carafate
Available as: 1 gram tablets, 1 gram/10 mL suspension.

Special notes:
- An adhesive polymer that binds to the stomach lining and promotes healing.
- May also bind to orally administered drugs, resulting in a lack of absorption of the drugs.

Laxatives

Laxative agents consist of four types:

- *Irritant (stimulant) laxatives*—These agents irritate the intestinal lining, causing secretions that soften the stool. Examples are *bisacodyl* and *senna* (a "natural" product).
- *Bulk laxatives*—These agents absorb water and are incorporated into the stool, which softens it. Examples are *psyllium husk (Metamucil)* and *citrus fiber (Citrucel)*.
- *Stool softeners (demulcents)*—These agents are oily substances that both bind water and make the stool softer, and thus more "slippery" and easier to pass. Examples are *docusate, glycerin,* and *mineral oil.*
- *Osmotics*—These agents cause water retention in the stool material by the process of osmosis. Examples are *lactulose* and *polyethylene glycol 3350* (MiraLax).

Laxative agents are sold in various preparations over the counter (e.g., Dulcolax contains bisacodyl and ExLax contains senna).

Antidiarrheals

These agents are sold over the counter or by prescription (C-V) and are opiates. These opiates do not cross the blood-brain barrier well, or, as in the case of over-the-counter drugs, do not cross at all. Opiates slow the bowel and are very effective in the therapy of diarrhea. Drugs available include:

Diphenoxylate with atropine
Brand name: Lomotil

Available as: Tablets: 2.5 mg of diphenoxylate and 0.025 mg of atropine; Liquid: 2.5 mg of diphenoxylate and 0.025 mg of atropine/5 mL. C-V.

Special notes:

- Diphenoxylate does not cross the blood-brain barrier well, but will accumulate in the brain in high doses, so the drug is potentially abusable.
- Atropine is added to discourage abuse—high levels of atropine can cause central nervous system and cardiac effects that are unpleasant (e.g., dry mouth, tachycardia, confusion).
- This drug is sold by prescription and is classified as class V.
- Overdosage: In case of overdosage, procedures for opiate overdose should be followed (e.g., respiratory support and the administration of opiate antagonists should be used, as appropriate). Atropine intoxication may also be seen, with symptoms including confusion, tachycardia, and dry mouth. This may be remedied by the administration of physostigmine.

Loperamide

Brand name: Imodium

Available as: 1 mg and 2 mg tablets (OTC); 2 mg/5 mL liquid.

Special notes:

- Loperamide does not cross the blood-brain barrier and is not abusable.
- This drug is sold over the counter.

Drugs for Use in Parasitic Infections

Two types of parasites seen most commonly are lice and roundworms. Lice are multi-legged creatures that attach to the skin in areas that have a large number of hair strands, and suck the blood from surface vessels of the skin. Because they attach to the skin and hide in the hair, they are difficult to reach and kill with a topical drug agent. In addition, the eggs are not affected by most agents. Thus, lice are difficult to eradicate. The preparations commonly used for lice infestations in days past were petroleum derivatives, such as gasoline and kerosene. We now have the less dangerous alternative of piperonyl butoxide (RID, A-200), which is available over the counter. Also marketed by prescription are the potentially toxic alternatives of organophosphate insecticides (e.g., malathion).

Nematode Infestations

Nematodes, such as roundworm and pinworm, are fairly common in the United States, especially among children. These parasites can be picked up from the soil, and are commonly picked up from infested pets. The mature worms lay eggs at the anus, which causes itching, as the tails of the worms move around. The person (or pet) begins to scratch, which eventually conveys the eggs to the mouth. Once swallowed, the eggs hatch in the intestine and mature, completing the cycle. Drugs used in the therapy of worm infestations are called *anthelmintics.* Anthelmintics presently on the market for nematode infestations are pyrantel pamoate (sold over the counter—Pin-X), as well as thiabendazole and mebendazole. These drugs act on nematode proteins called tubulin (or enzymes related to tubulin processing), paralyzing the organism, so that it cannot survive or breed. Because the eggs are impervious to outside influences (e.g., stomach acid, medication), these medications are only effective against the adult worms. Some of these drugs can act on mammalian tubulin as well (e.g., mebendazole), which can be detrimental to the patient, especially in pregnancy. Drugs available for the therapy of pinworm and roundworm infestations include:

Mebendazole
Brand name: Vermox

Classification: Anthelmintic, microtubule inhibitor

Available as: 100 mg chewable tablets.

Special notes:
- Mebendazole inhibits the formation of nematodal tubulin.
- It will also affect human tubulin and crosses the fetal-placental barrier.
- Contraindicated in pregnancy.

Thiabendazole
Brand name: Mintezol

Classification: Anthelmintic, enzyme inhibitor

Available as: 500 mg chewable tablets; 500 mg/5 ml suspension.

Special notes:
- More potent than mebendazole.
- May be used safely in pregnancy, as it does not cross the placenta.

Chapter Review Questions

1. Which of these drugs is a histamine receptor blocker?
   a. Imodium
   b. Axid
   c. Prilosec
   d. Nexium

2. Which of these drugs has interactions with drugs that are metabolized by cytochrome P_{450}?
   a. Tagamet
   b. Axid
   c. Lomotil
   d. both a and b

3. A patient has eaten spicy food and has heartburn. Which of these drugs would be the correct therapy?
   a. Tums
   b. Prilosec
   c. Lansoprazole
   d. Tagamet

4. Which of these drugs is available for injection?
   a. Prilosec
   b. Carafate
   c. Zantac
   d. Axid

5. Which of these drugs is a delayed-release formulation?
   a. Cytotec
   b. Tagamet
   c. Prevacid
   d. Mylanta

6. Which of the following may cause smooth muscle contraction and possibly premature labor?
   a. Carafate
   b. Misoprostol
   c. Nexium
   d. Citrucel

7. Docusate sodium and mineral oil are:
   a. demulcents
   b. laxatives
   c. proton pump inhibitors
   d. antacids

8. Which of the following contains an opiate?
   a. Prilosec
   b. Imodium
   c. Vermox
   d. Tagamet

9. Which of the following might cause tachycardia in high doses?
   a. Mebendazole
   b. Nexium
   c. Lomotil
   d. ExLax

10. Mintezol:
    a. is contraindicated in pregnancy
    b. is useful in nematode infestations (e.g., roundworm)
    c. is used for diarrhea
    d. is used for acid reflux disease

11. The patient profile for Amelda Jones contains the following drugs: Lomotil Verapamil, OxyContin. In addition, she is taking Tums over the counter. Which drugs should you call to the attention of the pharmacist?
    a. Lomotil and OxyContin
    b. Verapamil and the antacid
    c. Tums and OxyContin
    d. Verapamil and Tums

12. A patient is taking phenobarbital for seizures (phenobarbital is a weak acid, partially eliminated by the kidney). He takes a lot of Alka-Seltzer for his upset stomach. Which of the following could happen?
    a. he will develop a rash
    b. he will have abdominal pain
    c. his seizures will increase in frequency
    d. he will accumulate toxic levels of phenobarbital

13. A patient is taking Tegretol. Which of the following drugs in his patient profile might interfere with the drug?
    a. Lasix
    b. Calan
    c. Adalat
    d. Carafate

14. Which of the following is a proton pump inhibitor?
    a. Protonix
    b. Tagamet
    c. Dulcolax
    d. Imodium

15. Which of the following is a C-V drug?
    a. Dulcolax
    b. Lomotil
    c. Cytotec
    d. Pepcid

CHAPTER 29

Endocrine System and Reproductive System Agents

Quick Study

I.   Drugs used in the therapy of diabetes mellitus

    A.   Drugs used in type I diabetes—insulin and the various insulin formulations

    B.   Drugs used in type II diabetes mellitus

        1.   Sulfonylureas

        2.   Drugs that regulate blood sugar—meglitanides and thiazolinediones

    C.   Drugs useful in both type I and II diabetes mellitus

II. Drugs used in the therapy of hypothyroidism

III. Drugs used in the therapy of hyperthyroidism

IV. Reproductive hormone replacement and antagonists

Physiology Review

The endocrine system is a system of glands, which secrete chemical substances (hormones) into the blood. There are two classes of hormones—**peptide** hormones, which are essentially small proteins, and **steroid** hormones, which are lipid in nature. The majority of peptide hormones are secreted from the anterior pituitary, with the exception of insulin and glucagon, which are secreted from islet cells in the pancreas (the *endocrine pancreas*).

The Therapy of Diabetes Mellitus

Diabetes mellitus results from a lack of insulin effects. It may arise from two causes:

1. Lack of insulin. This is termed **type I diabetes** and results from too little insulin being secreted. This condition can either result from chemical toxicity or have a genetic basis and is treated with daily injections of insulin. Although it is not commonly used anymore, type I diabetes is sometimes referred to as insulin-dependent diabetes.

2. **Type II diabetes** results from a lack of functional insulin receptors. Insulin is secreted in response to a food stimulus. If a person secretes too much insulin, the receptors may compensate by desensitizing or decreasing in number ("down regulation") with time. Receptors may also be genetically defective. This type of diabetes is treated with drugs that may increase the sensitivity of the receptors, or slow carbohydrate absorption, etc. *Administration of insulin may not be appropriate for these patients in the early stages of the disease, but may eventually require insulin.*

INSULIN

Insulin is released from the endocrine pancreas in response to ingested sugars and amino acids. Low levels of insulin are constantly being secreted into the blood. Insulin serves two major functions in the body: the storage and utilization of sugars and promotion of tissue growth. It is required for maintenance of tissues, particularly vascular tissue, and without it small blood vessels begin to break down. This results in decreased oxygen delivery to tissues in the extremities (fingertips and toes, particularly), and to the retina. As a result, lack of insulin can cause gangrene of the fingertips and toes under the right conditions (lack of insulin in combination with infection) and can also cause blindness.

Therapy of Type I Diabetes

Type I diabetes is treated with insulin injections. Insulin is injected subcutaneously, using an insulin syringe and attached 28 – 31G needle. An easy-to-use *pen* form is also available for most insulins.

An insulin solution or suspension must be kept refrigerated, or it will lose potency. It should not be frozen. An opened bottle of insulin may be stored at room temperature for up to 28 days.

Types of Insulin

Complexing of the insulin with zinc or protamine (a protein) will increase the duration of action of the insulin.

There are now many types of insulin that have different sources and different durations of action.

Insulin products today are made by splicing human genes into bacteria, which then make the insulin ("cloned" human insulin). Beef and pork were original sources of insulin but are no longer used due to the advent of newer, safer technologies and quality control problems. Complexing of the insulin with zinc or protamine (a protein) will increase the duration of action of the insulin, as the insulin must be chopped off of the complex before it can be used (this complexing is like making a storage form, from which the insulin can be extracted as needed).

Forms of insulin available:

- Rapid-acting
- Short-acting
- Intermediates
- Long-acting
- Premixes

NPH insulin, or Neutral Protamine Hagdorn insulin, is insulin that has been complexed with protamine for a longer duration of action.

> **NOTE**
>
> *Complexed insulin, such as NPH insulin, is not useful in a crisis situation (e.g., diabetic coma), as the onset is delayed!* A rapid-acting insulin (e.g., insulin as part or normal insulin) must be used.

Dosage forms available:

- Solution for subcutaneous injection
- Pen injection with insulin cartridges of 3 mL each

Rapid-Acting Insulins

Insulin aspart
Brand name: Novolog

Available as: Solution for injection.

Storage: Vials of solution should be stored under refrigeration, but not frozen. Vials in use may be stored at controlled room temperature, away from direct heat or light, for up to 28 days. They should then be discarded.

Insulin lispro
Brand name: Humalog

Available as: Solution for injection, 100 units/mL.

Storage: Vials of solution should be stored under refrigeration, but not frozen. Vials in use may be stored at controlled room temperature, away from direct heat or light, for up to 28 days. They should then be discarded.

Special notes:
- It is an analog of human insulin (cloned from *E. coli*).
- It has a short duration of action.
- For use in combination with longer-acting forms of insulin.
- Potency is equal to that of human insulin, but onset is more rapid.
- Humalog is similar to insulin aspart in character.

Short-Acting Insulins

Human insulin
Brand names: Humulin R (zinc regular insulin)

- *Humulin R:* A complex of zinc with regular insulin. This type of insulin has a *rapid onset*, and *short duration*.

Special notes:
- Human insulin is well tolerated, with few allergic reactions. Allergic reactions may occur to agents coming from the bacteria that are used to make the insulin or something used in the method of preparation.
- The duration of action of the various insulin complexes is dependent on the dose and site of injection (e.g., the blood supply to the area being high or low), as well as other factors, such as physical activity and temperature.

Intermediate-Acting Insulins

Brand names: Humulin N, Novolin N
Available as: 100 units/mL, in 10 mL vials.

- *NPH insulin (isophane):* A complex of protamine, and insulin; an intermediate-acting insulin

Long-Acting Insulins

Insulin glargine (zinc complex)
Brand name: Lantus

Available as: Solution for injection, 100 units/mL, in 10 mL vials; 3 mL cartridges of 100 units/mL solution for use in the OPTI-PEN one insulin delivery device.

Storage: Vials of solution should be stored under refrigeration, but not frozen. Vials in use may be stored at controlled room temperature, away from direct heat or light, for up to 28 days. They should then be discarded. Cartridges installed in the OPTI-PEN device should not be refrigerated in the device.

Special notes:
- Used in both type I and type II diabetes mellitus, in adults and children over age 6.
- The potency of insulin glargine is approximately the same as that of human insulin.
- The long duration of action of insulin glargine depends on the route of injection. If the drug is not injected subcutaneously, the duration of action is reduced to approximately that of normal insulin.
- Intravenous injection may result in severe hypoglycemia.
- Not for use in the treatment of diabetic ketoacidosis.
- This type of insulin must not be diluted, or mixed with any other type of insulin (e.g., intra-syringe mixing).

Insulin detemir

Brand name: Levemir

Available as: Solution for injection, 100 units/mL, in 10 mL vials; 3 mL cartridges of 100 units/mL solution for use in the Pen-Fill insulin delivery device, FlexPen 3 mL.

Storage: Vials of solution should be stored under refrigeration, but not frozen. Vials in use may be stored at controlled room temperature, away from direct heat or light, for up to 42 days. They should then be discarded.

Special notes:
- Used in both type I and type II diabetes mellitus, in adults and children over age 6.
- This type of insulin must not be diluted, or mixed with any other type of insulin (e.g., intra-syringe mixing).

Premixes

- *Humulin or Novolin 70/30:* A 70/30 mixture of isophane insulin and regular human insulin; it is a *rapid-onset, intermediate-acting* insulin.
- *Humalog 50/50:* A 50/50 mixture of lispro protamine insulin and lispro insulin; it is a *rapid-onset, intermediate-acting* insulin.
- *Humalog 75/25:* A 75/25 mixture of lispro protamine insulin and lispro insulin; it is a *rapid-onset, intermediate-acting* insulin.

Drugs Used in the Therapy of Type II Diabetes Mellitus

Drugs used in the therapy of type II diabetes mellitus are presently classified in several groups.

Oral Sulfonylureas

Note that oral sulfonylureas can cause severe hypoglycemia! The degree of insulin release produced by these drugs is unpredictable and varies from patient to patient, making hypoglycemic effects unpredictable.

These drugs act by inhibiting the transport of potassium across the membrane of the islet cell. This makes the cell supersensitive, and increases the release of insulin, which may help to stimulate desensitized receptors. In addition, the drugs help to sensitize the insulin receptors.

Oral sulfonylureas have been grouped into two "generations," based on drug properties. The first-generation drugs are less potent and have less protein binding than the second-generation drugs. All drugs of this class are highly plasma protein bound.

> **NOTE**
>
> *These drugs are not useful in type I diabetes,* due to a lack of functioning beta cells.

Drugs Prescribed

There are several oral sulfonylureas are prescribed. These include:

- chlorpropamide
- tolazamide
- tolbutamide
- acetohexamide
- glimepiride
- glyburide
- glipizide

The most frequently prescribed are the second-generation sulfonylureas, as listed below.

Oral Sulfonylureas Most Frequently Prescribed

Glipizide
Brand names: Glucotrol, Glucotrol XL
Classification: Second-generation oral sulfonylurea

These drugs are highly protein bound, so concurrent administration of other drugs that bind to plasma proteins may cause displacement and increased plasma levels! This can result in severe hypoglycemia!

Available as: 5 mg and 10 mg tablets; 2.5 mg, 5 mg, and 10 mg extended-release tablets.

Special notes:

- Improves plasma glucose regulation.
- Reduces plasma concentrations of very low density lipoproteins (VLDLs), triglycerides, and plasma low-density lipoproteins (LDLs).

Glyburide

Brand names: DiaBeta, Micronase

Classification: Second-generation oral sulfonylurea

Available as: 1.25 mg, 2.5 mg, and 5 mg (non-micronized); 1.5 mg, 3 mg, and 6 mg (micronized) tablets.

Biguanides

These drugs increase the uptake of glucose into tissues (e.g., muscle and fat). They thus lower blood sugar and lower plasma lipids. They do not cause hypoglycemia.

Metformin

Brand name: Glucophage

Available as: 500 mg, 850 mg, and 1000 mg tablets and XR (timed-released) tablets.

Special notes:

- May cause lactic acidosis in patients with decreased kidney function (e.g., geriatric patients).
- It is the first-line drug for type II diabetics not responding to diet and exercise.
- It can be used in combination with many other diabetic medications.

Thiazolidinediones

These drugs are "insulin sensitizers." They stimulate a particular intracellular receptor thought to be involved in genetically decreasing insulin resistance. They may be used in the therapy of type II diabetes (either monotherapy or in conjunction with another antidiabetic drug).

Unlike oral sulfonylureas, these drugs enhance tissue sensitivity to insulin rather than stimulating insulin secretion. *Thiazolinediones do not cause hypoglycemia, and are ineffective in type I diabetes.* Troglitazone was the first drug of the class to be used; however, it was shown to cause

> Thiazolidinediones (e.g., pioglitazone) may be used in the therapy of type II diabetes (either monotherapy or in conjunction with another antidiabetic drug).

severe hepatotoxicity. It is no longer used, in favor of the newer drugs of the class.

Pioglitazone

Brand name: Actos

Available as: 15 mg, 30 mg, and 45 mg tablets.

Dosage: 15 or 30 mg qd (irrespective of meals)

Special notes:

- Used as an adjunct to diet in the therapy of type II diabetes mellitus.
- May be used in conjunction with oral sulfonylureas, metformin, or insulin to stabilize blood sugar.

Rosiglitazone

Brand names: Avandia, Tiltab, Avandamet (combination drug with metformin)

Available as: 2 mg, 4 mg, and 8 mg tablets.

Dosage: 4 mg/day in single dose or two divided doses increasing to 8 mg, as necessary; no dosage adjustment is required for geriatric patients.

Meglitinides

> *Meglitinides (e.g., repaglinide) stimulate insulin secretion. These drugs will not increase the secretion of insulin without adequate glucose present, and therefore will not cause hypoglycemia!*

These drugs affect potassium flow across the membrane of the beta cell. They are particularly useful, as they produce a pattern of secretion of insulin that mimics normal secretion. These drugs:

- have a rapid onset and short duration of action.
- stimulate insulin secretion in the presence of moderate concentrations of glucose, but not in the absence of glucose.

Repaglinide

Brand name: Prandin

Available as: 0.5 mg, 1 mg, and 2 mg tablets.

Dosage: Doses are individualized, and should be taken 15 to 30 minutes before each meal. Maximum dose—up to 80 mg/day has shown negligible adverse effects.

Special note:

- Contraindicated in patients with type I diabetes.

Alpha-Glucosidase Inhibitors

This class of drugs inhibits carbohydrate breakdown and thus slows the absorption of carbohydrates. Slower absorption of sugars and carbohydrates allows the patient to better assimilate them, with lower insulin activity.

- These drugs are not absorbed systemically, so they have virtually no adverse effects.
- They are used as adjunct therapy (along with another drug) or alone (monotherapy) in elderly patients.
- They must be taken immediately before meals.
- Two drugs of the class are available—miglitol and acarbose. They inhibit different enzymes and have slightly different effects—acarbose is more effective in slowing the breakdown of starches, and miglitol is more potent in the inhibition of sugar breakdown.

Drugs Prescribed

Thyroid hormone (thyroxine, or T_4) and triiodothyronine (T_3) regulate metabolism, and, in infancy, are necessary for proper brain development. Too little thyroid during development or infancy can cause cretinism, a form of mental retardation. Too little thyroid in an adult will cause weight gain, edema (puffy face, hands, and feet), fatigue, and lack of mental alertness.

Acarbose
Brand name: Precose

Available as: 25 mg, 50 mg, and 100 mg tablets.

Dosage: Starting dose is 25 mg tid. Dosage is individualized, but should not exceed the maximum dose of 300 mg/day (100 mg tid) for patients weighing over 60 kg (132 lb) or 150 mg/day for patients weighing less than 60 kg. Doses should be taken immediately preceding a meal (i.e., with the first bite of food).

Miglitol
Brand name: Glyset

Available as: 25 mg, 50 mg, and 100 mg tablets.

Dosage: Dosage is individualized; approximately 25–50 mg three times a day, taken with the first bite of each meal. Maximum dose is 100 mg, three times daily.

Special note:
- Miglitol does not cause hypoglycemia and may be combined with oral sulfonylureas.

Exenatide
Brand name: Byetta

Available as: 5 mcg/dose prefilled pen (60 doses); 10 mcg/dose prefilled pen.

Storage: Refrigeration is required. Do not freeze.

Special notes:

- It is not a substitution for insulin.
- Used as an adjunct to diet and exercise to improve glycemic control.

Sitagliptin
Brand name: Januvia

Available as: 25 mg, 50 mg, and 100 mg tablets.

Special notes:

- Januvia can be taken with or without food.
- It can be used as a monotherapy agent or in combination with other diabetic agents.

Drugs Used in the Therapy of Thyroid Disorders

Thyroid disorders may result from too little thyroid hormone being produced (*hypo*thyroidism), or too much being produced (*hyper*thyroidism).

Therapy of Hypothyroidism

Hypothyroidism is treated with the administration of thyroid hormone. Purified (or synthetic) thyroid hormone is now used, which is of known composition and activity. Desiccated thyroid from natural sources (e.g., pork thyroid) is no longer used, as the composition is too variable and the pharmacological results are unpredictable.

Preparations Available

Levothyroxine
Brand names: Synthroid, Levothroid,

Classification: Thyroid hormone replacement

Available as: 200 mcg and 500 mcg, powder for injection; 25 mcg, 50 mcg, 75 mcg, 88 mcg, 100 mcg, 112 mcg, 125 mcg, 137 mcg, 150 mcg, 175 mcg, 200 mcg, and 300 mcg tablets.

Liotrix
Liotrix is a 1:4 mixture of T_3 and T_4.

Brand name: Thyrolar

Available as: Thyrolar ¼ –3.1 mcg T_3 : 12.5 mcg T_4 (15 mg), Thyrolar ½ –6.25 mcg T_3 : 25 mcg T_4 (30 mg), Thyrolar 1–12.5 mcg T_3 : 50 mcg T_4 (60 mg), Thyrolar 2–25 mcg T_3 : 100 mcg T_4 (120 mg), Thyrolar 3–37.5 mcg T_3 : 150 mcg T_4 (180 mg).

Therapy of Hyperthyroidism

Recall that thyroid hormones are made from a large polymer molecule called thyroglobulin. Thyroglobulin within the thyroid follicle is exposed to free iodine and iodinated, then chopped up into tyrosyl residues. Whichever of these residues happen to have the proper number of iodine molecules attached in the proper places is the active thyroid hormone. The other residues are "recycled" back into thyroglobulin.

> Hyperthyroidism can be potentially life-threatening, as thyroid hormone sensitizes the heart to catecholamines (e.g., epinephrine and norepinephrine). Excess thyroid hormone can promote serious cardiac arrhythmias.

> **NOTE**
>
> There are two possible mechanisms of action of hyperthyroid agents: (1) to inhibit the recycling of thyroglobulin, so that the supply of thyroglobulin eventually runs out; and (2) to inhibit the incorporation of iodide into the thyroglobulin (iodide trapping). The majority of drugs in use today inhibit the incorporation of iodide into thyroglobulin. *These drugs can cause drug interactions with warfarin.*

Propylthiouracil (PTU)
Brand name: Propyl-Thyracil (PTU)
Available as: 50 mg tablets.

Special notes:
- This drug is an iodide-trapping agent.
- PTU is the preferred agent for the treatment of hyperthyroidism in pregnant women, as it does not cross into the placenta or enter breast milk.
- May cause agranulocytosis.

Methimazole
Brand name: Tapazole
Available as: 5 mg and 10 mg tablets.

Special notes:
- Methimazole carries less risk of agranulocytosis than PTU.
- The drug concentrates in the thyroid gland so it has a long duration and is eliminated slowly.
- Renal elimination.

- This drug is an iodide trapping agent.
- It can cause congenital defects.

Other drugs that may be used in the therapy of hyperthyroidism are Lugol's solution (iodine solution—an older therapy) and radioactive iodine (^{131}I, which is incorporated into the thyroid gland and destroys tissue by emission of radioactive particles). These drugs are given by injection, on an inpatient basis.

Drugs That Affect the Reproductive System

Estrogens

Estrogens work by inhibiting the release of hormones from the hypothalamus that stimulate the ovaries. This prevents the initial development of the ovum. Since they are only effective before the reproductive cycle begins, they must be taken for the first several days after the end of a cycle, and again at the beginning of a cycle (contraceptives are normally dispensed as a 28-day dose pack, in which the appropriate tablets are either drug or placebo, which contains no drug).

Beneficial effects:

- lower serum lipids and may increase bone density.

Adverse effects:

- increase the amount of clotting factors, which can lead to spontaneous clot formation and stroke or infarction.
- increase the risk of hormone-related cancers, such as uterine and breast cancers.
- have been shown to increase the incidence of *endometrial cancer* in postmenopausal women.
- should *not be used during pregnancy,* as damage to the fetus may occur. For example, female fetuses exposed to estrogens are several times more likely to develop certain cancers (e.g., cervical) later in life. Exposure of a male fetus to estrogens may cause feminization. In addition, they may precipitate spontaneous abortion.

> **NOTE**
>
> All estrogenic drugs must be dispensed with a mandatory patient package insert.

Conjugated Estrogens

Brand name: Premarin

Classification: Estrogen, natural

Available as: 0.3 mg, 0.625 mg, 0.9 mg, 1.25 mg, and 2.5 mg tablets; 25 mg/mL powder for injection; 0.625 mg/g vaginal cream.

Combination Drugs

These drugs are available as 2.5 mg and 5 mg tablets, packaged in a dispenser pack.

Brand names: Premphase, Prempro: Conjugated estrogens with medroxy-progesterone

Estradiol

Brand names: Estrace, Estring, Esclim, Vagifem (vaginal tablet)

Available as: 0.5 mg, 1 mg, and 2 mg tablets; 0.1 mg/g cream.

Transdermal patch formulations: Climara, Estraderm, Vivelle

- Patch formulations are available in surface areas of 10 cm^2 (4 mg estradiol—delivering 0.05 mg estradiol/day) and 20 cm^2 (8 mg estradiol—delivering 0.1 mg estradiol/day).

Combination Drugs

Brand names: Activella—estradiol 1 mg norethindrone acetate 0.5 mg

Dosage: 1–2 mg daily

- It is used in the therapy of osteoporosis, postmenopausal symptoms. Lunelle—estradiol cypionate with medroxyprogesterone actetate

- It is used as a contraceptive agent.

    Premphase, Prempro—conjugated estrogens (0.625 mg) medroxypro-gesterone (2.5 mg or 5 mg) tablets

- It is used as a contraceptive agent.
- Used in the treatment of osteoporosis, postmenopausal symptoms.

Estropipate

Brand names: Ogen, Ortho-est, Estropipate

Available as: 0.625 mg, 1.25 mg, and 2.5 mg tablets; 1.5 mg/gram vaginal cream.

Dosage: 10 mg tid for three months or more

Esterified Estrogens

Brand names: Menest, Estratab

Available as: 0.3 mg, 0.625 mg, 1.25 mg, and 2.5 mg tablets.

Estradiol cypionate

Brand names: Depo Estradiol Estradiol Cyp, Lunelle (with medroxyprogesterone acetate)

Ethinyl estradiol

Brand names: Nuvaring Vaginal Insert (with etonogestrel), Estrostep, Ortho-Novum (with norethindrone), Preven (with levonorgestrel), Levlite (with levonorgestrel)

Available as: Dose packs containing tablets with varying amounts of estradiol and progestin (TriPhasil), arranged in stages or "phases":

- Phase 1 consists of six brown tablets to be taken daily, each containing 0.050 mg of levonorgestrel with 0.030 mg of ethinyl estradiol.
- Phase 2 consists of five white tablets to be taken daily, each containing 0.075 mg of levonorgestrel and 0.040 mg ethinyl estradiol.
- Phase 3 consists of ten yellow tablets, each containing 0.125 mg levonorgestrel and 0.030 mg ethinyl estradiol.

Special notes:
- Ethinyl estradiol (Preven) is used as the "morning after" or *postcoital* contraceptive.
- It is combined with levonorgestrel.

Estrogen Antagonists (Anti-Estrogens)

These drugs bind to the estrogen receptor and prevent activation of the receptor by estrogen. They are competitive antagonists, for the most part. Adverse effects produced relate to the decrease in estrogenic effects and may include elevated serum lipids, alterations in libido, and temperature regulation, etc.

> **NOTE**
>
> Estrogen antagonists are mainly used in the therapy of estrogen-dependent cancers, although they may also be used in a reproductive context. Because of this use, some texts list them as *anticancer agents* (antineoplastic agents), which they really are not.

Anastrozole

Brand name: Arimidex

Available as: 1 mg tablet.

Primary Uses: Used in the therapy of advanced breast cancer, following tamoxifen therapy

Dosage: 1 mg taken once per day

Clomiphene citrate

Brand names: Clomid, Serophene

Available as: 50 mg tablet.

Dosage: Dosage is individualized, beginning with 50 mg daily for five days.

Special notes:

- Used in the therapy of ovulatory dysfunction during pregnancy, polycystic ovary syndrome.
- Indicated in patients with demonstrated ovulatory dysfunction.
- Clomiphene is used as a fertility drug.

Tamoxifen

Brand name: Nolvadex

Classification: Competitive antagonist of estradiol

Available as: 10 mg and 20 mg tablets.

Primary Uses: Used in the therapy of advanced breast cancer

Letrozole

Brand name: Femara

Available as: 2.5 mg tablet.

Primary Uses: Used as extended treatment in women who have received 5 years of tamoxifen therapy

Progestins

Progestin agents may be given to prevent miscarriage. However, recent evidence shows that use of these agents in the first trimester of pregnancy may cause fetal abnormalities, including the impression of male traits on a female fetus, and vice versa. In addition, use of these agents may prevent the spontaneous abortion of a nonviable fertilized ovum or defective ovum. They can also be used in birth control, stopping excessive vaginal bleeding, or to start a delayed menstrual cycle once confirmation is made that there is no pregnancy.

Progesterone
Brand name: Prometrium

Available as: 100 mg capsule.

Medroxyprogesterone acetate
Brand names: Provera, Depo-Provera

Available as: 2.5 mg, 5 mg, and 10 mg tablets; 400 mg/mL suspension for intramuscular injection (Depo-Provera) prefilled 1 mL syringes of 150 mg.

Hydroxyprogesterone caproate
Brand name: Delalutin

Classification: Competitive antagonist of estradiol

Available as: 125 mg/mL and 250 mg/mL solution for intramuscular injection.

Special note:
- Use of this drug in the first four months of pregnancy is not recommended.

Chapter Review Questions

1. Which of the following has the longest duration of action?
   a. Insulin complexed with zinc
   b. Regular insulin
   c. NPH insulin
   d. Lantus insulin

2. A patient is going into a diabetic coma. Which of the following would be best to administer?
   a. Micronase
   b. Humulin N
   c. Metformin
   d. Novolog

3. Lantus insulin is:
   a. a long-acting form of insulin
   b. a mixture of regular insulin and NPH insulin
   c. a mixture of semilente and ultralente insulin
   d. insulin complexed with zinc

4. A patient taking Micronase most likely has which of the following conditions?
   a. a bacterial infection
   b. breast cancer
   c. Type I diabetes
   d. Type II diabetes

5. Which of the following drugs should be taken just before a meal?
   a. Tapazole
   b. Prandin
   c. Diabeta
   d. Depo-Provera

6. A pregnant patient comes into the pharmacy; she has the following drugs in her patient profile. Which should you call to the attention of the pharmacist?
   a. Tapazole
   b. Isophane insulin
   c. PTU
   d. Acarbose

7. The advantage of using a 25/75 ratio of insulin aspart to NPH insulin is that:
   a. it mimics normal insulin secretion
   b. it has a delayed onset
   c. it has a fast onset and long duration
   d. it is inexpensive

8. Two methods of insulin dosing include:
   a. the oral tablet and subcutaneous injection
   b. the tablet and suppository
   c. the insulin syringe and cartridge pen
   d. the insulin syringe and suppository

9. A patient reports the occurrence of hives after taking his regular insulin. To remedy this situation, his doctor should have him:
   a. use an antihistamine cream on the hives
   b. switch to Humalog insulin
   c. use an oral sulfonylurea instead of the insulin
   d. stop taking it for a few days

10. Which of the following is an oral sulfonylurea?
    a. Roglitazone
    b. Glipizide
    c. Miglitol
    d. Acarbose

11. Which of the following may cause severe hypoglycemia?
    a. Glyburide
    b. Miglitol
    c. Glipizide
    d. both a and c

12. Glucotrol has an advantage over Micronase because it can also:
    a. lower blood sugar faster
    b. cause hypoglycemia
    c. lowers serum lipids
    d. be effective in type I diabetes as well as type II

13. Which of the following might be effective in both type I and type II diabetes?
    a. Micronase
    b. Levemir
    c. Prandin
    d. Actos

14. Prandin does not cause hypoglycemia, as it:
    a. does not affect blood sugar
    b. does not work unless sufficient glucose is present in the blood
    c. affects mainly lipids
    d. affects the breakdown and absorption of sugars, not sugar utilization

15. A patient experiences tachycardia and severe weight loss. Which of the following drugs might be to blame?
    a. Miglitol
    b. Synthroid
    c. Estrace
    d. Provera

16. Thyrolar is useful because it:
    a. has a fast onset
    b. has a long duration
    c. mimics the normal thyroid hormone profile of 1:4 T_3 to T_4
    d. is a potent inhibitor of thyroid synthesis

17. Propothiouracil and methimazole are both:
    a. used in contraception
    b. iodide-trapping agents
    c. used for hypothyroidism
    d. used for type II diabetes mellitus

18. Side effects of estrogens include:
    a. increased risk of clot formation
    b. increased risk of endometrial cancer
    c. decreased plasma lipids
    d. both a and b

19. The "morning after pill" is:
    a. quinestrol
    b. diethylstilbestrol
    c. ethinyl estradiol with levonorgestrel
    d. tamoxifen

20. Which of the following would interfere with the effects of an estrogen-based contraceptive?
    a. Liotrix
    b. Tamoxifen
    c. Ogden
    d. Estrovis

CHAPTER 30

Vitamins

Quick Study

I. Classification of vitamins

    A. Water-soluble vitamins—these are not stored in the body
        1. B vitamins—thiamine, riboflavin, niacin, pantothenic acid, cyanocobalamin, etc.
        2. Vitamin C

    B. Fat-soluble vitamins—these vitamins are stored in fatty tissue and can accumulate in the body, causing toxicity
        1. Vitamin A
        2. Vitamin D
        3. Vitamin E
        4. Vitamin K

II. Physiological roles of the various vitamins

    A. Symptoms of deficiency
    B. Symptoms of toxicity (fat-soluble vitamins)

III. Minerals necessary for proper body function

    A. Physiological roles of the various minerals
    B. Chemical symbols

Vitamins are classified into two types: water-soluble vitamins and fat-soluble vitamins. Water-soluble vitamins are not stored in the body—fat-soluble vitamins are. Thus, *fat-soluble vitamins have more potential for toxicity*, and have a longer duration of action.

Water-Soluble Vitamins

These drugs include the B vitamins and vitamin C. These drugs are not stored, so they must be taken daily, as they are quickly eliminated in the urine. Overdosage of these vitamins is unlikely.

> **NOTE**
>
> Alcoholics are particularly susceptible to deficiencies in water-soluble vitamins, due to the diuretic effect of alcohol. Persons taking diuretics may also be vitamin deficient for the same reason. Alcohol also decreases the absorption of these vitamins.

Vitamin B$_1$

Proper name: Thiamine

Available as: 50 mg, 100 mg, 250 mg, and 500 mg tablets; 100 mg/2 mL injection.

- Useful in the production of red blood cells, and particularly necessary for proper neurotransmission.

Dietary Sources:

- Legumes, beef, pork, whole grains, fresh vegetables, yeast.

Name of deficiency: Beri-Beri

Vitamin B$_2$

Proper name: Riboflavin

Available as: 25 mg, 50 mg, and 100 mg tablets.

- Useful in energy production (used to make the cellular chemical FAD, used in the mitochondria).
- Necessary for proper nerve maintenance and maintenance of connective tissue.

Dietary Sources:

- Beef liver, kidney, whole grain cereals, dairy, mushrooms, yeast, green vegetables, eggs.

Symptoms of deficiency:

- Scaly skin
- Sores on the mouth

- Sensitivity to light
- Itching, watery eyes
- Swollen tongue

Vitamin B₃

Proper name: Niacin

Available as: 50 mg, 100 mg, 250 mg, and 500 mg tablets; 125 mg, 250 mg, 400 mg, and 500 mg sustained-release capsules; 50 mg/5 mL elixir.

- It is useful in lowering serum lipids.
- It may cause cutaneous vasodilation and flushing of the skin and other areas. Given with aspirin may reduce the flushing.
- Poor patient compliance can occur due to uncomfortable side effects (e.g., severe "flushing").
- The niacinamide form does not cause flushing, but also *does not have beneficial effects* on the lipid profile.
- Niacin can cause liver toxicity, *particularly if the sustained release form is used*. This may be manifested by nausea and abdominal cramps.

Dietary Sources:

- Whole wheat, rice grains, liver, lean meats, peanuts, legumes, poultry, and fish.

Name of deficiency: Pellagra

Vitamin B₅

Proper name: Pantothenic acid

- Involved in the generation of energy; production of blood cells; and the synthesis of bile, fats, and steroid hormones.
- Deficiencies are rare, and are mainly seen with conditions of extreme starvation.

Dietary Sources:

- Vegetables, cereals, yeast, and liver.

Vitamin B₆

Proper name: Pyridoxine

Available as: 250 mg capsule; 25 mg, 50 mg, 100 mg, 250 mg, and 500 mg table; 100 mg/mL injection.

- Involved in immune function, nerve transmission, red blood cell synthesis, energy production.

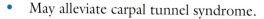

- May alleviate carpal tunnel syndrome.
- Can also relieve nausea associated with pregnancy.

Symptoms of deficiency:

- Mild neural dysfunction (can mimic carpal tunnel syndrome).
- Seizures—especially in infants..
- Muscle weakness.
- Depression and fatigue.
- Deficiency of pyridoxine is rare.

Dietary Sources:

- Whole grain cereals, lima beans, red meats, bananas, potatoes, yeast, and poultry.

Vitamin B$_9$

Proper name: Folic acid (folate)

Available as: 5 mg/mL injection; 400 mcg, 800 mcg, and 1 mg tablets.

- Essential for red blood cell formation and for the formation of DNA in general (the requirement for folate is greatest in rapidly dividing cells, such as blood cells).
- Large doses of folic acid for long periods of time may result in tingling of the hands and feet, and sedation. These are reversible with a decrease in intake of the vitamin.
- May mask the symptoms of vitamin B$_{12}$ deficiency.

Dietary Sources:

- Yeast, liver, kidney, green vegetables, and whole grains.

Vitamin B$_{12}$

Proper name: Cyanocobalamin

Available as: 1,000 mcg/mL injection; 500 mcg/0.1 mL nasal spray; 50 mcg, 100 mcg, 250 mcg, 1,000 mcg, and 5,000 mcg tablets.

- Involved in blood cell formation and also essential for formation of myelin.
- Necessary for myelination of the spinal cord.
- Required in *microgram* amounts.

Name of Deficiency: Pernicious anemia.

Symptoms of deficiency:

- Characterized by a loss of red blood cells.
- Spinal cord demyelination.

Dietary Sources:

- Liver, eggs, dairy, beef, pork, and fish.

Vitamin C

Proper name: Ascorbic acid

Available as: 100 mg, 250 mg, 500 mg, and 1,000 mg tablets; 100 mg, 250 mg, and 500 mg chew tabs; 90 mg/mL oral solution; 250 mg/mL and 500 mg/mL injection.

- Necessary for maintenance of tissues.
- Necessary for proper formation and orientation of collagen in bone and connective tissue.
- Supports immune system function.
- Antioxidant properties—vitamin C protects tissues from breakdown caused by free radical formation.
- Buffered forms (e.g., "nonacidic" vitamin C or "ester C") do not have the same beneficial effects.
- The maximum amount of vitamin C that can be absorbed per dose is 180 mg, so large dose formulations do not have a greater effect.
- Vitamin C is absorbed from the stomach, because it is an acid.

Name of deficiency: Scurvy

Symptoms of deficiency:

- Weight loss
- Bleeding gums, poor jaw and tooth development
- Poor wound healing
- Easy bruising
- Susceptibility to illness

Dietary Sources:

- Green plants, tomatoes, and citrus fruits.

Fat-Soluble Vitamins

Fat-soluble vitamins include vitamins A, D, E, and K. Toxicity may be seen with overdosage of these vitamins. The common unit of measure for these vitamins is the *international unit (IU)*.

Vitamin A

Brand name: Retinol, Vesanoid, Aquasol A, Retin-A

Available as: 10,000 IU and 25,000 IU capsules; 50,000 units/mL injection; Aquasol A oral solution; Retin-A cream/gel.

- This vitamin is a group of chemicals derived from beta carotene.
- Essential for the formation of retinal pigment (rods) and black-and-white vision.
- Retinol and other retinoids are the primary components of vitamin A.

Symptoms of deficiency:

- Dry skin and hair
- Nyctalopia (night blindness)

Toxicity:

- Headaches
- Insomnia
- Visual disturbances
- Dry skin
- Orange hue to the skin
- Nausea

Name of deficiency: Keratomalacia

Dietary Sources:

- Milk, butter, cheese, liver, fish oils, and yellow and dark green leafy vegetables.

Vitamin D

Vitamin D must be activated to vitamin D_3 before it is useful. This activation takes place when sunlight hits the skin, activating the vitamin in the dermis.

Proper name: Cholecalciferol, ergocalciferol, paricalcitol, calcitriol

Available as: 50,000 IU capsules (Drisdol); 0.25 mcg and 0.5 mcg capsules (Rocaltrol); 1.2 mcg/mL injection (Calcijex); 1 mcg, 2 mcg, and 4 mcg capsules; 5 mcg/mL injection (Zemplar).

- Vitamin D (cholecalciferol) is converted to an active form (1,25 dihydrocholicalciferol) in the upper layers of the skin. The activated form (vitamin D_3), or 1,25 dihydrocholicalciferol, is essential for the formation of bone. It must be present in order for calcium to be absorbed from the intestine and also works with parathyroid hormone to increase the storage of calcium in the bone.
- Persons who are infrequently exposed to sunlight will have low levels of activated vitamin D and fragile bones (less than 10–15 minutes throughout the week). This is most frequent with children (this condition is termed *osteomalacia*).

Symptoms of deficiency:

- Bone loss
- Ricketts
- Nervousness

- Diarrhea
- Insomnia
- Muscle weakness

Toxicity:

- Hypercalcemia (increased blood calcium) leading to headaches, nausea, muscle weakness, and abnormalities of the cardiovascular system.
- Calcium deposits may also form in major organs, causing organ toxicity.
- Dose limit—400 international units (IU)/day.

Name of deficiency: Ricketts

Dietary Sources:

- Butter, milk, egg yolks, cheese, and fish oils.

Vitamin E

Proper name: Alpha tocopherol (vitamin E is actually a group of tocopherols, of which tocopherol is the main compound)

Available as: Aquasol E—100 IU, 200 IU, 400 IU, 500 IU, 600 IU, and 1,000 IU capsules; oral drops 15 IU/0.3 mL.

- Vitamin E acts as a *fat-soluble antioxidant*. It decreases free radical damage in connective tissue and organ tissue, resulting in accelerated wound healing and protection of tissue from damage. It is stored in fatty tissue, and shows essentially no toxicity.

Dietary Sources:

- Liver, eggs, leafy greens, soybean oil, wheat germ, rice germ, cotton seed, nuts, corn, and butter.

Vitamin K

Proper name: Like vitamin A, this vitamin is a combination of similar chemicals—the primary one being a substance called *phytonadione*.

Available as: 10 mg/mL and 0.5 mg/mL injection (Aqua-Mephyton); 5 mg tablets (Mephyton).

- Vitamin K is essential for blood clotting—many clotting factors require activation by vitamin K.

Symptoms of deficiency:

- Excessive bleeding
- Bruising

Toxicity:

- Allergic reactions.

- Also, excessive clotting produced by vitamin K may lead to minor strokes or infarcts.

- This vitamin is not normally taken as a supplement, as there are ample stores in the liver and it is also made by bacteria in the intestinal tract. It is also readily available in food. Because required amounts are in the microgram range, supplementation is not required.

Dietary Sources:

- Leafy greens, wheat bran, and soybeans.

Mineral Supplements

Mineral supplements are used differently in the body than are vitamins. Most mineral supplements are essentially metals, and trace amounts of these substances are required for normal body function. Below is a table of mineral supplements and their present role in human physiology.

Mineral	Chemical symbol	Physiological role (s)
Calcium	Ca^{++}	Essential for proper muscle and nerve function
Chromium	Cr^{+++}	Aids in metabolism of sugars
Copper	Cu^{+}	Essential for proper blood formation
Iodine	I^{-}	Essential for proper thyroid function
Iron	Fe^{++}	Essential for red blood cell formation
Magnesium	Mg^{++}	Essential for muscle function
Potassium	K^{+}	Essential for proper heart and nerve function, and cellular homeostasis
Sodium	Na^{+}	Essential for nerve and muscle function, and cellular homeostasis (sodium is not regularly supplemented)
Sulfur	S	Essential for energy production and cellular function
Zinc	Zn^{++}	Essential for proper immune function

Chapter Review Questions

1. Which of the following is involved in blood formation?
   a. Folic acid
   b. Vitamin D
   c. Vitamin K
   d. Vitamin A

2. The vitamin required for myelination of nervous tissue is:
   a. B_1
   b. B_5
   c. B_{12}
   d. B_6

3. Cyanocobalamin is:
   a. a water-soluble vitamin
   b. Vitamin C
   c. Vitamin B_{12}
   d. both a and c are correct

4. ß-tocopherol would most likely be a component of which vitamin?
   a. Vitamin C
   b. Vitamin K
   c. Vitamin A
   d. Vitamin E

5. Retinol is a component of:
   a. Vitamin E
   b. Vitamin A
   c. Vitamin D
   d. Vitamin K

6. An example of a water-soluble antioxidant would be:
   a. Vitamin D
   b. Vitamin A
   c. Vitamin C
   d. Vitamin K

7. The vitamin required for the maintenance of bone is:
   a. Cyanocobalamin
   b. 1,25 Dihydrocholicalciferol
   c. Retinoic acid
   d. Thiamine

8. A fat-soluble antioxidant would be:
   a. Ascorbic acid
   b. Vitamin E
   c. Vitamin D
   d. Vitamin B_{12}

9. This vitamin is required for proper vision, particularly night vision.
   a. Cyanocobalamin
   b. ß-tocopherol
   c. Niacin
   d. Vitamin A

10. This vitamin is essential for the conversion of glucose to energy.
    a. Vitamin A
    b. Vitamin B_2
    c. Vitamin B_6
    d. Vitamin C

11. The chemical symbol for iron is:
    a. Na^+
    b. Fe^{++}
    c. K^+
    d. $Mg++$

12. The mineral that is essential for heart and nerve function is:
    a. sodium
    b. magnesium
    c. calcium
    d. potassium

13. Another name for pantothenic acid is:
    a. B_{12}
    b. D_3
    c. B_9
    d. B_5

14. Calcium is essential for:
    a. red blood cell formation
    b. metabolize sugars
    c. proper muscle and nerve function
    d. blood clotting

15. Excessive bleeding and bruising is a deficiency of:
    a. Vitamin K
    b. Vitamin C
    c. Vitamin E
    d. Vitamin B

CHAPTER 31

Pharmacology Review

1. A drug used for hypertension that would affect the vascular system is:
   a. Norvasc
   b. Timoptic
   c. Diamox
   d. Cefobid

2. Which of the following are antibiotics?
   a. Keflex
   b. Ceclor
   c. Polymox
   d. all of the above

3. Which of the following is a diuretic?
   a. Haldol
   b. Lasix
   c. Thorazine
   d. both a and b

4. Which of the following is contraindicated with antihistamines?
   a. Elavil
   b. Prozac
   c. Paxil
   d. none of the above

5. Which of the following directly affect(s) the cardiovascular system?
   a. Cardizem
   b. Cardura
   c. Catapres
   d. both a and b

6. Which of the following is an antifungal drug?
   a. Miconazole
   b. Cefamandole
   c. Tegopen
   d. Hydrocort

7. Which of the following is not a penicillin drug?
   a. Geocillin
   b. Geopen
   c. Pentoxifylline
   d. Beepen-K

8. Which of the following might be a long-lasting form of nitroglycerin?
   a. Nitro-Bid
   b. Nitrostat
   c. Nitro-Dur
   d. Nitropress

9. Which of the drugs is not a form of nitrogylcerin at all?
   a. Nitro-Bid
   b. Nitrostat
   c. Nitro-Dur
   d. Nitropress

10. Production of vitamin K could be reduced by which of these drugs?
    a. Aminophylline
    b. Keflex
    c. Singulair
    d. Adalat

11. The patient profile for Doug Holm shows that he is taking the following drugs. Which drugs would you call to the attention of the pharmacist?

   Drug list—Doug Holm (pt #234567)

Coumadin 2 mg bid	Percodan tabs 2 bid PRN
Tagamet 200 mg ac hs	Xanax 0.25 mg TID

   a. Coumadin and Xanax
   b. Tagamet and Xanax
   c. Coumadin and Percodan
   d. Coumadin and Tagamet

12. Nifedipine would likely have synergistic reactions with which of the following?
    a. Verapamil
    b. Nitroglycerin
    c. Alprazolam
    d. Propranolol

13. The physiological effects of Calan and those of atropine could be described as:
    a. synergistic
    b. antagonistic
    c. not related
    d. symbiotic

14. Major drug interactions exist between:
    a. Warfarin and Amoxicillin
    b. Carbamazepine and Phenytoin
    c. Torsemide and Digoxin
    d. Ethinyl Estradiol and Acetaminophen

15. Micronase and Diabeta are:
    a. tricyclic antidepressants
    b. oral sulfonylureas
    c. used in the therapy of type I diabetes
    d. antibiotics

16. Which of the following drugs will produce photosensitivity?
    a. Carbamazepine
    b. Tetracycline
    c. Digoxin
    d. both a and b

17. A patient is prescribed Lasix and Cardioquin by his cardiologist, and gentamicin by his internist. Which of these drugs might cause toxicity if used together?
    a. Lasix and Cardioquin
    b. Lasix and gentamicin
    c. Cardioquin and gentamicin
    d. No toxicity will be produced among these drugs

18. A patient is prescribed Tagamet, tetracycline, and Roxicet. He is taking Rolaids for his upset stomach. What problem is immediately noticeable to you, as an astute pharmacy technician?
    a. the Tagamet and Rolaids have synergistic effects
    b. the tetracycline cannot be taken with Tagamet
    c. the tetracycline cannot be taken with an antacid such as Rolaids
    d. the Roxicet will make the upset stomach worse

19. The ability of a drug to maintain its form and therapeutic value over time is termed:
    a. potency
    b. efficacy
    c. stability
    d. storage index

20. Lanoxin is a member of which class of drugs?
    a. Nonsteroidal anti-inflammatory drugs
    b. Sodium channel blockers
    c. Cardiac glycosides
    d. Tricyclic antidepressants

21. Cardioquin is a(n):
    a. digitalis glycoside
    b. sodium channel blocker
    c. antihypertensive agent
    d. pain reliever

22. A patient has an atrial arrhythmia and high blood pressure. Which of the following drugs would be effective for both conditions?
    a. Phenytoin
    b. Quinidine
    c. Verapamil
    d. Diphenoxylate

23. A patient is experiencing heart palpitations. Which of the following combinations of drugs might be at fault?
    a. Zocor and Lasix
    b. Clozapine and aspirin
    c. Prozac and Nardil
    d. Diphenhydramine and acetaminophen

24. Which of the following drugs should be avoided in a patient allergic to Ceclor?
    a. Gentamicin
    b. Diamox
    c. BuSpar
    d. Clavamox

25. Which of the following is an opiate sold over the counter?
    a. Sertraline
    b. Loperamide
    c. Buspirone
    d. Gentamicin

26. Lomotil is classified as a C-V controlled substance because:
    a. diphenoxylate is an opiate
    b. the drug contains atropine
    c. the dose is too small to abuse
    d. both a and b

27. Which of the following drug combinations should be brought to the attention of the pharmacist?
    a. Atropine and Synthroid
    b. Vicodin and Polymox
    c. Paxil and Lasix
    d. Nexium and lamotrigine

28. A patient taking Naprosyn for tennis elbow should be advised to take which of the following for a headache?
    a. Aspirin
    b. More Naprosyn
    c. Tylenol
    d. Percodan

29. Which of the following will synergize to produce severe orthostatic hypotension?
    a. Prazosin and Naprosyn
    b. Terazosin and carbamazepine
    c. Prazosin and Nitrostat
    d. Streptomycin and Lasix

30. Which is an anti-emetic used in chemotherapy treatment?
    a. Coumadin
    b. Lomotil
    c. Aspirin
    d. Reglan

Match the brand name with the generic name.

31. Ambien
32. Aricept
33. Avandia
34. Biaxin
35. Cardura
36. Celexa
37. Imodium
38. Lopid
39. Nolvadex
40. Pepcid
41. Reglan
42. Relafen
43. Rocephin
44. Singulair
45. Stadol
46. Taxotere
47. Vitamin B$_1$
48. Vitamin B$_{12}$
49. Vitamin B$_3$
50. Zestril

a. Butorphanol
b. Ceftriaxone
c. Citalopram
d. Clarithromycin
e. Cyanocobolamin
f. Docetaxel
g. Donezepil
h. Doxazosin
i. Famotidine
j. Gemfibrozil
k. Lisinopril
l. Loperamide
m. Metoclopramide
n. Montelukast
o. Nabumetone
p. Niacin
q. Rosiglitazone
r. Tamoxifen
s. Thiamine
t. Zolpidem

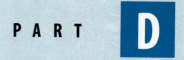

Pharmacy Law

CHAPTER **32**

State and Federal Regulations

Quick Study

I. The Federal Food, Drug, and Cosmetic Act guarantees the purity and appropriate labeling of drug products

II. The Controlled Substances Act

    A. Regulates narcotics and drugs of abuse

    B. Classifies prescription drugs into five classes, from Class I (highly abusable and no proven therapeutic benefit) to Class V (low abuse potential)

III. The Federal Hazardous Substances Act

    A. The Poison Prevention Packaging Act (PPPA) mandates childproof packaging on drug products. Exceptions include packaging for the elderly and handicapped.

    B. The Occupational Safety and Health Act (safety in the workplace)
- Safety regulations in the pharmacy
- Disposal of hazardous materials and proper procedure for cleaning of spills

IV. The Omnibus Budget Reconciliation Act includes provisions for:

- Mandatory patient counseling by the pharmacist, including instruction in self-monitoring techniques and explanation of drug actions and adverse effects
- Drug utilization review

V. The Health Insurance Portability and Accountability Act (HIPAA)

    A. HIPAA provides for the development of a health information system that protects patients' privacy through the establishment of standards for communication and the electronic transmission of health information. Security measures in place to protect patient privacy include:

- Code sets—encoding of procedures performed, diagnostic codes, and medical data
- Development of a health care clearinghouse to process identifiable information into standard data elements that are not identifiable with a particular patient
- Provision of clear definition of terms that tell which patient information may be disseminated to a third party
- Definition of the applicability of patient confidentiality regulations to various providers (e.g., health plans, primary care provider, etc.)
- Provision of minimum privacy standards for electronic exchange of patient information

Laws that govern pharmacies and pharmaceuticals are designed to protect the general public, as well as the individual patient. These regulations may be federally mandated or mandated at the state level. They set the minimum standards for conduct within the pharmacy, service to the patient, and the quality of drugs dispensed.

- The **Federal Food, Drug, and Cosmetic Act** guarantees a safe, effective, and unadulterated drug product that is appropriately labeled.

- The **Controlled Substances Act** serves to protect the public by regulating abusable drugs in an effort to prevent addiction and the destructive behavior that may be associated with these drugs.

- The *Federal Hazardous Substances Act* mandates safety measures to prevent accidental poisoning. This provides for the **Poison Prevention Packaging Act**, which establishes mandates for childproof packaging.

- The Consolidated **Omnibus Budget Reconciliation Act** provides protection to the patient in the form of mandates that provide for patient counseling and medical supervision, as well as monetary protection to the patient through mandates that prevent overcharging for pharmaceuticals.

- The **Health Insurance Portability and Accountability Act (HIPAA)** provides for patient privacy within the health care structure. Revised in 2002, 2005, and in 2009, it provides for stringent regulation of information sharing regarding a personally identifiable patient. (Personally identifiable means that sufficiently precise information has been communicated that the patient is able to be identified.) Particularly addressed in this statute are issues regarding the electronic transmission of patient information and the preservation of both the information shared and the patient's privacy.

The Federal Food, Drug, and Cosmetic Act

The Food, Drug, and Cosmetic Act is enforced and governed by the Food and Drug Administration (FDA). Manufacturers of drugs and drug products must comply with the regulations and manufacturing standards set by the FDA. The regulations provide that:

1. Drugs introduced for sale:
    *   *are effective.* This is documented by clinical trials and studies involving both animals and humans, from a wide cross-section of parameters that include age, general health, and gender.
    *   *fall within established parameters for safety.* The safety of a drug is normally established by means of a mathematical representation called the therapeutic index, which is a comparison of the lethal dose to the effective dose. The incidence of serious adverse effects is also considered.
    *   *are properly labeled.* This requires documentation of studies that demonstrate safety and efficacy, and provides that information on the product label is accurate. Any claims made by the product's manufacturer must be documented to be accurate. Any medical conditions for which the product is to be used and claims for its effectiveness in such conditions must also be documented and approved.
    *   *are pure.* According to FDCA 1938.

2. *Food and food products* (e.g., herbal supplements and vitamins) as well as medical devices are documented to be safe and *are properly labeled.* Currently, claims made on the label of a food product (e.g., "lowers risk of heart disease" or "increases memory") are not required to be documented by research studies as long as they do not make specific claims. Items like "treats depression" or "treats high blood pressure" are specific medical claims that must be supported by research. Studies are presently being done on herbal products to document safety and manufacturer's claims, and upcoming legislation may soon change federal requirements for labeling of these products.

3. Drugs and devices for investigational use are safe and effective. Documentation of research and clinical studies must be approved by the FDA, before dispensing an investigational drug or device to the patient. This is termed *premarketing government approval* of such drugs or devices.

4. Over-the-counter medications are safe, efficacious, and have no abuse potential. OTC drugs must be appropriately labeled for self-administration by the patient. Since these drugs are to be taken without medical supervision, their strength must be low to help prevent overdosage, and abuse potential must be negligible. They must also require little to no monitoring by a health care professional. (Some drugs are

> Since drugs sold over the counter are to be taken without medical supervision, their strength must be low to help prevent overdosage, and abuse potential must be negligible.

not abusable in and of themselves, but can be easily separated into individual components that may be abusable or chemically converted into an abusable substance.)

Product Labeling

Proper labeling of OTC products is extremely important, as the patient often relies on individual judgment to decide which products to take. The information on the label helps the patient to make an informed decision. This information is important because it may be potentially lifesaving (e.g., warnings and contraindications placed on the label). Thus, the product's various uses, as well as adverse effects, contraindications, and warnings, must be clearly stated on the label (see Figure 32-1).

Additional amendments to the Food, Drug, and Cosmetic Act are contained in a list of safeguards called the *Durham-Humphrey Amendments.* These require the following:

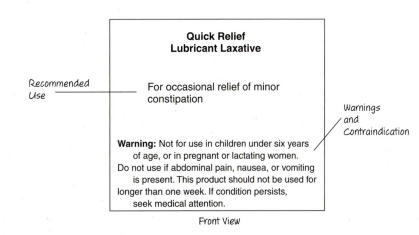

Quick Relief
Lubricant Laxative

Recommended Use —————— For occasional relief of minor constipation

Warning: Not for use in children under six years of age, or in pregnant or lactating women. Do not use if abdominal pain, nausea, or vomiting is present. This product should not be used for longer than one week. If condition persists, seek medical attention. —————— Warnings and Contraindication

Front View

Dosage:

Procedure for Dosing —— Adults and children over six years:

One teaspoon full (5 ml) at bedtime, followed by eight (8) ounces of water.

Children under six years: Consult a doctor.

Product Preparation Instructions —————— **SHAKE WELL BEFORE USING**

Back View

Figure 32-1

Delmar/Cengage Learning

A typical legend reads, "Federal law prohibits the dispensing of this drug without a prescription."	

The Prescription Order and Legend

- Prescription drugs must be dispensed by prescription order *only*. Thus, the label on the prescription as well as the manufacturer's label must bear the statement "Federal law prohibits the dispensing of this drug without a prescription" or bear "R$_X$" on container. This statement is called a "legend," which earns prescription medications, and some medical devices, the title of "legend drugs."

A transfer warning reads, "State or federal law prohibits the transfer of this drug to any person other than the person to whom it was prescribed."

The Transfer Warning

- Prescription drugs must be dispensed to and used *only* by the patient for whom they are prescribed. This mandate is on the prescription label in the form of a *transfer warning*, which reads, "State or federal law prohibits the transfer of this drug to any person other than the person to whom it was prescribed."

Documentation of Prescription Refills on the Prescription

- Prescription drugs may only be refilled according to the prescriber's authorization.

An electronic or verbally communicated prescription must be transcribed onto a prescription form. This may only be done by a licensed medical professional!

Written Prescriptions Must Be on File

- All prescriptions must ultimately be in written form and are filled under the supervision of the pharmacist. Thus, when prescriptions are called into the pharmacy by telephone or sent by e-mail, the information and explicit instructions must be accurately transcribed on a prescription form for filing. This may only be done by a licensed pharmacist, pharmacy intern, or, in a hospital setting, a nurse or other licensed professional in most states.

Any dispensing or sale of a drug without proper labeling shall be deemed "misbranding" of the drug and is in violation of federal statutes.

Containers Must Be Appropriately Labeled

- Both prescription and nonprescription drugs must be appropriately labeled with generic and trade names (if applicable), dosage form and strength, expiration date, and the name of the manufacturer. Instructions for patient dosage, as well as the preparation of the drug for dosing and any other necessary information, must also be included.

Purity of Drugs

Drugs must be offered for sale in a sanitary and unadulterated condition. *Any drug is considered adulterated if*:

- It contains poisonous or hazardous materials, putrid or decomposed materials, or has been intentionally exposed to radiation.
- A substance has been added or mixed with the drug that has no purpose except to increase the volume (bulk) of the drug (thus reducing its strength).

- The drug has been stored in an inappropriate manner (e.g., storage in improper temperature or in close proximity to toxic or decomposed substances).

- Any substance crucial to the drug's action has been omitted or substituted (thereby reducing its potency or bioavailability).

- Damage to the drug or inferior quality has been disguised in any manner.

- It contains an unsafe color additive.

- It contains a nonnutritive substance (e.g., resin, plastic).

The Controlled Substances Act

> Abusable drugs are classified into one of five groups, depending on the degree of abuse potential. These classifications are abbreviated as C-I to C-V (e.g., C-II) on the manufacturer's label.

The Controlled Substances Act regulates the manufacture, distribution, and dispensing of controlled substances (drugs of potential abuse). Abusable drugs are classified according to a *schedule* and are placed into one of five groups. These are designated as classes I to V, depending on the degree of abuse potential. These classifications are abbreviated as C-II to C-V on the manufacturer's label (drugs classified as C-I have no proven therapeutic value, so they are not sold commercially). Although the DEA determines the classes, minor differences in classification may occur from state to state. For example, in some states Talwin (pentazocine) is a schedule C-IV, but in other states it is a schedule II. The following are generally accepted classifications:

- **C-I:** These drugs have no proven therapeutic benefit and are highly abusable. This class includes drugs such as heroin, methamphetamine, and marijuana. THC (the abusable component in marijuana) is now commercially manufactured as the drug *dronabinol* (C-III) in some states.

- **C-II:** This class includes drugs that have a high potential for abuse, with severe psychological or physical dependence possible. Unlike drugs classified as C-I, drugs classified as C-II are therapeutically useful. Examples of this classification would be strong opiates such as morphine, codeine, and meperidine. Methadone, though not as psychologically addictive, is still physically addictive and also falls under this category.

- **C-III:** Drugs classified as C-III have proven therapeutic benefit and have less potential for abuse. These drugs may lead to physical or psychological dependence, but to a much lesser degree than drugs classified as C-I or C-II. Drugs classified as C-III are fairly widely prescribed and require less special documentation than drugs classified as C-II. Examples of this class include opiates that have been modified or formulated to have less abuse potential, such as hydrocodone with acetaminophen (Vicodin), or codeine with acetaminophen (Tylenol #3). These drugs may be prescribed on a regular prescription form, but they must be marked as a controlled substance prescription.

> The classification of individual drugs as C-III or C-IV may vary by state!

- **C-IV:** These drugs have much less potential for abuse and require less special documentation. Examples would be some benzodiazepines, such as alprazolam and lorazepam, and some opiates that do not cross easily into the central nervous system and are used as analgesics (e.g., propoxyphene [Darvocet]). These drugs may have been modified to decrease the potential for abuse, usually with the addition of acetaminophen. Without such a modification, the classification is increased to C-II.

- **C-V:** These drugs have a low potential for abuse. An example of a C-V drug would be the antidiarrheal Lomotil (diphenoxylate with atropine). Diphenoxylate is an opiate that crosses into the CNS poorly. As an additional safeguard, atropine is added in order to discourage dosage-related abuse (high doses of atropine have very unpleasant effects).

Documentation for Dispensing of Controlled Substances (Schedule Drugs)

Storage and Dispensing of Schedule II Drugs

Drugs that are classified Schedule I and Schedule II require special documentation and special storage. Schedule II drugs must be stored in a locked cabinet in the pharmacy or patient floor, or in a locked area of the medication cart. Prescription of controlled substances, particularly Schedule II drugs, requires special forms and handling. Normally, C-I drugs are not prescribed, so special dispensation may be required in order to consider a request for these drugs. In general, to dispense a Schedule II drug, the prescription received must be written on a duplicate or triplicate prescription form depending on the state. The prescription must be written *in ink* to discourage tampering. No refills are allowed on a prescription for a Schedule II drug.

Disposal of Schedule II Drugs

Both the ordering and disposal of Schedule II drugs also require the use of forms that can only be obtained from the DEA. These forms may only be obtained and used by a person approved by the DEA to handle such drugs. (The supervising pharmacist usually has applied for and been granted the approval to order and dispose of controlled substances.) The ordering of Schedule II drugs requires completion of DEA Form 222, and their disposal requires a request for approval to the State Bureau of Controlled Substances and to the DEA, made on DEA Form 41.

Storage and Dispensing of Drugs Classified as C-III and C-IV and C-V

Drugs that are classified C-III and C-IV and C-V may be prescribed on a regular prescription form, but they should be noted as controlled substances (by printing a red "C" on the prescription form, or simply noting the "C" class). They may be filed with regular prescriptions in some states; however, it is a good idea to file all prescriptions for controlled substances separately, in case of a federal audit.

The Federal Hazardous Substances Act

This regulation is enforced by the Consumer Product Safety Commission, and it protects the consumer from accidental exposure to potentially dangerous substances. The official records of investigations done by the commission are public record and may be examined by request, according to the *Freedom of Information Act*. The Federal Hazardous Substances Act encompasses the following:

The Poison Prevention Packaging Act

The Poison Prevention Packaging Act (PPPA) is an amendment to the Federal Hazardous Substances Act. It was enacted in 1970 to aid in the prevention of accidental poisoning. This act specifies that certain substances available for home use must be packaged in child-resistant packaging. This packaging is intended to be significantly difficult for children under five years of age to open within a reasonable time, but not difficult for the average adult to open. Exceptions to mandatory childproof packaging may be made for the elderly and handicapped who might have difficulty opening such containers. Drugs may be dispensed in regular (noncomplying) packaging for the sake of these individuals, provided the container carries a warning that it is not recommended for use in households with children.

Exemptions from Mandatory Child-Resistant Packaging

1. Prescription drugs may be dispensed from the pharmacy in non-child-resistant packaging upon the specific request of the prescribing doctor or the patient. Often, this requires the signing of a waiver by the patient, releasing the pharmacy and pharmacist from liability.

2. Certain prescription drugs are exempt from mandatory childproof packaging. These include drugs with a low potential for toxicity and those that are used in life-threatening acute conditions (e.g., nitroglycerin for angina, prednisone for severe allergic reactions), where the added time needed to remove a childproof cap could put the patient's life at risk.

    Some examples of exempt drugs include:

    *   Sublingual nitroglycerin (used in acute attacks of angina)
    *   Sublingual (or chewable) isosorbide dinitrate
    *   Oral contraceptives packaged in a dispenser package, which contain less than 27 mg of conjugated estrogens and/or less than 50 mg of norethindrone
    *   Medroxyprogesterone tablets

- Corticosteroids such as prednisone and methylprednisolone in dosages used for the treatment or prophylaxis of severe allergic reactions

3. OTC products when it is labeled that the container is not child resistant.

4. Situations where the patient is institutionalized and medication is administered to the patient.

The Occupational Safety and Health Act

This legislation was passed to ensure the safety of the worker in the workplace. Under this act, the Occupational Safety and Health Administration was formed.

The Occupational Safety and Health Administration (OSHA) was designed to protect employees in the workplace. OSHA has standards of safety and sanitation that must be met. It conducts periodic site visits or inspections to ensure that the pharmacy and its employees are complying with appropriate safety guidelines.

OSHA regulations state that:

- The floors in the work area must be clean and dry, and the pharmacy aisles should be free of boxes or other clutter.

- The exits and fire doors should be clearly marked and accessible—no boxes, barrels, or equipment should block them.

- Sharp objects and utensils should be put away when not in use. This includes sharps and needles as well as small spatulas, which could cause injury if they flip off a bench and land on a foot, on a hand, or in an eye.

- Flammable or caustic substances should be properly stored when not in use. They should not be left on the pharmacy bench. Flammable substances should be stored in specially vented "flammable" cabinets or, if necessary, in an explosion-proof refrigerator.

- Acids and bases, such as hydrochloric acid and sodium hydroxide, should never be stored in the same cabinet. If the two were to mix, a violent reaction would occur.

- OSHA-approved personal protective equipment should be worn when working with hazardous chemicals or drugs. This may include safety glasses and goggles. Closed-toe shoes and clothing that covers the arms and legs should also be worn.

Disposal of Hazardous Waste

Hazardous waste includes needles, syringes, and toxic chemicals (drugs).

- Needles or syringes should never be thrown in the trash. Syringes and needles can pose a health hazard to anyone using or disposing of the trash and could wind up in landfills or other public places. Both needles and syringes should be placed into an autoclavable sharps container for autoclaving (high-heat treatment) and disposal.

- Toxic substances, especially those such as cancer chemotherapeutics, should never be disposed of through the regular trash. Nor should the material be poured down the drain, because this would contaminate the water supply of the area. Instead, these substances should be placed into a biohazard bag or container for destruction.

Sanitation Management

Rinsing or washing equipment for liquid measure and wiping off dispensing trays and tablet counters should be done before and after each use. If the device is used and then used again without proper cleaning, residue from one prescription may be incorporated into another prescription, causing cross-contamination of drugs. Depending on the drug, this could be fatal to the patient. For example, many pharmacies have a separate, designated counting tray for penicillins.

Spills

Procedures must exist for the proper cleanup of substances spilled in the work area. Many substances used within a pharmacy are toxic, not only drugs (especially antineoplastics) but other substances as well, such as phenol and mercury (e.g., from a broken thermometer).

Flammable materials: Spills of flammable materials, such as alcohol, should first be contained so that the material does not contact electrical outlets on the floor or bench. Since it is the fumes (vapors) that ignite, proper ventilation must be provided. Electrical appliances such as portable fans should not be used for this purpose, due to sparks, which could ignite the fumes. After containment, an absorbent material is placed on the spill. Once absorbed, the material is swept away and disposed of in a well-ventilated area.

> Because of the potential of a strong chemical reaction, only weak acids or bases should be used to neutralize, such as acetic acid or sodium bicarbonate.

Caustic materials: Acids and bases are dangerous because they can dissolve most materials, including human skin. (Indeed, caustic agents like phenol are used to dissolve calluses on the feet and cauterize wounds.) Therefore, if an acid or base is spilled, it must first be neutralized before the spill is cleaned. When a substance of the opposite pH is added (e.g., a weak acid to neutralize a base), the spilled substance becomes a salt, which is not hazardous to clean up or dispose of. Once neutralized, the substance can be cleaned with disposable towels or wipes and thrown in the paper trash. It may also be disposed of down the drain.

Mercury

Mercury is an extremely toxic substance. At room temperature, it exists in a liquid form; at higher room temperature, it goes directly into a vapor (sublimation). It can then be inhaled through the respiratory tract as well as absorbed through the skin. Mercury is a very toxic substance that the body cannot eliminate once it has been absorbed. Therefore, it is essential that these spills be cleaned up immediately.

Cleaning mercury spills: To clean a spill of mercury, a spill kit is used that contains a porous sponge, which traps the small spheres of mercury and prevents dissemination throughout the area. The sponge should be used in a gentle blotting motion to avoid breaking up the spheres into smaller spheres, thus increasing the probability of sublimation. Mercury also reacts very quickly with gold, so be sure to remove any jewelry before attempting to clean a mercury spill.

Antineoplastic Drugs

Spills of antineoplastic drugs should be cleaned according to proper procedure and disposed of properly. Should the spill come in contact with the skin, the drug should be brushed from the skin (if it is in powder form) and removed as much as possible *before* washing thoroughly, to prevent absorption of the drug through the skin. If the spill is in liquid form, care must be taken not to rub the affected area, which would drive the drug into the skin. Liquid drug on the surface of the skin should be gently blotted off before the skin is washed thoroughly. Affected clothing should be removed immediately. It is also wise to wear a mask, goggles, and two sets of gloves when cleaning a spill.

> Wearing protective gloves will not protect you from toxic drugs if you touch your face, eyes, or mouth with the contaminated glove!

When working with antineoplastic drugs, you must be careful never to touch the area around the eyes, nose, or mouth. Working with gloves may protect the hands from exposure but will not prevent the drug from entering the body if the contaminated, gloved hands come in contact with the mucous membranes of the eyes, nose, or mouth. Reflex actions of rubbing an itching eye or nose should be avoided when working with antineoplastic drugs.

The Consolidated Omnibus Budget Reconciliation Act

This legislation was enacted in 1990, to improve the overall effectiveness of pharmaceutical therapy.

Mandatory Counseling of Patients

> Patient counseling may only be done by a licensed medical professional (e.g., pharmacist or pharmacy intern).

Under this act, pharmacists are now *required* by law to offer to counsel patients regarding every drug dispensed to them by the pharmacy. This entails describing the drug to the patient, including the generic and various brand names, correct dosage and correct method of dosing, and what actions are to be taken if a duplicate dose is taken by mistake or if a dose is missed. The patient is informed of the therapeutic uses of the drug and what adverse effects may be expected. Also included may be special instructions for storage, use, and preparation of the drug (if any). Techniques for **self-monitoring** of drug therapy are also taught at this time.

For example, when taking digitalis glycosides, the heart rate must be monitored with each dose, as bradycardia (slow heart rate) is a symptom of impending toxicity. Thus, the patient or caregiver must be advised to monitor the pulse rate with each dose, and, if necessary, shown how to accurately measure the pulse rate.

The Drug Utilization Review—Monitoring the Patient

As a consequence of this act, the drug utilization review was also established to ensure that records are kept of all medications dispensed to or regularly taken by the patient. The patient profile is a part of this review process. The patient profile contains information that allows the pharmacist to check for possible drug-drug interactions and improper use of prescription or nonprescription drugs. Possible adverse reactions that may occur as a result of drug allergies to similar drugs and possible interactions of a drug with an existing physiological condition are also considered.

The use of the information in the profile also allows detection of **therapeutic duplication**. A drug duplication occurs when two or more preparations contain the same drug, or same class of drug—either both are exactly the same drug (e.g., under different brand names), or both contain a percentage of the same drug. For example, the antidiarrheal Lomotil and the antispasmodic Chardonna both contain the drug atropine, even though they are different drug combinations and prescribed for different conditions. Combination therapy with both drugs may cause adverse effects from the increased dose of atropine.

> In order to ensure proper medication of the patient, the Consolidated Omnibus Budget Reconciliation Act mandates counseling of the patient with each prescription obtained from the pharmacy, as well as a drug utilization review by the pharmacist.

> The patient profile is an important part of the drug utilization review process!

> Therapeutic duplication is when two or more drugs taken by the patient contain the same, or similar, drug.

The Health Insurance Portability and Accountability Act (HIPAA)

The Health Insurance Portability and Accountability Act (HIPAA) was implemented in 1996. The original plan included provisions that were designed to encourage electronic transactions and that required that new safeguards be implemented to protect the security and confidentiality of health information being transferred electronically.

The first-ever federal privacy standards to protect a patient's medical record and other health information took effect in the form of new revisions to the HIPAA and were implemented in April 2003. Developed by the federal Health and Human Services division, these new standards provide patients with access to their medical records and afford the patient more control over how their personal health information is used and disclosed. The new HIPAA statutes are a *federal* mandate and do not affect privacy laws within a particular state.

The new privacy regulations provide each business the opportunity to set up a consistent process for the protection of patient privacy by limiting the ways that agents other than the primary care provider may interpret and use a patient's medical information. Previously, the privacy mandates provided for the regulation of information sharing only by the primary health care provider and his or her immediate staff, along with others such as laboratory workers and accounting personnel. With the new amendments, patient privacy also extends to the dissemination, interpretation, and handling of patient information by other parties involved in the care of the patient (e.g., pharmacies and insurance companies). The new mandates limit the ways that health plans, pharmacies, and hospitals can use a patient's personal information.

Key points in the revised HIPAA regulations include the following:

- Any personally identifiable information must now be protected as confidential. This includes written information (e.g., patient charts, laboratory results, and summaries of test results), verbal information, and any information stored on computers or peripherals (e.g., storage devices or media).

- Patients will now be allowed to access and request copies of their medical records. Previously, patients were not allowed easy access to their own medical charts, laboratory results, or other confidential medical records. With the new HIPAA mandates, patients are allowed to see and obtain copies of their medical records (in the case of a pharmacy, this would include the patient profile and dispensing records). These copies must be provided within 30 days of the patient's request. The patient is also allowed to make corrections in the records, should he or she find an error.

- Health care providers and involved organizations must now provide a written statement to the patient that states how personal medical information will be used by the provider. An explanation of the patient's rights of confidentiality (the privacy policy) must be provided. This statement should include information about the filing of complaints regarding privacy issues, and must be provided to the patient on the first visit. Patients will be required to sign or initial a form acknowledging receipt of the written privacy policy. Patients have the right to request that their personal information be more strictly regulated than the privacy policy, but the health care provider is not required to comply with this request.

- The use of personal medical information is now limited. The new privacy rules set limits on how health plans and other providers may use personally identifiable health information. The communication among doctors, nurses, pharmacists, and other health professionals is not limited by the new regulations, in order to provide for optimum health care. Organizations not directly involved in health care, such as insurance companies, banks, or marketing agencies to whom such information might be sold or exchanged, are no longer allowed access to privileged medical communications or information, unless the patient signs a waiver expressly allowing the dissemination of such information.

- Patients are now entitled to a free and complete discussion of health care options and treatment options from the health care provider.

- Patients may now request that confidential communications be done in a manner that they feel is appropriate. For example, he or she may request that any calls regarding medical issues be made to a work number or home number.

Responsibilities of the patient-care provider, as provided under the revised HIPAA regulations, are as follows:

- Any organization or practice involved in patient care must have a written privacy procedure, including a description of the particular staff who have access to confidential information.

- Organizations involved in health care must educate their staff on proper procedures for maintaining confidentiality. In addition, a single responsible individual (the privacy officer) must be designated to ensure that these procedures are followed by the staff.

- Health care providers are permitted, but not obligated, to disclose confidential medical information for the purposes of public health or to disclose limited information in other necessary circumstances, such as judicial or administrative proceedings, assistance in the identification of a deceased person, national defense issues, or the oversight of hospital administration or health care personnel.

- In 2005, the second portion of HIPAA was enacted which deals with maintaining the security of patient information.

- Updates were recently enacted in 2009. With technology always changing, updates and revisions will be an ongoing task.

Complaints Regarding Privacy Issues

A patient may file a complaint against a health care provider regarding privacy issues at any time, either by making the complaint directly to the provider or by filing a complaint with the Office for Civil Rights (OCR). The OCR is responsible for investigating complaints about privacy issues and enforcing the new privacy regulations. Information on the filing of a complaint may be found online at www.hhs.gov/ocr/hipaa.

Chapter Review Questions

1. A drug product is assumed to be free of contaminants, due to the following legislation:
   a. the Poison Prevention Packaging Act
   b. the Federal Hazardous Substance Act
   c. the Consolidated Omnibus Budget Reconciliation Act
   d. the Federal Food, Drug, and Cosmetic Act

2. Childproof packaging would be required on:
   a. a bottle of low-dose aspirin sold over the counter
   b. a bottle of Viagra
   c. a bottle of Celebrex dispensed to an elderly, arthritic person
   d. both a and b

3. The Food, Drug, and Cosmetic Act provides for documentation of the safety and efficacy of drugs by reviewing:
   a. safety and efficacy data provided by the manufacturer
   b. data from clinical trials and animal studies
   c. patient reports
   d. manufacturing data

4. In order for a drug to be sold over the counter:
   a. it must have a low abuse potential
   b. it must be low in strength to help prevent overdosage
   c. it must be approved by the FDA
   d. b and c only

5. A drug classified as Schedule I would have:
   a. high therapeutic efficacy
   b. low abuse potential
   c. no proven therapeutic benefit
   d. a low risk-to-benefit ratio

6. An example of a Schedule II drug would be:
   a. morphine
   b. meperidine
   c. heroin
   d. both a and b

7. A prescription for Xanax (alprazolam) might be:
   a. written on a regular prescription form
   b. notated with a red "C" before filing
   c. written on a triplicate form only
   d. a and b are correct

8. Mandatory patient counseling:
    a. may be done by the technician
    b. is only applicable to the elderly
    c. is not given to the caregiver, only the patient
    d. is required with all new and refill prescriptions

9. The words "This medication is intended for use only by the person for whom it was prescribed" might be found on a drug label. This would be termed:
    a. a warning label
    b. a precautionary statement
    c. a transfer warning
    d. a margin statement

10. The warning "Not recommended for use in households with children" might be found on a label for which product?
    a. a bottle of aspirin dispensed without a childproof cap
    b. a bottle of cough syrup
    c. a vial of morphine
    d. a bottle of Viagra

11. The label on a drug sold over the counter must carry:
    a. instructions for use and dosage
    b. contraindications and warnings
    c. pediatric dosage (if applicable) or contraindications
    d. all of the above

12. Counseling of the patient includes _____ and may be done by the _____.
    a. an explanation of the drug's mechanism of action—pharmacist
    b. an explanation of the drug's proper usage—technician or pharmacist
    c. teaching the patient self-monitoring techniques—pharmacist
    d. an explanation of the importance of proper dosage interval—technician or pharmacist

13. An example of a therapeutic duplication might be when a patient:
    a. is prescribed aspirin and Naprosyn
    b. is prescribed codeine and Tylenol #2
    c. is prescribed Metamucil and gemfibrozil
    d. receives prescriptions from more than one prescriber

14. Accurate records of patient demographics, drug history, and therapeutic profile must be kept, due to the mandates of the:
    a. Federal Hazardous Substances Act
    b. Controlled Substances Act
    c. Consolidated Omnibus Budget Reconciliation Act
    d. Poison Prevention Packaging Act

15. Therapeutic monitoring:
    a. involves regular assessment of the patient profile
    b. assures that the right drug is dispensed to each patient
    c. involves the pharmacy and therapeutics committee
    d. is done by the pharmacist

16. Which is the best way to dispose of a syringe and needle?
    a. cut both the syringe barrel and needle in half and discard them
    b. place both the syringe and needle in an autoclavable sharps container
    c. cut the needle off of the syringe and discard them
    d. place both syringe and needle in a biohazard (red) bag

17. When working with antineoplastic (anticancer) drugs, you should wear:
    a. clothing that has long sleeves and covers the legs
    b. a protective cloth coat
    c. a paper coat, hat, shoe covers, and goggles
    d. both a and c

18. The first step in cleaning an alcohol spill should be:
    a. absorbing the material
    b. protecting exposed electrical outlets
    c. turning off any open flames or electrical appliances
    d. both b and c

19. A patient requests that all telephone conversations regarding medical issues be directed to his cell phone. The staff of the pharmacy is obligated to comply with this request because of provisions in which law?
    a. the Consolidated Omnibus Budget Reconciliation Act
    b. the Controlled Substances Packaging Act
    c. the Health Insurance Portability and Accountability Act
    d. the Occupational Safety and Health Act

20. According to the new HIPAA regulations, a written privacy procedure for a health care provider must:
    a. contain a list of personnel who will have access to confidential information
    b. be available to the patient and staff
    c. be enforced by a designated person on the staff
    d. all of the above

CHAPTER 33

State and Federal Regulatory Agencies

Quick Study

I. Federal regulatory agencies

    A. The U.S. Food and Drug Administration (FDA)
- Regulates the manufacture, distribution, and quality of drugs sold within the United States
- Regulates the admission of new drugs and devices into the U.S. market
- Regulates the manufacture of drugs and devices
- Regulates proper product labeling
- Mandates the inclusion of package inserts
- Investigates complaints against manufacturers and distributors of drug products

    B. The U.S. Consumer Product Safety Commission (CPSC)
- Protects the consumer against unreasonable risk of injury associated with consumer products
- Mandates standards of safety for consumer products
- Investigates product-related deaths and injuries
- Administers the:
  1. Consumer Product Safety Act
  2. Flammable Fabrics Act
  3. Federal Hazardous Substances Act
  4. Poison Prevention Packaging Act
  5. Refrigerator Safety Act

II. State regulatory agencies

    A. The State Board of Pharmacy
- Regulates standards of professional knowledge and care
- Regulates the quality of drugs dispensed from pharmacies within the state

    B. Regulation of hospital and long-term care facilities

III. Regulation at the institutional level

A. The pharmacy and therapeutics committee
- Sets standards within an institution for pharmacy operations
- Chooses the drug formulary and mandates procedures

B. The Joint Commission
- Sets standards for institutional care
- Institutional compliance is voluntary
- Legal issues

A number of regulatory agencies have been established to ensure the safety and viable therapy of the patient. The most familiar of these agencies are federally controlled, such as the Food and Drug Administration and the Consumer Product Safety Commission. A number of agencies are administrated at both the state and institutional levels. These include the State Board of Pharmacy, the American Society of Health System Pharmacists (a professional organization), and The Joint Commission.

Federal Regulatory Agencies

The U.S. Food and Drug Administration

The U.S. Food and Drug Administration (FDA) regulates the drug products on the market in the United States. It was founded to protect the consumer by ensuring the purity, potency, efficacy, and safety of drug and food products.

Developing a New Drug

New drugs that enter the market must comply with a standard of procedures that document their efficacy and safety. They must go through a long series of *clinical trials* in both animals and humans in order to generate enough data on their safety, therapeutic efficacy (how well the drug works), and *toxicity*. These trials help to establish recommended dosage parameters, drug interactions, and a therapeutic index. These are necessary to satisfy the requirements of the FDA regarding the safety and efficacy of the drug.

The NDA and Clinical Trials

Manufacturing companies must first file a *New Drug Application* (NDA), which documents the composition and action of the drug product, including supporting animal studies. They are then allowed to apply for *clinical trials*. Clinical trials normally proceed in stages, called *phases*.

- *Phase I* is the initial trial that documents the drug's safety profile.
- *Phase II* documents its safety and efficacy in an expanded pool of patients.
- *Phase III* continues to use human subjects to document efficacy and dose potency of the drug versus placebo (a dosage form with no drug). At this stage, the drug is considered investigational, and the manufacturer files an Investigational New Drug (IND) form with the FDA.

These procedures must be followed not only when a new drug enters the market, but also when an existing drug is being investigated for use in a new way. Example: The anticancer drug methotrexate is also useful in the treatment of autoimmune diseases, such as rheumatoid arthritis, due to its secondary effects on the immune system. In order for methotrexate to be approved for use in the treatment of autoimmune disease, it had to undergo clinical trials *for this purpose,* even though its properties were already well documented when it first came on the market as an antineoplastic anticancer agent.

An exception occurs when there is no cure for a disease and the drug may provide a benefit to the patient, which no other drug does.

Drug/Food Classifications

The classifications of drugs by the FDA fall into two general categories: therapeutic drugs and food supplements. The regulations on drugs and drug products are extremely stringent, while those on food supplements are less so. Most herbal drugs are presently classified as food supplements, primarily in order to avoid the years of clinical testing necessary for the marketing of these products as drugs. This may be changing in the near future, as the number of drug interactions, hospitalizations, and deaths related to the unregulated use of these herbal drug products is increasing.

Product Labeling

The FDA has recently established a division for product labeling, which regulates the information placed on a drug label. Any claims made by the manufacturer on a product label must be substantiated by clinical studies, and the proper warnings, contraindications, and listing of adverse effects must be included.

> A lack of cleanliness could lead to cross-contamination of drug products. This might be potentially lethal, should the patient be allergic to the contaminating drug!

Regulation of Drug Manufacturing Sites

The FDA is responsible for inspecting drug manufacturing sites to ensure cleanliness, purity of ingredients, and a lack of cross-contamination of drugs. For example, cross-contamination of drugs would be seen if a volatile powdered drug was being manufactured adjacent to and then mixed in with a cream. Another example would be if the machinery used in the manufacturing and packaging of one drug was not cleaned thoroughly before using it to manufacture or package a second drug; some of the first drug might be incorporated into the second.

Investigation of Complaints

The FDA is responsible for investigating claims of drugs that are adulterated, misbranded, and sold even after they have expired. Drugs found to be adulterated or misbranded are immediately seized and fines or sanctions levied on the manufacturer or supplier at fault.

Package Inserts

> Package inserts contain safety information, study results, potential adverse effects, interactions, and contraindications associated with the drug, as well as information documenting its efficacy.

The FDA mandates that package inserts be included with all drug products. Package inserts are required to contain important information, such as:

- Safety data
- Results of studies done on the drug
- Adverse effects of the drug
- Drug interactions and contraindications
- Data that documents the efficacy of the drug

This information assists the pharmacist in counseling the patient and monitoring the patient's drug profile. It should be noted that *any* adverse effect must be recorded, even if it is reported in only one patient.

Dispensing of Patient Package Inserts (PPIs)

> A PPI is required to be dispensed to any patient receiving estrogen, and must be given to the patient before the first dose of medication is administered or dispensed to the patient.

In the case of some drugs, one example is contraceptives, patient package inserts (PPIs) are required to be dispensed to the patient along with the drug. *A PPI is required to be dispensed to any patient receiving estrogen.* It must be given to the patient before the first dose of medication is administered or dispensed, and *every time the prescription is refilled* during therapy. The PPI describes the benefits and adverse effects of the medication, and is written in terms that a layperson can understand. Distribution of this document is the responsibility of the person dispensing the drug (e.g., the pharmacist and technician, in the outpatient setting, or the nurse, in the inpatient setting).

The Bureau of Alcohol, Tobacco, and Firearms

The Bureau of Alcohol, Tobacco, and Firearms is a federal agency that has jurisdiction over the dispensing of tax-free alcohol. This agency oversees the dispensing of alcohol from the hospital pharmacy.

The Consumer Product Safety Commission

The Consumer Product Safety Commission (CPSC) is an independent regulatory agency that functions under the provisions of the Consumer Product Safety Act (CPSA). It consists of five members who are appointed by the president and serve for terms of seven years. The purposes of the commission under the CPSA are:

1. To protect the public against unreasonable risks of injury associated with consumer products.
2. To assist consumers in evaluating the comparative safety of consumer products.
3. To develop uniform safety standards for consumer products and to minimize conflicting state and local regulations.
4. To promote research and investigation into the causes and prevention of product-related deaths, illnesses, and injuries.

The Consumer Product Safety Commission administers the following five acts:

1. The Consumer Product Safety Act
2. The Flammable Fabrics Act
3. The Federal Hazardous Substances Act
4. The Poison Prevention Packaging Act
5. The Refrigerator Safety Act

Agencies Controlled at the State Level

> Should regulations conflict between state and federal mandates, the more stringent law should be followed.

In addition to federal regulations and federally mandated agencies, there are regulatory agencies established at the state level. It is important to note that *should regulations conflict between state and federal mandates, the more stringent of the two laws will apply.* Regulatory agencies vary from state to state—some have much more stringent laws regarding the dispensing of pharmaceuticals than others (New York, for example). In most states, the dispensing of pharmaceuticals and regulation of professional conduct is governed by the State Board of Pharmacy.

The State Board of Pharmacy

The State Board of Pharmacy exists to ensure that the welfare of the patient is best served. It mandates strict codes of professional conduct by the pharmacist. In addition, it oversees the quality of the drugs dispensed from the state's pharmacies to ensure proper potency, purity, and labeling of the drug product. The State Board of Pharmacy functions to:

- *Ensure the proper education and level of knowledge of the pharmacist,* through licensing examinations. The board also grants licensure only to pharmacists who meet strict criteria for ethical and educational standards.
- Handle *consumer complaints* and provide appropriate disciplinary action against a pharmacist or pharmacy when warranted.

- Set the *policies and procedures regarding the filling and labeling of prescriptions.* Regular inspections may be performed by representatives of the State Board of Pharmacy to ensure compliance with the policies.

Regulation of Hospital and Long-Term Care

The care of patients in a long-term care facility is also regulated by the state. To a certain extent, the pharmacy service is also regulated by federal laws, since a variety of criteria must be met in order for the facility to be eligible to accept federal aid, such as Medicare and Medicaid.

The state board of pharmacy oversees the pharmacy's quality of care, which includes ensuring the quality of drugs, mandating of prescription filling policies, and licensure.

Accountability of Drug Distribution within an Institution

The pharmacy is accountable for all drug products within the long-term care facility, from the initial dispensing of the drug to its transfer to the nurse or resident and subsequent administration to the patient. This includes:

- Monitoring of patient records
- Monitoring of patients and evaluation of the prescribed drug regimen
- Responsibility for the proper care of the drugs, including the ultimate administration or destruction of the medications administered
- Maintaining records of the disposition of the drugs dispensed and documenting their ultimate fate (e.g., whether they were administered to the patient or destroyed—hopefully, the drugs will not simply disappear!)

Regulation at the Institutional Level

There are a variety of committees and commissions formed outside of state and federal regulations that function to ensure competent and proper health care. These include the **Pharmacy and Therapeutics Committee**, which is formed within an institution, and **The Joint Commission**, which is a nongovernmental agency composed of members of health care organizations that oversees hospital care.

The Pharmacy and Therapeutics Committee

This organization is formed within a health care institution and consists of pharmacists, nurses, and physicians. It may also include members of the hospital's financial division. The role of this committee is to *set guidelines for the practice of pharmacy within the institution.*

The pharmacy and therapeutics committee chooses *the drug formulary for the pharmacy,* as the diverse types of expertise of the various members of the committee contribute to the inclusion of the best possible drugs in the hospital formulary. The pharmacy and therapeutics committee also *devises and enforces hospital policy with regard to the pharmacy* and pharmacy administration.

The Joint Commission

The Joint Commission is a nonprofit organization that sets standards for proper hospital administration and policies. Compliance with The Joint Commission is voluntary; however, compliance may ensure both the reputation of the institution and a recognized standard of care, in case of legal action. Failure to meet The Joint Commission standards may result in a loss of prestige or public trust in a hospital, and also may result in a lack of the ability to attract the best health care professionals. Consequently, the staff may be less competent.

To ensure that the standard of health care is being adhered to, representatives of The Joint Commission make periodic visits to hospitals and review records, policies, and procedures. The team may then make patient-floor visits, where interviews of caregivers, managers, and patients are conducted to assess the quality and consistency of care. A dedicated (especially reserved) visit to the pharmacy and a review of the pharmacy services is conducted. An assessment is then made of the ability of staff members to perform their jobs competently and meet patient needs.

Chapter Review Questions

1. Which of these organizations is a state regulatory agency?
   a. The U.S. Food and Drug Administration
   b. The Joint Commission
   c. The U.S. Consumer Product Safety Commission
   d. The State Board of Pharmacy

2. Which of the following is regulated by the FDA?
   a. the purity and efficacy of drug products
   b. proper labeling of drug products
   c. the standards of manufacture of drug products
   d. all of the above

3. Claims of misbranded drugs would be handled by the:
   a. Pharmacy and Therapeutics Committee
   b. Joint Commission on Accreditation of Healthcare Organizations
   c. U.S. Consumer Product Safety Commission
   d. U.S. Food and Drug Administration

4. A package insert:
   a. must be included by the manufacturer with all drugs and drug products
   b. must contain safety information, toxicity, and adverse effects
   c. contains the results of scientific studies done on the drug
   d. all of the above are true

5. The patient package insert is:
   a. required to be given with every refill of the drug preparations containing estrogen
   b. required to be delivered to the patient at the time of the first dose of a drug containing estrogen
   c. available to the patient on request, but delivery is not required
   d. both a and b are correct

6. An elderly person buys acetaminophen at the grocery store. He has a severe headache, so he takes ten tablets (5 gr) in the course of six hours. He is taken to the hospital several hours later, diagnosed with acute liver failure, and dies. His case might be investigated by:
   a. the FDA
   b. the U.S. Consumer Product Safety Commission
   c. the State Board of Pharmacy
   d. the local police

7. Which of the following agencies mandates the Poison Prevention Packaging Act?
   a. The Pharmacy and Therapeutics Committee
   b. The Joint Commission on Accreditation of Healthcare Organizations
   c. The U.S. Consumer Product Safety Commission
   d. The U.S. Food and Drug Administration

8. Evidence that a hospital is performing with competent personnel and maintaining a good standard of care would be:
   a. accreditation of the pharmacy by the State Board of Pharmacy
   b. accreditation of the hospital by The Joint Commission
   c. a lack of complaints investigated by the FDA
   d. a lack of complaints investigated by the U.S. Consumer Product Safety Commission

9. Herbal products are currently considered:
   a. OTC drugs
   b. food supplements
   c. prescription drugs
   d. none of the above

10. The Pharmacy and Therapeutics Committee chooses:
    a. the drug formulary for the hospital pharmacy
    b. the pharmacy staff
    c. the Director of Pharmacy
    d. all the above

CHAPTER 34

Law and Ethics in the Practice of Pharmacy

Quick Study

I. The legal definition of pharmacy

    A. Therapeutic monitoring
    B. Patient counseling

II. Recognizing a legally valid prescription

- Who is legally authorized to prescribe?
- What are the legal limitations on drug prescription?

III. Verifying the prescription

    A. A prescription for a legend drug—valid for one year
    B. A prescription for a controlled substance—valid for three days (C-II) to six months, (C-III to C-IV) depending on the state

IV. Prescriptions generated by electronic means—controlled substance laws versus regular legend drugs

V. Drug refills—regular drugs versus controlled substances, C-II versus C-III to C-V

VI. Controlled substance registration—the DEA number:

- Who gets one?
- How to recognize a valid DEA number

VII. Handling regular prescriptions and controlled substances

    A. Dispensing
    B. Record-keeping
    C. Documentation
    D. Transferring prescriptions between pharmacies

VIII. Liability and ethics

   A. The ultimate liability falls on the pharmacist

   B. Patient confidentiality and ethical standards

The Legal Definition of Pharmacy Practice

> Drug monitoring or drug utilization review includes the proper education of the patient to the extent that the patient is able to properly self-medicate. This is accomplished by mandatory patient counseling.

The legal definition of pharmacy practice is an occupation whereby one maintains drug substances for therapeutic use, reviews prescriptions for legality and propriety, and selects the appropriate drug product to fill such prescriptions. In addition, the legal definition of pharmacy includes the practice of drug monitoring in the scope of medicinal therapy. This includes creating and monitoring patient profiles, screening medications dispensed for potential drug interactions or physiological interactions, and ensuring appropriate therapy. Drug monitoring or drug utilization review also includes the proper education of the patient to the extent that the patient is able to properly self-medicate. This is accomplished by mandatory patient counseling.

Patient counseling includes education of the patient as to:

> Patient counseling is required when dispensing any prescription drug directly to a patient. This includes mail order and Web-based pharmacies as well!

- drug action
- basic physiology
- potential adverse effects to be expected
- foods and drinks to be avoided
- the importance of a proper dosage regimen

Counseling also must include a discussion of self-monitoring of physiological reactions (e.g., blood pressure, heart rate) as appropriate to alert the patient to potential drug toxicity before it becomes a problem.

> Patient counseling in the pharmacy may be done only by the pharmacist or by a pharmacy intern under the direct supervision of the pharmacist!

Receiving Prescriptions

Recognizing a Legally Valid Prescription

A prescription is *legally valid* only if written by a licensed medical professional or veterinarian. In addition, the *prescription is only valid if written for a drug or drug product that is used within the scope of the prescriber's normal practice.*

> **EXAMPLE**
>
> A patient comes to the pharmacy window with a prescription for Ambien written by her family dentist. Legally, this prescription would not be valid, as a sleeping pill is not common therapy in dentistry. (Some of us think that they should hand out such drugs at the door in a dentist's office, but that is beside the point.) Similarly, a prescription for contraceptives that is written by an optometrist would not be accepted at the pharmacy window, as it is not a legally valid prescription.

Licensed medical professionals who are allowed to prescribe medication include the:

- medical doctor (MD)
- doctor of osteopathic medicine (DO)
- doctor of dentistry (DDS)
- nurse practitioner (NP, ARNP)
- physician's assistant (PA)

Medical and dental students are allowed to prescribe medication within the scope of their institution (e.g., while on rotation in a hospital). Prescriptions written by veterinarians may be filled at retail pharmacies, as long as the medication is intended for and labeled for veterinary use. Again, a prescription that is written by a veterinarian for a drug that is clearly intended for human use would not be legally valid.

Verifying the Prescription

If a prescription is to be accepted at the pharmacy window, the prescription must be accurately written and verifiable. A prescription for a regular drug or device should contain:

- The date of prescription.
- The patient's name.
- The generic or proprietary name of the drug.
- The strength, dose, and instructions for administration.
- The quantity or days supply required.
- Instructions for preparation or special instructions as appropriate.
- The name and address of the prescriber and a *verifiable* DEA number (in most states). In addition to the verification of the DEA number by letters and numerical equation (Chapter 1), the DEA will also confirm validity by telephone.

- A valid signature *in ink* (no stamps or facsimiles).
- A date that the prescription is written.
- Must be presented for filling within six months to one year (depending on the state) from the date on the prescription, can be refilled up to one year from the date on the prescription; six months for controlled substances (C-III–C-V).

Verification of Controlled Substance Prescription

A prescription for a C-II controlled substance should contain all of the above, plus:

- The prescription should be on a triplicate form if required by the state.
- The prescription should be completely filled out at the time of acceptance.
- No corrections should be present.
- The prescription must be written and signed in ink.
- The technician should examine the prescription form for possible additions or changes (e.g., #10 becomes #100, 5 mg becomes 25 mg, etc.).
- The identity of the patient should be verified.

The prescription label for a controlled substance should contain a transfer warning statement, which indicates that it is a punishable crime to give such medication to another person. Transfer warnings are now preprinted on all prescription labels.

Prescriptions Generated by Electronic Means

Prescriptions may now be submitted by telephone, fax, or e-mail (with the exception of those for Schedule II drugs). These prescriptions must be taken by the pharmacist, or by a pharmacy intern under the direct supervision of the pharmacist.

When received, electronic orders must be printed off or written on a paper prescription form in order to have a hard copy for filing. *Schedule II drugs are not allowed to be submitted by electronic means.* The presentation of a hard-copy prescription to the pharmacy is required. In some states, this should be on a triplicate form.

Emergency Situations

In the event of an emergency, an order for a Schedule II drug *may* be taken by telephone. The telephone order must be received by the pharmacist and transcribed onto a prescription form that is clearly dated and marked

"Authorization for Emergency Dispensing." In addition, the verbal order must be followed by a written prescription from the prescriber within 72 hours. The written prescription is then permanently attached to the transcribed telephone order taken by the pharmacist.

Drug Refills

> The length of time between refills is not influenced by the frequency of dosage. For example, drugs taken "as needed" cannot be refilled as they are used.

Prescriptions for regular drugs may be refilled up to the number of refills authorized on the original prescription, but not beyond one year from the original date of the prescription. However, for certain drugs it is appropriate to dispense more than one refill at a time, if the insurance provider will allow it. (It is often cheaper for the patient to buy the drug in bulk, particularly if it is something to be taken every day for a long period of time, such as an anticonvulsant drug or an anti-inflammatory drug taken for arthritis.) Once all the refills on a prescription have been dispensed, it is necessary to obtain a new prescription. In some cases, the pharmacist may call for a *refill authorization*.

Refilling Prescriptions for Controlled Substances

> If the entire amount necessary to fill an order for a C-II drug is not available when the order is presented, the remaining amount must be dispensed within three days (72 hours).

Prescriptions for controlled substances of Classes III and V may have up to five refills. The prescription is no longer valid after six months. *No refills are allowed on a prescription for a C-II drug.* Prescriptions for C-II drugs are only valid for a short length of time. If the entire amount is not available at the time of presentation, the remainder must be dispensed within 72 hours. If the drug is not dispensed within that time, the prescription has expired and the balance is voided. Bear in mind that these regulations may differ somewhat by individual state law.

Dispensing of Drugs and Drug Products Without a Prescription

Normally, legend drugs are not dispensed without a prescription. The exception is when an institutional pharmacy dispenses drugs to be used as floor stock, which will be stored in a secure area or pharmaceutical supplies container (e.g., medication cart).

Controlled Substance Registration

Persons who prescribe a legend drug and any institution that dispenses them are required to register with the Drug Enforcement Agency (DEA). Once registered, the person or institution receives a registration number or **DEA number.**

Only prescribers, wholesalers, and health care institutions can receive a DEA number. Since the pharmacist does not prescribe drugs, but only dispenses them according to the instructions of the prescriber, no DEA number is necessary—the registration under which the pharmacist dispenses drugs is that of the institution. This may be changing with the advent of the PharmD (doctor of pharmacy) degree in clinical practice, as laws are being considered that would allow pharmacists to give injections and prescribe medications within the scope of their practice.

Handling Controlled Substances

Controlled substances may be handled only by those persons or institutions approved by the DEA to do so. This requires the submission and approval of an application to handle controlled substances. The exceptions to this rule are as follows:

- Nurses, physician's assistants, and medical residents—these personnel are allowed to handle controlled substances under the authority of the institution in which they work. Prescriptions for controlled substances may be written by those licensed to do so under the authority of the institution.

In a hospital setting, medical interns and residents are considered trainees and are assigned DEA numbers based on the DEA number assigned to the hospital. All interns and residents use the same DEA number, which has additional letters/numbers attached on the end to designate a specific person.

> **EXAMPLE**
>
> The hospital DEA is BU1654929. Dr. Yannis's DEA would be BU1654929 CLP S145 and Dr. Bon Jovi would be BU1654929 CLP A485.

- Pharmaceutical sales representatives—these persons have no formal license, but are allowed to handle controlled substances under the scope of their position as salespeople. They are allowed to dispense small quantities of such substances to licensed physicians as samples, but they must maintain appropriate records.

Record-keeping

All drugs dispensed from the pharmacy require a hard copy for filing that shows the amount dispensed and the date that the prescription was received. Prescriptions for regular drugs remain valid and may be refilled for a period of one year from the date of writing. Should a prescription be transferred from one pharmacy to another, the expiration date of the prescription and the number of refills available do not change.

Controlled Substance Records

> In a hospital pharmacy, control sheets are to be maintained that indicate the time of administration of Schedule II drugs, as well as the patient to whom they were administered.

Especially accurate records must be kept of controlled substances and their disposition. This includes records of inventory as well as dispensing records. An inventory of controlled substances is to be performed by the institution according to their policies.

The dispensing records of Schedule II drugs must be kept separately from those of other drugs. The records of drugs falling under Schedules III–V may be filed with those of other prescription drugs, depending on the state. These must be clearly designated as records for controlled substances (e.g., by stamping a red "C" on the prescription form where it is clearly visible). It is best to keep the records of all controlled substances dispensed separate from those of other prescription drugs, mainly because the records of controlled substances are subject to periodic audits by the DEA, and separating records makes this much easier.

> When a prescription is transferred from one pharmacy to another, the accepting pharmacy is required to keep the prescription on file for a period of one year after transfer.

Some drugs classified as Schedule V may be sold over the counter in some states and are considered Exempt Narcotics. If such drugs are sold over the counter, a "Legend Book" must be maintained. When they are purchased, the sale must be recorded in the Legend Book, with the name of the purchaser, the address of the purchaser, the quality of the drug, and the price. The purchaser must be 18 years of age. Consequently, to avoid the additional record-keeping, most pharmacies simply choose not to carry Schedule V drugs that can be sold over the counter, or choose not to sell them without a prescription.

Liability and Ethics

> The dispensing records of Schedule II drugs must be kept separate from those of other drugs. Records of drugs falling under Schedules III–V may be filed with those of other prescription drugs.

Federal laws govern the manufacture of drugs and ensure their safety, efficacy, and potency. State laws govern how these drugs will be dispensed, and by whom. This includes mandates on the filling and refilling of prescriptions. As a technician, you should request a copy of the state laws from your State Board of Pharmacy to ensure that your practice of pharmacy is legally valid. The supervising pharmacist is legally liable for the actions of the pharmacy technician. Therefore, technicians have an obligation and responsibility to follow the state and federal laws to the best of their ability. As a technician, you may be subject to legal action, even though you are working under the pharmacist's license. You may also be subject to civil judgments.

Patient Confidentiality

As a technician, you will work with a large amount of information, much of it personal and confidential. This may include a patient's financial records, medical records, and other confidential information. The recently passed HIPAA regulations strictly govern patient confidentiality (the Freedom of Information Act does *not* cover this area). Any discussions of the patient's confidential information should be conducted *only* with the pharmacist and *only* within the scope of pharmacy practice. Such information is not to be discussed in public areas and may not be given out, even to a close family member, without the express *written* consent of the patient.

Chapter Review Questions

1. Dr. Dan Dee walks into the pharmacy. He is an optometrist who has written himself a prescription for Valium. You should:
   a. fill the prescription
   b. alert the pharmacist
   c. deny the prescription, as it is not a legal prescription
   d. both b and c are correct

2. A patient is on tranylcypromine, an MAO inhibitor. Patient counseling might include:
   a. a discussion of the drug's action
   b. a warning to stay away from certain foods
   c. a warning to see a physician if certain symptoms, such as rapid heart rate and restlessness, are exhibited
   d. all of the above

3. A medical student may prescribe drugs:
   a. only in the scope of his or her studies within the hospital
   b. using his or her DEA number
   c. only in the hospital, using the hospital's DEA number
   d. both a and c are correct

4. In October 2010, a customer brings in a prescription for Keflex. The prescription is dated 2/10/2010. Legally, the prescription:
   a. will only be valid until 2/10/2011
   b. will only be good for two refills, instead of the three originally prescribed
   c. must be filled immediately
   d. cannot be filled, as it is over six months old

5. A prescription for Demerol:
   a. must be received on a triplicate form, according to federal law
   b. may be called or faxed in
   c. may be obtained by telephone in an emergency
   d. both a and c are correct

6. You receive a prescription for meperidine (classified as a C-II). It contains a corrected date. You should:
   a. alert the pharmacist
   b. ask the patient why the date was corrected
   c. ignore the change in date and fill the prescription
   d. refuse to fill the prescription and give it back to the patient

7. Which of the following is true regarding a prescription for Valium?
   a. It requires a triplicate form
   b. It is only valid for six months
   c. no more than five refills are allowed
   d. both b and c

8. Mrs. Jones has a prescription for hydromorphone (classified as C-II), written for ten tablets. The pharmacy has only five in stock. You have the tablets on order for next week. You should:
   a. fill the prescription for five and mark the other five on the form as a refill
   b. fill the prescription for five tablets and tell the patient to come in next week for the rest
   c. refuse to fill the prescription
   d. tell the patient that she can only have five unless she goes to another pharmacy

9. Which of the following people, all of whom handle controlled substances, do not require a controlled substance registration?
   a. a nurse
   b. a physician
   c. a pharmacist
   d. a sales representative for a pharmaceutical company

10. A patient brings in a prescription, dated 2/25/2010, to Hill Road Pharmacy on that same day. The prescription is for Ceclor (a very pricey drug) and has five refills authorized. He receives a refill on 4/15/2010. On 5/12/2010, the patient discovers that Dale pharmacy is cheaper and has the prescription transferred there. Dale pharmacy:
    a. will only fill two of the remaining four refills
    b. will be able to fill refills on the prescription until 2/25/2011
    c. will have to get a refill authorization in order to fill the remaining refills
    d. cannot fill this prescription

Maintaining Medication and Inventory Control Systems

THIS SECTION of the book reviews the content in the second functional area, as tested in the ExCPT or PTCB exam. This comprises 23% (ExCPT) and 22% (PTCB) of the examination questions. This section includes:

Stocking the Pharmacy

Quick Study

I. The drug formulary

    A. The national formulary
    B. The pharmacy formulary

II. Choice of drugs to be stocked—based on use, efficiency, adverse effects, cost, and storage requirements

    A. Drug cost, efficacy, and frequency of prescription (drug demand)
    B. Therapeutic uses, adverse effects, and storage requirements

III. Ordering and receipt of drugs and devices

    A. Use of the *purchase order* and "want book"
    B. Information to be specified when ordering drugs and devices:
- The drug or device name (generic or proprietary)
- Strength and dosage form of the drug (or size, if ordering a device)
- Type of packaging and quantity per package of drug dosage forms
- Quantity ordered of bottles, packages, or devices

IV. Ordering of controlled substances: Schedules II–IV

The Drug Formulary

The list of drugs that reflects what the pharmacy routinely stocks is called a **formulary**. There are literally hundreds of individual drugs available for dispensing by the pharmacy, so the pharmacy cannot possibly stock all available drugs. The pharmacy must choose which drugs to stock based on cost, efficacy, and demand. The national formulary is a listing of all drugs marketed in the United States. The letters "NF" after a drug name indicate that the drug is included in the *national* formulary.

The drug formulary within an institution is derived from a joint effort by the pharmacist and the institution. In a hospital pharmacy, an organization within the hospital called the **Pharmacy and Therapeutics Committee** decides which drugs to stock in the pharmacy. This committee is made up of the pharmacists and representatives of the various healthcare fields: physicians, nurses, and dietitians. This is necessary to present all views on a drug's ease of use and efficacy, in order to choose the best drugs to stock. For example, a drug may be just as efficacious as another, but it may be very difficult to administer or not well tolerated by the patient. The pharmacist does not actually administer the medication to patients, so other professionals are needed to accurately assess the drugs.

The formulary is a very selective list of drugs. These drugs have been selected because they have been determined to be *the best drugs at the lowest cost*. More than one proprietary (brand) name of a drug is available for most drugs, and many different generic brands are available as well. However, only one brand name and one generic per drug are normally stocked in a pharmacy, as stocking more than one brand of the same drug (called **drug duplication**) takes up valuable shelf space and resources. Two brands may be stocked if there is sufficient justification for carrying both in the formulary.

We choose which of the available drugs to stock in the pharmacy according to:

- *Cost*: the best drug at the lowest cost
- *Efficacy*: only drugs proven to be efficacious are stocked
- *Demand*: drugs frequently prescribed are routinely stocked

Other factors involved in the selection of drugs are their uses, side effects, and storage requirements. The storage requirements determine how much it will cost the pharmacy to keep the drug stocked (the "carrying costs"). For example, if a particular drug is stored on the pharmacy shelf and another must be refrigerated, the one stored on the shelf would cost less to maintain.

> The formulary is a selective listing of drugs that have been determined to be the best medications at the lowest cost.

> **NOTE**
>
> The drug formulary is under constant revision as new drugs and dosage forms are constantly being produced and as more information is gathered about older drugs; some may be removed from the market due to unforeseen problems.

Automated Ordering Systems

Automated ordering systems are an important part of keeping a pharmacy's costs down and still maintaining adequate inventory. Since the drugs are ordered and replenished only when an established lower limit is reached (i.e., the preset automatic reordering or **"PAR" level**), the size of the pharmacy's inventory and associated costs of maintaining drugs in peak condition is substantially decreased.

Maintaining the PAR Level

The inventory amount at which a drug is automatically reordered is called the PAR level. When automated systems are used, the amount of a particular drug available for dispensing is electronically monitored. When the inventory level of that drug falls below the preset automatic reorder level, it is electronically reordered. If the automated system is a computerized unit, such as the Pyxis, Omnicell, or Sure-Med unit, the automated order is then sent to the parent facility (if the institution retains a company to provide the automated filling service), the main pharmacy, or a satellite pharmacy to be filled. The drug(s) are then taken to the unit dose cart for restocking.

Pharmacies may also utilize automated reordering systems to maintain inventory on the pharmacy shelves. In this case, the automatic order would be sent to a supplier (vendor) for filling. Depending on the arrangement between the pharmacy and the supplier, the drugs may be shipped to the pharmacy or sent to the pharmacy by courier.

Ordering and Receipt of Drug Products and Devices

All drugs may be ordered electronically by fax, e-mail, or computer. Some states still have restrictions on C-II drugs being ordered electronically. The order is normally made on a form called a **purchase order**. The decision as to when to reorder a drug or item depends largely on how well it sells in the pharmacy. For example, when the amount of a popular drug that sells quickly falls to 1,000 tablets on the shelf, the drug may be reordered. The amount of a less popular drug may have to be substantially lower before reordering (e.g., a balance of 100 tablets remaining). Pharmacies may have a list (a "want book") of drugs and devices that routinely need to be ordered. When the supply of a drug or device falls to the reorder point, it is entered into the "want book" for reorder. (Ordering may be done routinely on a certain day of the week, for example, not whenever the stock of a drug falls low.) With the modern computerized ordering of drugs and devices, however, the "want book" is now falling into disuse.

> The list of drugs and supplies for reorder and stocking (the "want book") is now computerized.

Obtaining Drugs and Devices for Resale in the Pharmacy

The Wholesaler and Prime Vendor

Drugs ordered for stocking in the pharmacy may be obtained from different sources. Drugs for normal dispensing (e.g., FDA-approved drugs) may be obtained from the manufacturer or distributor (wholesaler). Often, a wholesaler carries a selection of drugs and drug products, so it may be more efficient for the pharmacy to use a particular wholesaler that carries a large number of drugs contained in the pharmacy's formulary. The vendor may give the pharmacy a discounted price in exchange for preferred use. Thus, the pharmacy may order almost exclusively from this wholesaler, so it then becomes the **prime vendor** for the pharmacy.

Investigational Drugs and Devices

Occasionally, a drug or device is dispensed for investigational use. These drugs are normally dispensed for use in a controlled study that is sponsored by a particular drug company or agency. In rare cases, special dispensation may be granted by the FDA to use the drug for the treatment of a patient who has exhausted all other treatment options (this is rare, and requires much paperwork and legal complexities).

The use of an investigational drug in a controlled study may involve the pharmacy, in that the drugs are dispensed from the pharmacy and pharmacy records may be used as supporting documents to validate the study. The investigational drugs are obtained from the agency that sponsors the study (the sponsor), in limited quantities. These drugs should be kept separate from the standard drugs to be dispensed, and accurate dispensing records should be kept for the sponsor. When the study is completed or terminated, any remaining investigational drug is to be inventoried and returned to the sponsor.

Ordering Drugs and Devices—Stocking the Pharmacy

A **purchase order** may be required when ordering drugs or devices. This form contains the information discussed above, as well as other information such as the vendor (the company selling the drug), price, shipping information, and date of order. The purchase order is usually assigned a number (the purchase order number) for tracking the shipment. The order is transmitted to the company, which generates a bill or *invoice* that tells the pharmacy how much to pay. The information on the invoice should be carefully checked against the purchase order to be sure that the drug ordered and the drug that the pharmacy is being billed for are exactly the same in name, strength, and quantity.

When the drug or device ordered arrives at the pharmacy, the information on the manufacturer's label should match the information contained on the invoice. The drug label and invoice should be compared to ensure that the proper drug or device was received, as ordered.

The following information needs to be specified when ordering (and should be checked between the manufacturer's label and the invoice, when the drug is received):

- The drug or device name and manufacturer. For a drug product, the generic or brand (trade) name must be specified.
- The strength and dosage form of the drug (or size, if ordering a device).
- The quantity of drug dosage forms per package (e.g., bottle of 100, package of two).
- The type of packaging.
- The number of bottles, packages, or devices being ordered.

> Drugs and supplies should be ordered in an organized and timely manner.

The usual time for delivery should be taken into account when ordering drugs and devices. If the supplier takes three weeks to send a shipment of drugs to the pharmacy, the supply at the time of the order cannot be so low that the pharmacy will run out before the shipment is received.

Alternate Vendors

In case of emergency, when drugs or supplies are needed quickly, the technician must know of other sources from which to obtain the materials. In a pharmacy chain, this may be another pharmacy within the chain. In a hospital situation, drugs or urgent supplies may be borrowed from another hospital and replaced when reordered.

Ordering Controlled Substances (Schedule Drugs)

The technician may order regular drugs and devices for sale but may not order Schedule II drugs. This may only be done by the pharmacist and requires a special triplicate form for ordering, called a DEA 222, which must be obtained from the Drug Enforcement Agency (DEA).

The DEA Form 222 may only be obtained by a licensed health professional, such as a pharmacist, physician, or dentist. These forms are regulated and numbered, and the DEA keeps records of the numbers and to whom a particular 222 form was given. This security measure is intended to help prevent unauthorized persons from ordering controlled substances.

Chapter Review Questions

1. The listing of drugs that are stocked in the pharmacy is called a(n):
   a. inventory
   b. formulary
   c. want list
   d. dispensing list

2. The pharmacy contracts to buy the majority of its formulary from a particular wholesaler. This is called a:
   a. preferred agreement
   b. preferential agreement
   c. prime vendor agreement
   d. preferred vendor contract

3. When a clinical study of an investigational drug is concluded, the drugs are to be:
   a. removed from the pharmacy shelves and destroyed
   b. removed from the pharmacy shelves, inventoried, and stored
   c. removed from the pharmacy shelves, inventoried, and returned to the sponsor
   d. removed from the pharmacy shelves and returned to the FDA

4. When the PAR level is reached, the medication:
   a. is fully stocked
   b. should be taken off the shelves
   c. is automatically reordered
   d. should be discarded

5. The ordering of morphine tablets:
   a. may be done by the technician
   b. is done by the nursing staff
   c. requires a special form
   d. must be done within five days of running out

CHAPTER 36

Maintenance of Pharmaceutical Products

Maintenance of Drug Products in Inventory

Once the drugs are received, they are placed in inventory. This means that the drug name, strength, and quantity of each drug must be entered into the computer system. Drugs are identified using a series of numbers printed on the manufacturer's label, called a **national drug code (NDC) number**. This number identifies the drug, the specific dosage form, the strength, and the manufacturer. The amount of tablets (or number of milliliters, etc.) must be entered into the records, and the amount dispensed is normally deducted from inventory electronically.

Mandatory Physical Inventory

Drugs in inventory must be accounted for at all times—particularly controlled substances. Thus, an inventory of a pharmacy's entire drug stock is required to be conducted at regular intervals. *A physical inventory is conducted one to two times a year.* Documentation for controlled substances is more stringent than that for other prescription drugs. Thus, a complete inventory of *controlled substances* must be made every two years.

Proper Storage of Drug Products in Inventory

During the time that drugs remain in inventory, they must be stored properly, in a way that maintains the drug's integrity. Drugs and drug products must be stored in a climate-controlled environment. Climate control includes low levels of light and humidity as well as proper temperature. Drug stock is normally stored in opaque or amber plastic containers on the pharmacy shelf, in order to protect the drugs from the effects of light, which may degrade the drug. Drugs for injection are stored dry (e.g., powder for injection), as the addition of water tends to decrease the shelf life of the drug. Drug and salt solutions for injection are normally stored in the cold (e.g., a cold room) or refrigerated (as appropriate), as cold temperatures slow both the growth of bacteria and the rate of breakdown of a drug in solution. Any repackaging of injectable drugs must be done in plastic containers (as appropriate) that are **pyrogen-free** (pyrogens are fever-causing agents that can range from certain chemicals to organisms such as bacteria and viruses).

Proper Storage Conditions and Expiration Dates

During storage, drugs must be kept clean, sanitary, and up to date. This means that the drug containers should be free of dust and kept away from light and humidity. Drugs in inventory must also be checked at regular intervals for proximity to expiration dates. Those that are close to expiration should be removed from inventory.

Returning Unit Dose Medications to Inventory

Often, unit doses of medication are placed in medication carts and not administered to the patient (e.g., the patient was discharged before administration).

In this case, if the packaging has not been opened, the drug can be returned to inventory in the pharmacy. The charges for these drugs are then refunded back to the patient's account.

Rotation of Stock

It is important when adding new inventory to place the newest product toward the back of the storage area so that the older drugs, which are closer to expiration, will be dispensed first. This is called *rotation of stock*, and it helps to keep drugs from getting too close to their expiration dates before they are dispensed.

Storage of Controlled Drugs (Schedule Drugs)

It is important to remember that although regular drugs may be stored on the pharmacy shelf or in areas with free access, drugs under Schedule II must be kept in a locked cabinet or storage area. This is a security measure to prevent access to such drugs by unauthorized personnel. Pharmacies that have perpetual inventory machines assign access codes to track entrance into and dispensing of these controlled substances. Since the pharmacist is legally responsible for any discrepancies in inventory when the records of the pharmacy are audited, the pharmacist usually retains the master key to all locked storage areas.

Handling Expired Medications and Drug Recalls

Medications in inventory must be routinely checked for proximity to their expiration dates. Once a product is within a few weeks of its expiration date (usually around four weeks), it should be removed from the shelves.

Legally, a drug can be sold up to its date of expiration. However, it is good practice to remove drugs from the pharmacy shelves prior to that date, as the patient may retain the drug for as much as a month or more before finishing the prescription, during which time the drug could pass its expiration date. Expired drugs may be discarded with proper documentation but are often returned to the manufacturer for credit. The disposal of controlled substances requires documentation for the DEA and is done by the pharmacist with the use of form 41. There are also private companies now that will process and dispose of expired medications for retail pharmacies and institutions.

The Expiration Date

When a drug is manufactured, a set length of time that the drug retains optimum potency is established. Stability and efficacy tests are conducted, and the length of time that the drug remains potent and efficacious under

> The expiration date reflects the amount of time that the drug remains potent and safe to use. It serves as a guideline to the pharmacy for when the drug should no longer be sold.

various environmental conditions is translated into the *expiration date*. The expiration date is used by the pharmacy to determine when the drug can no longer be sold. The established date of expiration is important, as some drugs (tetracycline, for example) not only lose potency with time but also degrade into toxic chemical products.

Occasionally, a drug product may be contaminated, produced improperly, or deemed to have unexpected or detrimental side effects. In this case, the Food and Drug Administration (FDA) mandates a *recall* of the drug or a specific drug lot found to have a problem. Not only is the drug pulled from the shelves and returned to the manufacturer with appropriate documentation, but dispensing records must also be examined to determine which patients have received some of that particular lot of drug. These patients must be contacted and advised to return their prescriptions to the pharmacy for exchange. Returned drug products are then documented and returned to the manufacturer for credit. In addition to the patients who received the drug, the prescribers must also be notified of the problem in order to halt prescription of the recalled drug. An example of this type of recall would be the Tylenol poisonings in the 1980s.

Classification of Drug Recalls

Drugs may be recalled for different reasons. Recalls are classified based on the health threat posed to patients. The input of the pharmacist (e.g., reporting of adverse effects experienced by patients taking the drug) is a major factor in these recalls.

There are three basic classifications of drug recalls:

- *Class I*: This is the most serious cause for recall. Drugs under this classification have been associated with serious adverse health consequences (e.g., organ toxicity) or death.
- *Class II*: Drugs under this classification may have caused adverse effects, but the effects were reversible upon withdrawal of the drug. The probability of toxic effects (i.e., "serious adverse consequences") to the patient's health is relatively small.
- *Class III*: Drugs in this class are not likely to have caused adverse health consequences. It is more likely that the drug was recalled due to inappropriate labeling or other publicized misinformation.

Drug Recapture and Disposal

In a retail pharmacy, drugs and devices may not be returned once they leave the control of the pharmacy. However, in an institutional setting, the pharmacy may receive returned drugs from unit dose medications that were not used. These medications, if unopened, may be replaced in inventory (drug "recapture"). Drugs that have been opened, such as drug vials from which medication has been removed for a patient, are discarded according to procedure. The disposal of drugs is the responsibility of the pharmacy department, as the drugs are toxic and an environmental hazard if not disposed of properly.

Chapter Review Questions

1. When a drug is recalled, which of the following might occur?
   a. the patients using the drug should be notified
   b. the providers prescribing the drug should be notified
   c. the drug supply with the appropriate lot number should be removed from inventory and returned to the supplier
   d. all of the above

2. Unused unit dose medications:
   a. are always discarded
   b. are reused for the next patient
   c. may be placed back into inventory if unopened, and the charges credited back to the patient
   d. may be distributed to floor nursing staff for emergency use

3. A complete inventory of regular prescription drugs:
   a. should be done every two years
   b. should be done weekly
   c. must be done one to two times a year
   d. should be done before every inspection by the DEA

4. Schedule II controlled substances must be:
   a. kept in a locked cabinet
   b. documented carefully, with no mistakes or strikeovers
   c. inventoried every two years
   d. all of the above

5. Drugs on the shelf are stored in opaque bottles because:
   a. the drugs are sensitive to heat
   b. the drugs are sensitive to humidity
   c. the drugs are sensitive to light
   d. they are easier to handle that way

Administration and Management of Pharmacy Practice

THIS SECTION of the book reviews the content in the third functional area as tested in the ExCPT or PTCB exam. This comprises 25% (ExCPT) and 12% (PTCB) of the examination questions. This section includes:

CHAPTER 37

Using Computers in the Pharmacy

Quick Study

I. Uses of computers

    A. Repetitive tasks such as inventory, billing, pricing, and maintenance of patient records

    B. Education of pharmacy personnel

    C. Assistance in procedures for preparation of drug products

    D. General communication

    E. Communication of drug orders to the pharmacy

    F. Tracking of laboratory results and access to patient information

II. Components of a computer and their functions

    A. Hardware
  - Memory storage units and circuitry—the central processing unit (CPU) and hard disk
  - Peripheral units (printer, monitor, etc.)

    B. Software—A set of instructions for the computer to follow

III. Input devices feed information into the computer

    A. Examples: Light pen, optical scanner, keyboard

IV. Output devices export information from the computer

    A. Examples: Monitor, printer, modem, etc.

V. Information storage

    A. Permanent storage in bits and bytes (ROM: read-only memory)
- CD-ROM
- Fixed disk
- USB device

    B. Temporary storage (RAM: random-access memory)

The Components of a Computer

The working computer consists of two main divisions: **hardware** and **software**. The hardware is the circuitry, storage units, and peripheral ("add on") units of the computer, whereas the software is a set of instructions for the computer to follow that enables it to perform a specific function. The software is usually stored on a CD and installed onto the hardware (hard drive). The hardware portions of the computer consist of the following:

- The **central processing unit (CPU)** is a compact unit that contains the computer's memory, components used in data storage (such as the fixed, or "hard," disk and memory chips), communication (the modem), and sound generation. Most importantly, the CPU processes data before displaying it on the monitor screen or printer. The CPU may connect to a peripheral disk drive, which writes to a high-storage-capacity disk, CD, or USB device for additional data storage.

- The monitor is a "television set" that allows the operator to see data and information displayed by the computer. This is an output device, meaning that information from the computer goes *out* to the device to be displayed for the user.

- The printer is an output device that allows information to be printed out as a hard copy rather than viewed on a screen.

- The light pen and optical scanner are two input devices that carry information to the computer. This information is used by the computer to calculate charges, access information, and so forth. These devices are able to "read" bar-coded information on drug packaging and relay it to the computer's processor. The keyboard is another example of an input device whereby information is typed in by the user for the computer to process.

Storage of Information

Information may be *permanently* stored on the fixed disk (hard disk), a small, flat disk of hard plastic that contains grooves, much like a record. The more grooves that the disk has and the closer together they are, the more capacity the disk has to store information. Storage area is measured in *bits*, which are grouped into larger *bytes* (8 bits 1 byte). A *kilo*byte is 1,000 bytes, a *mega*byte is 1 million bytes, and a *giga*byte is 1 billion bytes. A CD or USB device is similar to the hard disk but is able to store less information. Both types of disks must be formatted by the disk operating system (DOS) software before they can be used with the system. Formatting prepares the disk to be used and also erases any information already stored on it.

Information can be temporarily stored in the computer's memory, or *buffer*. When you are working on the computer, the program in use as well as the information entered into the computer are all stored in the buffer. This is why, if the computer loses power or is shut off, information that was entered but not saved to disk is lost.

Due to the chance of mechanical failure, safeguards should be taken to preserve information. Information should be saved periodically as it is entered (rather than only when you are finished entering the data), and a hard copy of patient and pharmacy records should be printed out at regular intervals (e.g., daily). Information stored on the hard disk should also be copied (backed up) onto a removable disk (e.g., CD-ROM or USB device) at regular intervals, in case of computer failure. These copies and disks should be treated as sensitive information (in accordance with HIPAA confidentiality regulations) and stored in a secure place.

Memory

There are two types of memory: **read-only memory (ROM)** and **random-access memory (RAM)**. ROM comes from a disk that is protected, so that it cannot be written on (no additional information can be stored on it). It is only able to show information (i.e., the information cannot be erased or destroyed by formatting). This information goes to the computer in a specific sequence that tells the computer what to do. An example of ROM would be a compact disk (CD-ROM) with stored information. The hard disk has ROM but is able to accept information for storage.

RAM is found in the computer or printer buffer, where data is temporarily stored. Movement of this information into the buffer is defined by the user. The storage of data is temporary, so the information contained in it must be permanently stored or it will be lost when the power supply is interrupted or turned off, or when the program is terminated.

Use of Computers in Pharmacy Practice

Computers are almost indispensable in the pharmacy. With computers we can keep track of drug inventory, narcotics use, changes in the drug formulary, and personnel. Computers are used for patient billing, insurance billing and verification, pricing, maintenance of patient profiles, generation of the medication administration record, and a number of computational and repetitive tasks.

Using Computers in Continuing Education

Networks of databases provide a large number of resources—both online and downloaded to CD-ROM. There are Internet sites that present the latest drug information and monographs as well as sites that present the latest research results (e.g., MEDLINE). There are also Web pages for nearly all major scientific journals that contain both recent and archived journal articles and can be easily searched. In addition, other sources provide reference material that can be searched, downloaded, and obtained online or at the local library. This makes the computer an excellent tool for the ongoing education of pharmacy personnel. In addition, computers can provide the pharmacist and technician with information on a particular topic, references, communication with researchers and pharmaceutical companies, and the like.

Using Computers in Clinical Practice

The amount of information used in the pharmacy is huge. In addition to keeping up with the rapid changes in the field, with new drugs and new delivery systems added every day, computers and computer programs are useful in utilizing new drug information. Within the pharmacy, the computer simplifies ordering as well as drug information storage and retrieval. The rapid communication of patient information and prescriptions is also possible, allowing a patient with a prescription at Pharmacy X in Chicago to pick up a refill prescription, while on vacation in Hawaii, at another Pharmacy X location.

Computers can help to reduce medication errors with programs that are designed to alert the user of possible medication interactions or allergies, dose limitations, drug duplications, and other warnings. Computers are invaluable in hospital practice as well. For example, a properly programmed computer can suggest the proper diluting agent (diluent) to use in preparing an IV. (Some drugs are more compatible with a particular diluent—for example, NS as opposed to water or D_5W as opposed to NS, etc.) The computer may even suggest a procedure for dilution or compounding. Computer programs may also alert the pharmacist to potential drug-drug interactions and drug-physiology interactions, which help to safeguard the patient and are used in automated delivery and ordering systems (e.g., the Pyxis med carts).

The pharmacist and physician may also use computers (e.g., the portable palm computers) to track a patient's laboratory results or monitor drug levels. Information can also be passed back and forth from the physician to the pharmacist via these portable computers, making for optimal patient therapy.

Communication by Computer

Computers are useful in communicating (see Chapters 1–3) from the prescriber to the pharmacy and vice versa. They can also be useful in obtaining information related to a patient or a patient's condition from poison control centers, research centers, and other organizations that are highly computerized.

The Local Area Network (LAN)

Communication within an institutional or retail setting is also optimized by computers. Computers are often connected by a local area network (LAN), which allows communication between pharmacies and prescribers in a variety of settings.

> **EXAMPLE**
>
> The LAN allows pharmacists in a retail setting to communicate with other pharmacies of the same chain (e.g., Walgreens, CVS) in order to retrieve information. It may be necessary to retrieve information from the patient profile of a patient who requests a refill on a prescription that was previously filled at another pharmacy within the chain. LANs also facilitate communication with other businesses. For example, communication with insurance companies regarding patient coverage may also be accomplished using a LAN.

The LAN is also useful within an institutional setting for communication between the pharmacy and physicians or nurses. It also allows communication between the main pharmacy in the institution, satellite pharmacies, or outside providers.

Chapter Review Questions

1. Temporary storage of data occurs in the:
   a. random-access memory
   b. disk operating system
   c. read-only memory
   d. temporary memory

2. Which of the following is not an output device?
   a. monitor
   b. printer
   c. optical scanner
   d. plotter

3. Which of the following is not considered computer hardware?
   a. hard disk
   b. modem
   c. processor
   d. disk operating system

4. Which of the following is not a use for computers in the pharmacy?
   a. maintaining patient information
   b. billing
   c. generating prescriptions
   d. identifying drug-drug interactions

5. An example of an input device would be a:
   a. light pen
   b. printer
   c. modem
   d. monitor

CHAPTER 38

Communications within the Pharmacy

Quick Study

I. Role of the technician in communication

   A. Communication regarding routine requests
   B. Communication with third-party payors to verify payment
   C. Answering of general questions (to limitations of your knowledge)
   D. Verification of prescription orders
   E. Providing support to the patient

II. Role of the pharmacist in communication

   A. Patient consultation
   B. Medical advice and instruction, recommendation of emergency procedures
   C. Receipt of prescriptions generated by electronic means
   D. Accepts refill authorizations

III. Customer service—communicating with the patient

   A. Positive communication leads to smoother transactions and improved care
   B. Understanding the needs of the patient—dealing with anger and frustration
      • Education leads to understanding of drug effects
      • Education leads to understanding of specific illnesses and their symptoms and progression
      • Monetary concerns
      • Supporting the caregiver
   C. Exchanging information—verbal and nonverbal communication
   D. How actions influence communication as well as words

E. Communication with patients of varied backgrounds
   - Dealing with cultural bias
   - Factoring in age and gender in communication
   - Communication at various educational levels—the importance of making information understood

F. Gathering information—organizing questions makes for more efficient communication

G. Avoiding putting patients on the defensive, through respect and trust

Communication is defined as giving or exchanging information. In the pharmacy, we communicate by telephone, e-mail, fax, or in person. Only a part of communication is made up of words—the way in which the words are *perceived* makes up a large part of the message communicated. For example, the words "Here is your medication, Mr. Johnson" delivered with a smile and the same words accompanied by the tossing of the prescription on the pharmacy counter convey entirely different meanings.

Communication in the pharmacy is varied and the role of the technician is often crucial. The technician may interact with patients, vendors, and third-party payors, as well as with the pharmacist, prescribers, and caregivers. A positive perception in communication helps to facilitate proper dispensing of the medication and proper use by the patient. In addition, the technician can facilitate accurate communication with neat and precise handwriting, good note-taking skills, and a pleasant demeanor. A pleasant telephone voice and good verbal skills are also desirable, and a knowledge of medical terminology will ease communication with physicians and other health professionals.

At present, the legal role of the technician is strictly defined. The role of the technician may, however, be expanded to one of greater responsibility in the near future, depending on the laws of the individual state in which he or she practices.

Legally, the technician may:

- Communicate with patients, prescribers, and caregivers regarding routine requests.

- Communicate with third-party payors to ensure payment to the pharmacy.

- Refer patients to the pharmacist for consultation. If the questions or potential problems that the patient may have regarding a medication or condition require advice and professional judgment, the patient *must* be referred to the pharmacist. The technician is not qualified to address these questions, and to do so may cause the pharmacist to lose his or her professional license.

- Clarify prescription orders with the prescriber, if necessary. If the prescription is illegible or the instructions ambiguous, the technician is allowed, at the discretion of the pharmacist, to clarify the prescription order with the prescriber.
- Communicate with other pharmacy personnel and technicians.
- Answer general questions about medication and dosing, to the limits of his or her knowledge, provided that the answers do not require any professional judgment by the technician.
- Offer support to the patient. This may include recommending reading material or other resources to patients, should they require it.

The technician may *not:*

- Offer any advice to the patient regarding drug products.
- Counsel the patient in *any* way.
- Answer questions about drug interactions or physical interactions with a drug product.
- Recommend procedures of any kind, such as the induction of vomiting with overdose, supplementary medication, etc.
- Accept verbal or electronic prescription orders (e.g., from another computer by modem or by telephone) depending on the state.

Role of the Pharmacist in Communication

The role of the pharmacist is to dispense advice, answer all questions or address all problems requiring professional judgment, and handle any emergency situations. Patients frequently call the pharmacy with questions about a drug that has been prescribed for them or an over-the-counter drug that they are taking. Occasionally, a patient may even call the pharmacy in an emergency (a child has taken the medication, for example, or the patient has overdosed) and ask what to do. These calls should *immediately* be referred to the pharmacist. The pharmacist has the ability to screen these calls and dispense the proper advice. The technician is not trained to do so, and for the technician to dispense advice, however accurate, is technically illegal. The role of the technician *is* changing, however, with the advent of the national certification exam, formal training of technicians, and, in some states, licensure of technicians.

Effective Means of Communication—Overcoming Barriers

Effective communication is based on understanding. If you can understand the patient, how he or she feels, and the basis for his or her behavior, you are much more likely to communicate well. Most patients who come to the

466 Section III: Administration and Management of Pharmacy Practice

pharmacy are ill. Caregivers, though not ill, are stressed and possibly confused and upset. In any case, patients are seeking competent, professional care, and fast service. No one likes to wait for something that will make them feel better. Understanding the patient's needs and emotions helps to promote positive communication and good customer service.

Things to consider include:

- *Ethnic background or cultural bias*: Many cultures are uncomfortable giving private information to a stranger, particularly someone of the opposite sex. Some cultures do not view women as competent professionals and will prefer to speak with a man. Still other patients will view competence as a function of skin color, or even size and shape. (For example, a very short person may not be taken seriously, and an overweight person may be considered stupid and lazy, just by his or her appearance!)

- *Education level*: Patients should be given information appropriate to their level of education. Most patients are poorly educated in the sciences and may have only a high school education or less. The technician and pharmacist must give information in a way that is thoroughly understood by the patient.

- *Age and gender*: Many patients, especially those who are older patients, have been brought up to think that the giving of information or advice by a young person to an older person is not appropriate. Others may view the giving of information from a woman to a man as inappropriate. Your best effort should be made to accommodate the beliefs and feelings of a patient, regardless of your personal feelings on age or gender bias.

There are many ways that communication can be improved. Organizational skills become important, as does experience. With experience, you can anticipate the questions of a patient and be ready with answers. The organization of questions to be asked of the patient also becomes second nature, with experience. Some helpful principles to be adopted include:

- Organizing the questions to be asked of the patient in a way that will allow the most accurate information to be gained in the shortest amount of time.

- Attention to detail—listen carefully to all that the patient tells you (and doesn't). Subtle changes in body language and voice inflection may indicate a lack of accuracy. It may be that the patient is embarrassed about giving personal information and is trying to avoid divulging certain information. It may also be true if the person is trying to obtain medication under false pretenses.

- Listen carefully to what the patient tells you. Avoid distractions from other patients and pharmacy employees.

- Show respect and concern for the patient. Poorly educated people may feel especially intimidated by the environment and subjects that they do not understand. It is easy for them to feel "put down," and they may become defensive. Respect and concern build trust, and the patient is more likely to listen and to divulge personal information, which is necessary for them to use a medication properly.

- Be acutely aware of patient confidentiality. This not only includes the confidentiality of patient records but at the pharmacy window, as well. For example, speaking in a loud voice so that everyone in the waiting area can hear is not a good tenet of confidentiality. The HIPAA confidentiality principles should always be adhered to.

- Be aware of the psychological stages of illness—these include denial, anger, bargaining, and depression, before finally accepting the condition.

As a communicator in the pharmacy, your job is to answer questions, support the patient and the pharmacist, and focus on the patient and patient care. In addition, you will be required to interface with drug vendors, suppliers, regulatory agencies, and the general public, in addition to the patient. As a pharmacy professional, it is important to build confidence in the patient. This confidence is built on self-assurance (but not arrogance or condescension), courtesy, and a broad base of knowledge. Not only should you be aware of drugs and what they are used for, but also their adverse effects and what worsens or decreases these effects. You should also be prepared to answer any questions put to you, within the limits of the laws of the state in which you practice. This includes questions on over-the-counter drugs as well as prescription drugs. You should also be knowledgeable about the use of medical devices sold in the pharmacy (e.g., canes, walkers, blood glucose monitors, test strips, etc.). The more knowledge you can gain, the more trust you will inspire in the patient, and the more effective a pharmacy professional you will be.

> **Competence and knowledge build credibility!**

In addition to knowledge about drugs and devices, it is helpful to be knowledgeable about various illnesses: what it affects, its progression, and how it is treated. A familiarity with the patient profile and what the information means will also help to effectively answer the patient's questions. Most importantly, respect, courtesy, and humility will help to foster patient trust and effective communication.

Knowledge, competence, and the approach to the patient are very important factors in communication. There are, however, nonverbal aspects of communication that the technician must attend to. One of the most important of these is physical appearance. To be respected, a technician should dress neatly and professionally. No sloppy clothing, such as T-shirts, sweatshirts, or shorts should be worn, and the hair and skin should be clean and well groomed. Fingernails should be clean and trimmed. If nail polish is worn, it should be neat and simple, and of a quiet shade. (Green and black fingernails do not inspire confidence, particularly in the elderly.) The hair should be neat and tied back. Hair is a source of contamination anyway, so a neat appearance not only conveys professionalism and confidence to the patient, but also means that there is less chance of hair falling in the prescription. Makeup, perfume, or cologne, should be minimal. Jewelry should also be conservatively chosen, not only for appearances' sake but because it could also snag on containers or fall into the prescription. Appearances are important and communicate to the patient your attitude and level of care.

The Influence of HIPAA Regulations on Communication

The HIPAA regulations implemented in 2003 impact greatly on communication in the pharmacy. A patient or his or her therapy can no longer be discussed in any area where the discussion might be overheard, whether that area is the pharmacy window, a hallway, or an elevator. Patients may not be called out by name along with their medication name when their prescriptions are ready (Mrs. Jones, your Xanax is ready), and any discussions regarding their drug or therapy must be conducted in such a way that the discussion will not be overheard.

Information regarding a particular patient may only be freely communicated to a person or business that has a direct involvement with the patient (e.g., a physician or insurance provider), without the express written consent of the patient. Information may only be disseminated to a distantly involved business (e.g., a pharmaceutical company collecting information on the use and adverse effects of a particular drug) on a basis that does not personally identify a patient. In addition, a written privacy policy must be generated and a copy delivered to each patient, who must sign a statement indicating that he or she received a copy of the policy.

Chapter Review Questions

1. A patient calls to say that her young son has taken her medication by mistake and may have overdosed. You should:
   a. tell her to call 911
   b. refer her to the nearest poison control center
   c. attempt to comfort her
   d. refer her to the pharmacist

2. The technician is *not* allowed to:
   a. call the prescriber to clarify a prescription order
   b. offer support to the patient
   c. tell the patient not to take aspirin with her Coumadin prescription
   d. tell the patient that the pharmacy carries a generic drug for her prescription that is considerably cheaper than the proprietary (brand-name) drug

3. A patient has a question about a drug you know a lot about. You should:
   a. answer her questions
   b. refer her to the pharmacist
   c. refer her to information in the library
   d. tell her that you are not allowed to give out this information

4. Communication between two computers over telephone lines is accomplished by the use of a:
   a. fax machine
   b. printer
   c. modem
   d. computer monitor

5. Which of the following fosters good communication?
   a. knowledge
   b. a condescending attitude
   c. a neat appearance
   d. both a and c

6. You are a female technician trying to get information from a new patient for the patient profile. The patient becomes uncooperative and angry. This could be because:
   a. he resents giving out personal information
   b. he is in denial about his illness
   c. he doesn't like being questioned by a woman
   d. any of the above could be true

7. The patient asks you a question about the drug that she is taking. Under current law:
   a. you must refer her to the pharmacist
   b. you may answer the question to the limitations of your knowledge
   c. you must refuse to answer the question
   d. you should tell the patient that you do not know the answer to the question

8. A pharmacy technician discusses the proper care of an antibiotic suspension with a patient. The discussion is heard in the waiting area. The technician is in violation of which of the following regulations?
   a. The Confidentiality Act of 1996
   b. State statutes
   c. The HIPAA amendments implemented in 2003
   d. The Consolidated Omnibus Budget Reconciliation Act

9. Which of the following should be considered when talking to customers?
   a. ethnic background
   b. educational level
   c. gender
   d. all the above

10. A technician may:
    a. talk to third-party payors regarding payment
    b. recommend procedures and supplements for customers
    c. counsel patients
    d. take refill authorizations from physicians

Top 200 Prescription Drugs

Table A-1 lists the top 200 drugs by prescription.

Table A–1	Top 200 Drugs by Prescription	
Number	**Generic Name**	**Trade Name**
1	hydrocodone w/APAP	Lortab
2	atorvastatin	Lipitor
3	amoxicillin	Trimox
4	lisinopril	Prinivil, Zestril
5	hydrochlorothiazide	Diaqua, Esidrix
6	atenolol	Tenormin
7	azithromycin	Zithromax
8	furosemide	Lasix
9	alprazolam	Xanax
10	metoprolol	Toprol XL
11	albuterol	Proventil
12	amlodipine	Norvasc
13	levothyroxine	Synthroid
14	metformin	Glucophage, Glucophage XR
15	sertraline	Zoloft
16	escitalopram	Lexapro
17	ibuprofen	Motrin
18	cephalexin	Keflex
19	zolpidem	Ambien
20	prednisone	Deltasone
21	esomeprazole magnesium	Nexium

(continued)

Table A–1 (continued)

Number	Generic Name	Trade Name
22	triamterene	Dyrenium
23	propoxyphene	Darvon-N
24	simvastatin	Zocor
25	montelukast	Singulair
26	lansoprazole	Prevacid
27	metoprolol tartrate	Lopressor
28	fluoxetine	Prozac
29	lorazepam	Ativan
30	clopidogrel	Plavix
31	oxycodone w/APAP	Percocet
32	salmeterol	Serevent
33	alendronate	Fosamax
34	venlafaxine	Effexor, Effexor XR
35	warfarin	Coumadin
36	paroxetine hydrochloride	Paxil
37	clonazepam	Klonopin
38	cetirizine	Zyrtec
39	pantoprazole	Protonix
40	potassium chloride	K-Lor
41	acetaminophen/codeine	Tylenol-Codeine
42	trimethoprim/sulfamethoxazole	Septra, Bactrim
43	gabapentin	Neurontin
44	conjugated estrogens	Premarin
45	fluticasone	Flonase
46	trazodone	Desyrel
47	cyclobenzaprine	Flexeril
48	amitriptyline	Elavil, Enovil
49	levofloxacin	Levaquin
50	tramadol	Ultram
51	ciprofloxacin	Cipro
52	amlodipine/benazepril	Lotrel
53	ranitidine	Zantac
54	fexofenadine	Allegra
55	levothyroxine	Levoxyl
56	valsartan	Diovan
57	enalapril	Vasotec
58	diazepam	Valium
59	naproxen	Anaprox, Naprosyn

(continued)

Number	Generic Name	Trade Name
60	fluconazole	Diflucan
61	lisinopril/HCTZ	Zestoretic
62	potassium chloride	Klor-Con
63	ramipril	Altace
64	bupropion	Wellbutrin, Wellbutrin XL
65	celecoxib	Celebrex
66	sildenafil citrate	Viagra
67	doxycycline hyclate	Vibra-Tabs
68	ezetimibe	Zetia
69	rosiglitazone maleate	Avandia
70	lovastatin	Mevacor
71	valsartan/hydrochlorothiazide	Diovan HCT
72	carisoprodol	Soma, Rela
73	drospirenone/ethinyl estradiol	Yasmin 28
74	allopurinol	Alloprin
75	clonidine	Catapres
76	methylprednisolone	Medrol
77	pioglitazone hydrochloride	Actos
78	pravastatin	Pravachol
79	risedronate sodium	Actonel
80	norelgestromin/ethinyl estradiol	Ortho Evra
81	citalopram hydrobromide	Celexa
82	verapamil	Calan
83	isosorbide mononitrate	Ismotic
84	penicillin V	Penicillin VK
85	glyburide	Micronase
86	amphetamine sulfate	Adderall
87	mometasone furoate	Nasonex
88	folic acid	Folacin
89	quetiapine fumarate	Seroquel
90	losartan potassium	Cozaar
91	fenofibrate	Tricor
92	carvedilol	Coreg
93	methylphenidate hydrochloride	Concerta
94	ezetimibe	Vytorin
95	insulin glargine	Lantus
96	promethazine hydrochloride	Phenergan
97	meloxicam	Mobic

(continued)

Table A–1 (continued)

Number	Generic Name	Trade Name
98	tamsulosin hydrochloride	Flomax
99	rosuvastatin	Crestor
100	glipizide	Glucotrol XL
101	norgestimate/ethinyl estradiol	Ortho Tri-Cyclen Lo
102	temazepam	Restoril
103	omeprazole	Prilosec
104	cefdinir	Omnicef
105	albuterol	Ventolin
106	risperidone	Risperdal
107	rabeprazole sodium	AcipHex
108	digoxin	Digitek
109	spironolactone	Aldactone
110	valacyclovir hydrochloride	Valtrex
111	latanoprost	Xalatan
112	metformin	Fortamet
113	losartan potassium/ hydrochlorothiazide	Hyzaar
114	quinapril	Accupril
115	clindamycin	Cleocin
116	metronidazole	Flagyl
117	triamcinolone	Atolone
118	topiramate	Topamax
119	ipratropium bromide/ albuterol sulfate	Combivent
120	benazepril	Lotensin
121	gemfibrozil	Lopid
122	irbesartan	Avapro
123	glimepiride	Amaryl
124	norgestimate/ethinyl estradiol	Trinessa
125	estradiol	Alora, Climara
126	hydroxyzine	Atarax
127	metoclopramide	Maxolon, Reglan
128	fexofenadine/pseudoephedrine	Allegra-D 12 Hour
129	doxazosin mesylate	Cardura
130	warfarin	Jantoven
131	glipizide	Glucotrol
132	diclofenac sodium	Voltaren
133	raloxifene hydrochloride	Evista
134	diltiazem	Cardizem, Tiazac

(continued)

Number	Generic Name	Trade Name
135	tolterodine tartrate	Detrol, Detrol LA
136	meclizine	Antivert, Bonamine
137	glyburide/metformin	Glucovance
138	atomoxetine	Strattera
139	duloxetine hydrochloride	Cymbalta
140	nitrofurantoin	Furadantin
141	promethazine/codeine	Phenergan with Codeine
142	olmesartan medoxomil	Benicar
143	mirtazapine	Remeron
144	bisoprolol/HCTZ	Ziac
145	desloratadine	Clarinex
146	oxycodone	OxyContin
147	minocycline	Arestin, Minocin
148	sumatriptan	Imitrex
149	nabumetone	Relafen
150	olanzapine	Zyprexa
151	lamotrigine	Lamictal
152	cetirizine/pseudoephedrine	Zyrtec-D
153	polyethylene glycol	Glycolax
154	acyclovir	Zovirax
155	propranolol	Inderal
156	triamcinolone acetonide	Nasacort AQ
157	donepezil hydrochloride	Aricept
158	butalbital/acetaminophen/ caffeine	Fioricet
159	niacin	Niaspan
160	azithromycin	Zmax
161	divalproex sodium	Depakote
162	buspirone	Buspar
163	norgestimate/ethinyl estradiol	Tri-Sprintec
164	methotrexate	Amethopterin, MTX
165	oxycodone	Roxicodone
166	budesonide	Rhinocort Aqua
167	olmesartan medoxomil hydrochlorothiazide	Benicar HCT
168	terazosin	Hytrin
169	metaxalone	Skelaxin
170	clotrimazole/betamethasone	Lotrisone
171	tadalafil	Cialis

(continued)

Table A–1 (continued)

Number	Generic Name	Trade Name
172	irbesartan/hydrochlorothiazide	Avalide
173	fexofenadine	Telfast°
174	norgestimate/ethinyl estradiol	Ortho Tri-Cyclen
175	bupropion hydrochloride	Wellbutrin, Zyban
176	benzonatate	Tessalon
177	olopatadine hydrochloride	Patanol
178	quinine	Quinamm, Quiphile
179	diltiazem hydrochloride	Cartia XT
180	insulin lispro, rDNA origin	Humalog
181	paroxetine	Paxil CR
182	levonorgestrel and ethinyl estradiol	Aviane
183	digoxin	Lanoxin
184	amphetamine	Adderall XR
185	famotidine	Pepcid, Pepcid AC
186	digoxin	Lanoxicaps
187	levothyroxine	Levothroid
188	nifedipine	Adalat, Procardia
189	nortriptyline	Aventyl
190	hydrocodone polistirex/ chlorpheniramine polistirex	Tussionex
191	nitroglycerin	NitroQuick
192	phenytoin	Dilantin
193	budesonide	Endocet
194	etodolac	Lodine, Lodine XL
195	atenolol/chlorthalidone	Tenoretic
196	phentermine	Fastin
197	tramadol/acetaminophen	Ultracet
198	tizanidine	Zanaflex
199	cetirizine hydrochloride/ pseudoephedrine	Virlix-D
200	divalproex sodium	Depakote ER

Commonly Used Medical Abbreviations

a	artery
aa	of each
ABG	arterial blood gas
ac	before a meal
ad	right ear
ad lib	as desired
ad sat	to saturation
a.m.	in the morning
ant	anterior
app.	applicator full
aq	water
aq dist	distilled water
as	left ear
ATC	around the clock
au	each ear
AV	atrioventricular
bid	twice a day
BM	bowel movement
BS	blood sugar
BUN	blood urea nitrogen
c	with
Cap	capsule
CBC	complete blood count
cc	cubic centimeter
dc	discontinue
dil	dilute
disp	dispense
dr	dram
DW	distilled water

(continued)

477

D_5W	5% dextrose in water
$D_{10}W$	10% dextrose in water
D_5LR	5% dextrose in lactated Ringer's solution
D_5NS	5% dextrose in normal saline
Dx	diagnosis
ECF	extracellular fluid
elix.	elixir
ESR	erythrocyte sedimentation rate
et	and
F	female
FEV	forced expiratory volume
fl	fluid
fl dr	fluid dram
fl oz	fluid ounce
GI	gastrointestinal
gr	grain
Grad	gradually
gtt.	drops
h, hr	hour
HA	headache
Hgb	hemoglobin
h.s. (hor som)	hour of sleep (bedtime)
HTN	hypertension
ID	intradermal
IM	intramuscularly
qd	daily
Inj.	injection
Instill	instillation
IU	international unit (rarely used anymore)
IV	intravenously
IVP	intravenous push
IVPB	intravenous piggyback
Lot	lotion
mEq	milliequivalent
MS	morphine sulfate
N/V	nausea and vomiting
NMT	not more than
NPO	nothing by mouth
NS	normal saline
1/2 NS	half strength NS (0.45% NaCl)
NTE	not to exceed
NTG	nitroglycerin
OD	right eye

(continued)

Oint.	ointment
OS	left eye
OU	both eyes (each eye)
pc	after meals
pm	afternoon
po	by mouth
prn	as needed
pwd	powder
q	every
qam	every morning
qd	every day
qh	every hour
qhs	at bedtime every night
q2h, q4h . . .	every two hours, every four hours, etc.
qid	four times a day
qod	every other day
qs	a sufficient quantity
R	rectal
Rep	repeat
s	without
Sig	label (v.)
SL	under the tongue
SOB	shortness of breath
Soln	solution
sq (sc)	subcutaneously
ss	½ (one half)
stat	immediately
supp	suppository
susp.	suspension
syr	syrup
tab	tablet
tbsp	tablespoon
t.i.d	three times a day
top	topical
TPN	total peripheral (parenteral) nutrition
tr	tincture
tsp	teaspoonful
ud	as directed
ung	ointment
URI	upper respiratory infection
UTI	urinary tract infection
Vag	vaginally
Wk	week

(continued)

APAP	acetaminophen
ASA	acetylsalicylic acid (aspirin)
Ca	calcium
CDPX	chlordiazepoxide
DCN	Darvocet
DES	diethylstilbestrol
DSS/DOS	docusate sodium
EES	erythromycin ethylsuccinate
FA	folic acid
Fe ($FeSO_4$)	iron (ferrous sulfate—a common oral form of iron)
HCTZ	hydrochlorothiazide
INH	isoniazid
MOM	milk of magnesia
NTG	nitroglycerin
PB	phenobarbital
PCN	penicillin
SMZ/TMP	sulfamethoxazole with trimethoprim
TCN	tetracycline

Pretest with Answers

Chapter 1

1. Which of the following would be found on a hospital medication order but not a retail prescription?
   a. generic authorization
   b. prescriber's signature
   c. times of administration
   d. drug name, strength, and form

2. Which of the following must be present on the written prescription at the time of acceptance?
   a. drug allergies
   b. the exact name, strength, and form of the drug
   c. the age of the patient
   d. all of the above

3. Which of the following tasks may not be performed by the technician?
   a. accept refill requests by telephone
   b. authorize refills
   c. accept verbal prescriptions from a physician
   d. both b and c

4. Prescriptions received by electronic means:
   a. may be filled directly
   b. may be accepted and filled by the technician with the pharmacist's authorization
   c. must be transferred to paper (a hard copy) before being filled
   d. all of the above

5. You receive a prescription for Roxicet. The following must be present on the prescription form:
   a. the address of the patient
   b. the age of the patient
   c. the name, strength, and form of the drug, written in ink
   d. all of the above

6. In a hospital setting, the pharmacy technician:
   a. fills the medication order, once it has been checked by the pharmacist
   b. generates the Medication Administration Record
   c. compounds a new dosage form for a specific patient
   d. both a and b

Chapter 2

7. The following might be found on a patient profile:
   a. prescription drugs dispensed
   b. over-the-counter drugs such as Tylenol and cold medications
   c. herbal "food supplements" taken by the patient
   d. all of the above

8. A patient profile must be created for:
   a. a hospital patient
   b. any patient at an outpatient pharmacy
   c. a regular pharmacy customer
   d. anyone who receives prescription medications from any pharmacy

9. A former patient comes to the pharmacy with a prescription. His address has changed. You should:
   a. take the new information and update his patient profile
   b. call the pharmacist to take care of the situation
   c. put him in as a new patient and create a new profile
   d. ignore the information, because the address is not important

10. A patient comes to the pharmacy with a new prescription and says that he experienced a severe rash from the prescription that he had filled a few days ago. You should:
    a. make note of the problem in the "allergies" section of his patient profile
    b. alert the pharmacist
    c. both a and b
    d. recommend the Benadryl in aisle 8

11. The following would be found on a patient profile in the retail setting but not in the hospital setting:
    a. patient identification
    b. diagnosis and lab test results
    c. concurrent medications
    d. drug allergies

12. An example of a therapeutic duplication is:
    a. a prescription for Tylenol #3, when the patient is taking acetaminophen tablets
    b. a prescription for Lasix when the patient is taking an herbal diuretic
    c. a prescription for an antihistamine for a patient taking aspirin
    d. both a and b

Chapter 3

13. A bottle labeled "mannitol solution" appears to contain a solid material. This most likely means that the solution:
    a. is contaminated
    b. has been exposed to heat
    c. has been exposed to extreme cold
    d. has been mislabeled and is not mannitol

14. A prescription for Timoptic reads "1 gtt ou bid." The instructions to the patient would be:
    a. take one drop twice a day
    b. take 1 mL twice a day
    c. insert one drop in each ear twice a day
    d. instill one drop in each eye twice a day

15. In an institutional setting, a prescription for Tagamet would be:
    a. automatically filled generically
    b. filled with Tagament only
    c. filled with a similar drug (e.g., Zantac) if the pharmacy is out of Tagamet
    d. filled with Tagamet unless the prescriber has indicated on the MAR that a substitution is permissible

16. You receive a prescription for Amoxil, ordered "dispense as written." You check the stock and find Trimox. You:
    a. fill the prescription with the available stock
    b. fill the prescription but adjust the dosage according to the label on the bottle
    c. tell the patient that the prescription cannot be filled
    d. fill the prescription with Trimox, since it is the same thing

17. Which of the following is a solid dosage form?
    a. the suppository
    b. the lozenge
    c. the suspension
    d. the cream

18. A diskhaler utilizes:
    a. a prepared solution of drug
    b. a drug spray
    c. a packet of finely ground drug powder
    d. a drug cartridge

Chapter 4

19. A prescription for lamotrigine includes the instructions "i tab qd w/meal." What auxiliary label might be affixed to the dispensing container?
    a. take with food
    b. drink with plenty of water
    c. may cause drowsiness
    d. for the eye

20. The dosage strength of the medication dispensed is not required on the label if:
    a. the strength is below 10 mg
    b. the drug is a combination drug
    c. the drug only comes in one strength
    d. both b and c are correct

21. Which of the following are involved in the practice of aseptic technique?
    a. clean hands
    b. alcohol disinfection
    c. the use of masks and gloves
    d. all of the above

22. Aseptic technique is used for parenteral injections only, because:
    a. sterility is more important in drugs that enter directly into the bloodstream
    b. patients feel more comfortable knowing that the drugs entering the body are clean
    c. bacteria and other organisms multiply rapidly once in the bloodstream and could cause death
    d. both a and c are correct

23. The first segment of the NDC number represents the:
    a. type of drug
    b. drug's manufacturer
    c. dosage form
    d. relative safety of the drug

24. Which of the following types of injections are administered by slow infusion?
    a. intramuscular injection
    b. subcutaneous injection
    c. intra-arterial injection
    d. intravenous piggyback

Chapter 5

25. You receive a shipment of medication. To determine whether the drug should be stored on the shelf, you should:
    a. ask the pharmacist
    b. refer to the *United States Pharmacopoeia*
    c. try different ways of storage
    d. refer to the manufacturer's label

26. The stability of a drug is determined by:
    a. whether it turns a different color from exposure to light
    b. whether the drug can be stored on the pharmacy shelf
    c. how long it remains potent and in its present form
    d. how it should be stored

27. A reconstituted drug in suspension:
    a. is always stored on the pharmacy shelf
    b. will eventually settle to the bottom of the container
    c. will slowly break down over time
    d. Both b and c could be correct

28. You have a bottle of drug solution. The label does not state the concentration of the drug in the solution, just the amount of drug and the volume of liquid in the container. To dispense 30 mg of this drug, you can:
    a. go to the *United States Pharmacopoeia* for additional information
    b. estimate the amount of drug to be dispensed by the volume needed for injection
    c. calculate the concentration from the information given on the label
    d. The order cannot be filled, because the concentration is not given

29. You are a retail pharmacy technician and receive a prescription for cimetidine, written by Dr. John Smith. The DEA number is AS3284066. You should:
    a. fill the prescription
    b. alert the pharmacist, as this person is not authorized to prescribe outside of a hospital
    c. refuse to fill the prescription
    d. refuse the prescription, as the DEA number is not valid

Chapter 6

30. An example of a third-party payor would be:
    a. medicare
    b. a major insurance company
    c. a man ordered to pay medical expenses as a result of a lawsuit
    d. both a and b

31. The selling price of a medication is based on the:
    a. patient's income
    b. amount the insurance will pay
    c. overall cost to the pharmacy
    d. dispensing fee

32. An insurance affidavit is required when:
    a. medication is paid for by an insurance company
    b. the patient pays for the medication out of pocket and must submit proof of purchase to the insurance company for reimbursement
    c. the patient does not produce an insurance card
    d. the drug is not covered under the co-pay plan

Chapter 7

33. 100×0.002
    a. 0.2
    b. $-\dfrac{1}{50}$
    c. $\dfrac{1}{5}$
    d. both a and c are correct.

34. $\frac{1}{4} + \frac{1}{2} =$
   a. $\frac{3}{4}$
   b. 0.75
   c. 0.5
   d. both a and b

35. $\frac{3}{4} \div \frac{1}{2} =$
   a. $\frac{3}{2}$
   b. $\frac{3}{8}$
   c. 1.25
   d. both a and c

36. xxi + xiv =
   a. xxxv
   b. xxiiv
   c. 35
   d. both a and c

Chapter 8

37. 1:1,000 = ___ mg/mL
   a. 5
   b. 2
   c. 1
   d. 10

38. 2% = ___ mg/mL
   a. 20
   b. 2
   c. 12
   d. 200

39. 0.5 L = ___ mL
   a. 500
   b. 50
   c. 5
   d. 5,000

40. How many grams of drug are in 10 mL of a 7% solution?
   a. 70
   b. 7
   c. 700
   d. 0.7

41. How many milligrams of drug are in 5 mL of a 1:100 solution?
   a. 5
   b. 50
   c. 500
   d. 100

42. 5°C = ___°F
    a. 35
    b. 41
    c. 37
    d. 28

43. How many milligrams of epinephrine are in 0.5 mL of a 1:100 solution?
    a. 5
    b. 20
    c. 50
    d. 25

Chapter 9

44. A solution contains 0.5% drug. If a patient uses 0.2 mL of solution, what is the dose?
    a. 10 mg
    b. 1 mg
    c. 0.05 mg
    d. 5 mg

45. You have 10 mL of a 1% solution and need to dispense a 2 mg dose. How many doses are in the bottle?
    a. 20
    b. 30
    c. 50
    d. 500

46. A suppository contains 5% zinc oxide. How much zinc oxide is contained in a 5 g suppository?
    a. 0.5 g
    b. 0.25 g
    c. 150 mg
    d. 500 mg

47. A cream contains 0.5% phenylephrine. How much cream is needed to give a dose of 50 mg phenylephrine?
    a. 2 g
    b. 5 g
    c. 10 g
    d. 25 g

Chapter 10

48. When using a graduated cylinder made of glass, an accurate reading of the amount of fluid measured would be made by looking at the:
    a. top of the fluid in the cylinder
    b. sides of the meniscus
    c. bottom of the meniscus
    d. marking on the cylinder that is closest to the fluid

49. To measure 15 mL of cough syrup, a _____ should be used.
    a. 10 mL graduated cylinder used twice
    b. 10 mL syringe used twice
    c. 20 mL graduated cylinder
    d. 50 mL graduated cylinder

50. When using a double-pan balance to weigh material for compounding, the:
    a. sample and weights should be placed in the middle of their pans
    b. weights should not be touched
    c. sample to be weighed should not be more than the total of the counterweights
    d. all of the above

51. A prescription balance would be used to weigh which of the following amounts?
    a. 100 g
    b. 500 g
    c. 0.05 mg
    d. 6 mg

52. A suspension of insulin was removed from the refrigerator, and a dose of 100 units was withdrawn to fill an order for patient Hill. The suspension was then left out on the counter for an hour, and the same amount was withdrawn for patient Smith. The dosage for patient Hill:
    a. would be equal to that for patient Smith
    b. would be less than that for patient Smith
    c. would be greater than that for patient Smith
    d. would be slightly less than that for patient Smith

53. An order is received for 10 mL of 0.2% calcium gluconate solution, which is to be taken orally. You would measure the solution using:
    a. a 50 mL graduated cylinder
    b. a 20 mL graduated cylinder
    c. a 10 mL oral syringe
    d. any of the above would be acceptable

Chapter 11

For each question, determine the number of tablets dispensed to fill the order.

54. Your order is for prednisolone 0.05 g po q6h. You have 25 mg tablets in stock. How many will be dispensed for one dose?
    a. $\frac{1}{2}$ tablet
    b. two tablets
    c. $\frac{3}{4}$ tablet
    d. four tablets

55. A daily dose for the prescription in Problem 54 would be:
    a. two tablets
    b. one tablet
    c. four tablets
    d. eight tablets

56. Your order is for Digibind 200 mcg po. Your stock is 0.1 mg tabs, scored in fourths.

    a. $\frac{1}{2}$ tablet
    b. $\frac{1}{4}$ tablet
    c. two tablets
    d. cannot be dispensed

57. Your order is for morphine gr ss. Your stock is 30 mg tabs.

    a. $\frac{1}{2}$ tablet
    b. $\frac{1}{4}$ tablet
    c. two tablets
    d. one tablet

58. Your order is for penicillin 600,000 units po. You have 250 mg tablets in stock. The label says that one 250 mg tablet contains 400,000 units. The tablets are scored in half.

    a. $\frac{1}{2}$ tablet
    b. $1\frac{1}{2}$ tablets
    c. two tablets
    d. cannot be dispensed

Chapter 12

59. Your order is for digoxin elixir 0.25 mg qid. Your stock is 0.5 mg/10 mL. Amount dispensed per dose =

    a. 2 mL
    b. 5 mL
    c. 10 mL
    d. 0.5 mL

60. Your order is for sulfisoxazole susp. 300 mg po stat. You have a solution in stock that is 250 mg/5 mL. Amount dispensed =

    a. 3 mL
    b. 5 mL
    c. 6 mL
    d. 1.2 mL

61. Your order is for cyclosporine 150 mg po. You have a solution in stock that is 100 mg/mL. Amount dispensed =

    a. 0.75 mL
    b. 0.35 mL
    c. 1.5 mL
    d. 3 mL

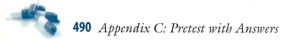

Chapter 13

62. Your order is for ethambutol 10 mg/kg for a child weighing 88 lb. One dose =
   a. 800 mg
   b. 200 mg
   c. 400 mg
   d. 880 mg

63. The adult dose of diazepam is 10 mg/m^2. One dose for a child with a BSA of 1.25 m^2 would be:
   a. 12.5 mg
   b. 6.25 mg
   c. 7.3 mg
   d. 10 mg

64. An adult dose of Keflin is 1 g. What is the dose for a child weighing 50 lb?
   a. 500 mg
   b. 333 mg
   c. 750 mg
   d. 170 mg

65. You receive an order for amoxicillin 250 mg for a 12-year-old child who weighs 88 lbs. The adult dosage is 500 mg. You call the prescription to the attention of the pharmacist because:
   a. the dosage is too high, according to Young's Rule
   b. the dosage is too high, according to the child's weight
   c. the dosage is under therapeutic dosage
   d. It is not necessary to alert the pharmacist, the prescription is fine.

Chapter 14

66. Your order is for Demerol 20 mg IM. Available stock is 50 mg/5 mL. Dispense:
   a. 5 mL
   b. 20 mL
   c. 2 mL
   d. 10 mL

67. Your order is for Lanoxin 0.6 mg IV. Available stock is 500 mcg/2 mL. Dispense:
   a. 2.4 mL
   b. 0.24 mL
   c. 1.2 mL
   d. 12 mL

68. Your order is for morphine gr ss. Available stock is 6 mg/mL. Dispense:
   a. 4 mL
   b. 2 mL
   c. 5 mL
   d. 8 mL

69. Your order is for heparin 2,000 units SC. Your stock of heparin is 10,000 units/5 mL. Dispense:
    a. 5 mL
    b. 2 mL
    c. 1 mL
    d. 0.2 mL

70. Your order is for 1 mg of epinephrine. Your stock is a 1:1,000 solution. Dispense:
    a. 10 mL
    b. 0.1 mL
    c. 1.5 mL
    d. 1 mL

71. You need to make 100 mL of a 2% calcium gluconate solution. Your stock is a 1:5 solution. How much stock solution will you need to make the 2% solution?
    a. 50 mL
    b. 20 mL
    c. 10 mL
    d. 5 mL

Chapter 15

72. 1 L of saline is administered over 5 hours. The infusion set states that the drop factor is 15 gtt/mL. The flow rate in gtt/min is:
    a. 35
    b. 50
    c. 15
    d. 150

73. 500 mL of D_5W runs for 4 hours. Calculate the flow rate in mL/min.
    a. 125
    b. 51.6
    c. 2.08
    d. 20.8

74. 1 L of NS runs for 16 hours 40 min. Calculate the flow rate in mL/hr.
    a. 100
    b. 120
    c. 60
    d. 220

75. You have an order for aminophylline 250 mg in 500 mL NS to run for 8 hours. The drop factor is 60 gtt/mL. What is the flow rate in drops per minute?
    a. 12.5
    b. 63
    c. 6
    d. 56

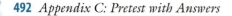

76. 1 L of NS is infused at 100 mL/hr. How long will the infusion go?
    a. 5 hours
    b. 10 hours
    c. 1 hour
    d. cannot be determined

77. In 5 hours 300 mL of lactated Ringer's solution is infused. The flow rate is 15 gtt/min. What is the drop factor in gtt/mL?
    a. 60
    b. 10
    c. 15
    d. cannot be determined

78. A 500 mL IV bag is prepared, containing 1 g of cephalexin. At a rate of 50 mL/hr, how long will it take half of the dose to infuse?
    a. 1 hour
    b. 2 hours
    c. 10 hours
    d. 5 hours

Chapter 16

79. Aminophylline 250 mg in 500 mL NS is to run for 4 hours. The flow rate is 100 mL/hr. What is the dose of drug administered?
    a. 200 mg
    b. 250 mg
    c. 100 mg
    d. 150 mg

80. You add 10 mL of 10% calcium gluconate to a 1 L bag of D_5W. What is the concentration of calcium gluconate in the bag?
    a. 10 mg/mL
    b. 100 mg/mL
    c. 1 mg/mL
    d. 0.1 mg/mL

81. You dilute a vial of drug with 2.5 mL of saline. The vial contains 2,500,000 units of drug. What is the final concentration of drug in the vial?
    a. 1,000,000 units/mL
    b. 250,000 units/mL
    c. 100,000 units/mL
    d. 10,000 units/mL

82. A patient receives 500 mL of D_5W that contains 100,000 units of heparin. The flow rate is 50 mL/hr. What is the hourly dose of dextrose?
    a. 5 g
    b. 10 g
    c. 2.5 g
    d. 50 g

83. You add 1,000,000 units of penicillin to a 500 mL IV bag. Using an infusion set calibrated for 10 gtt/mL, what is the hourly dose if the flow rate is 20 gtt/min?
    a. 100,000 units
    b. 240,000 units
    c. 4,000 units
    d. 24,000 units

Chapter 17

84. An IV solution of heparin contains 10,000 units in 500 mL and takes 2 hours to infuse. The amount of drug infused in 30 minutes is:
    a. 500 units
    b. 1,000 units
    c. 2,500 units
    d. 200 units

85. The solution in Problem 84 is to be infused so that the patient gets 1,000 units of heparin per hour. The flow rate in mL/hr is:
    a. 50
    b. 100
    c. 200
    d. 150

86. You add 5 mL of a 20% solution of calcium gluconate to a 500 mL IV bag. The flow rate is 30 gtt/min with an infusion set labeled 15 gtt/mL. How much drug does the patient get per hour?
    a. 60 mg
    b. 240 mg
    c. 600 mg
    d. 300 mg

Chapter 18

87. You need to make 5 L of diphenhydramine lotion. The procedure states that the cream contains 0.5% diphenhydramine. How much diphenhydramine do you need?
    a. 50 g
    b. 100 g
    c. 25 g
    d. cannot be determined

88. If 20 g of glycerol is needed to make 1 L of calamine lotion, how much glycerol is needed to make 240 mL of lotion?
    a. 2 g
    b. 4.8 g
    c. 5.6 g
    d. 12 g

89. You need 100 mL of a 4% solution of calcium hydroxide. How much calcium hydroxide do you need?
    a. 5 g
    b. 2.5 g
    c. 4 g
    d. 8 g

Chapter 19

90–91. You have a 5% solution of calcium gluconate, priced at $1 per 10 mL. There is a 200% markup on the drug product. Your order is for 1 g of calcium gluconate in a saline drip.

90. What would the patient be charged for the drug?
    a. $2
    b. $8
    c. $6
    d. cannot be determined

91. How much profit would the pharmacy make on this dose?
    a. $2
    b. $4
    c. $6
    d. $10

92–93. You have a vial of ampicillin sodium for injection that contains 5 g of drug. You dilute it to 500 mg/mL. The cost of the vial is $15 and its markup is 200%.

92. The entire vial sells for:
    a. $15
    b. $30
    c. $150
    d. $45

93. The amount of profit made on the one vial is:
    a. $15
    b. $25
    c. $30
    d. $150

94. A pharmacy sells a tube of Ben-Gay for $6.90, with a 200% markup. The cost of the Ben-Gay to the pharmacy was:
    a. $3.20
    b. $2.30
    c. $3.30
    d. cannot be determined

95. The pharmacy pays $200 for a bottle of 1,000 tablets of Tegretol. Assuming a 200% markup and a $5 dispensing fee, how much would a patient be charged for his prescription of 100 tablets?
    a. $50
    b. $75
    c. $65
    d. $125

Chapter 21

96. Which of the following drugs have a major drug-drug interaction?
    a. isoproterenol and furosemide
    b. digitalis and mannitol
    c. secobarbital and alcohol
    d. aspirin and diazepam

97. The action or potency of which of the following would be affected by concurrent use of antacids such as calcium carbonate (Tums)?
    a. aspirin
    b. ibuprofen
    c. doxycycline
    d. none of the above

98. Nimodipine and nifedipine are drugs that belong to the same class. This means that they:
    a. act exactly the same
    b. have the same mechanism of action
    c. have similar adverse effects
    d. both b and c

99. An example of a drug's mechanism of action might be:
    a. the glucose-lowering effect of a drug
    b. a decrease in heart rate produced by the drug, resulting in decreased blood pressure
    c. blockade of sodium channels produced by the drug
    d. any of the above

100. The binding of a drug to plasma proteins would be an example of:
    a. drug absorption
    b. drug metabolism
    c. drug distribution
    d. drug elimination

101. A drug such as phenobarbital, with a long half-life:
    a. will be absorbed slowly
    b. will have a delayed effect
    c. would have a long duration of action
    d. is eliminated quickly

102. A patient with decreased hepatic or renal clearance, such as a geriatric patient, might require:
    a. more frequent dosing
    b. a change in drug choice
    c. a lower dosage
    d. no special consideration would be made

103. You receive an order for sulfasalazine 400 mg qd. The normal maintenance dose is 200 mg qd. You should:
    a. alert the pharmacist
    b. refuse to fill the prescription, as the patient might die
    c. recognize that the 400 mg is a loading dose and fill the prescription
    d. call the prescriber

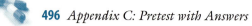

Chapter 22

104. Which of the following is used for treating depression?
    a. Tofranil
    b. Prozac
    c. Paxil
    d. all of the above

105. Which of the following directly affect(s) the cardiovascular system?
    a. Cardizem
    b. Cardura
    c. Catapres
    d. both a and b

106. Which of the following is an antifungal drug?
    a. Miconazole
    b. Cefamandole
    c. Tegopen
    d. Hydrocort

107. Fluoxetine and tranylcypromine:
    a. are antidepressant agents
    b. are monamine oxidase inhibitors
    c. may be safely used together
    d. are anticonvulsant agents

108. Which of the following, in high levels, may produce symptoms that mimic Parkinson's disease?
    a. tranylcypromine
    b. chlorpromazine
    c. fluoxetine
    d. divalproex sodium

109. Which antidepressant is related to a phenothiazine antipsychotic?
    a. imipramine
    b. amitryptiline
    c. amoxapine
    d. phenylzine

110. Which of these drugs, when combined with atropine, will produce excessive sedation?
    a. amitryptiline
    b. Paxil
    c. Pargiline
    d. Neurontin

111. Which of the following affects dopamine?
    a. Halcion
    b. Xanax
    c. Levodopa
    d. Paxil

Chapter 23

112. Which of the following has the most antithrombotic action?
    a. Celebrex
    b. Vioxx
    c. aspirin
    d. Tylenol

113. Which of the following is contraindicated in a patient who is in renal failure?
    a. valsartan
    b. Capoten
    c. Toprol
    d. atropine

114. Which of the following drugs would be inappropriate to administer to a patient with hepatitis?
    a. sulindac
    b. ibuprofen
    c. Vicodin
    d. Percodan

115. Which of the following drugs has no anti-inflammatory action?
    a. ibuprofen
    b. ketoprofen
    c. sulindac
    d. acetaminophen

116. Which of the following drugs might be most likely to promote stomach ulcers?
    a. sulindac
    b. acetaminophen
    c. ibuprofen
    d. aspirin

Chapter 24

117. A drug such as candesartan:
    a. would be useful in the therapy of high blood pressure
    b. would decrease the production of angiotensin II
    c. would increase memory retention
    d. is contraindicated in congestive heart failure

118. A venodilator such as isosorbide dinitrate would be most useful in the therapy of:
    a. angina
    b. hypertension
    c. arrhythmias
    d. congestive heart failure

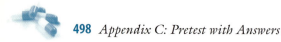

119. A drug that increases the force of contraction of the heart would be a(n):
    a. beta receptor blocker
    b. inotropic agent
    c. diuretic
    d. antianginal agent

120. Which of the following antagonizes the autonomic nervous system?
    a. isoproterenol
    b. phenylephrine
    c. atropine
    d. Lasix

Chapter 25

121. Which of the following is useful in an acute attack of asthma?
    a. Serevent
    b. Theo-Dur
    c. Aldomet
    d. Proventil

122. A patient reports swelling of the face and extremities after starting a new drug. The drug responsible might be:
    a. Serevent
    b. prednisone
    c. montelukast
    d. zafirlukast

123. Which of the following drugs is a powder formulation marketed for inhalation?
    a. Singulair
    b. formoterol
    c. epinephrine
    d. Theo-Dur

124. Which of the following is an inhibitor of leukotrienes?
    a. Serevent
    b. Singulair
    c. Ascendin
    d. none of the above

125. Which of the following is for prophylactic use only?
    a. zafirlukast
    b. formoterol
    c. isoproterenol
    d. both a and b

Chapter 26

126. Which of the following might cause photosensitivity?
     a. CefoBid
     b. doxycycline
     c. penicillin
     d. cefaclor

127. Gentamicin:
     a. is a bactericidal antibiotic
     b. may cause hearing loss
     c. is a tetracycline
     d. both a and b

128. CefoBid:
     a. may cause hypersensitivity reactions in penicillin-allergic patients
     b. is an antifungal drug
     c. is administered by IV drip only
     d. is useful in Enterobacter infections

129. Which of the following prescriptions should be called to the attention of the pharmacist?
     a. Amoxil 500 mg PO
     b. Ceclor 400 mg TID
     c. Penicillin G-K 100,000 Units IV
     d. Ilosone 250 mg PO

130. Milk or antacids would be contraindicated with:
     a. tetracycline
     b. doxycycline
     c. minocycline
     d. both b and c

Chapter 27

131. Which of the following drugs may suppress the immune system?
     a. Oncovin
     b. methotrexate
     c. Platinol
     d. Mitomycin

132. Which of the following drugs is contraindicated with alcohol?
     a. mitomycin
     b. procarbazine
     c. Platinol
     d. ifosfamide

133. Which of the following is contraindicated with anti-gout agents (e.g., probenecid)?
    a. methotrexate
    b. cladribine
    c. carboplatin
    d. 6-thioguanine

Chapter 28

134. Which of the following is used in the therapy of acid reflux disease and must be absorbed before it has therapeutic action?
    a. Tums
    b. Mylanta
    c. Axid
    d. Carafate

135. Which of the following is a histamine receptor blocker?
    a. Imodium
    b. Axid
    c. Prilosec
    d. Nexium

136. Which of the following has interactions with drugs that are metabolized by cytochrome P_{450}?
    a. Tagamet
    b. Axid
    c. Lomotil
    d. both a and b

137. Which of the following might cause tachycardia in high doses?
    a. mebendazole
    b. Nexium
    c. Lomotil
    d. Ex-Lax

Chapter 29

138. Propothiouracil and methimazole are both:
    a. used in contraception
    b. iodide-trapping agents
    c. used for hypothyroidism
    d. used for type II diabetes mellitus

139. Which of the following might be effective in both type I and type II diabetes?
    a. Micronase
    b. Precose
    c. Prandin
    d. Actos

140. Which of the following may cause severe hypoglycemia?
    a. glyburide
    b. miglitol
    c. glipizide
    d. both a and c

141. Which of the following forms of insulin is rapid-acting?
    a. insulin glargine
    b. insulin aspart
    c. NPH insulin
    d. lente insulin

142. A patient is taking Nuvaring. Possible effects of this drug include:
    a. an increased risk of cervical cancer
    b. an increased risk of clotting
    c. a lower blood level of cholesterol (LDL)
    d. all of the above

Chapter 30

143. Minerals necessary for proper nerve function include:
    a. potassium
    b. sodium
    c. calcium
    d. all of the above

144. The chemical symbol for sodium is:
    a. K^+
    b. Na^+
    c. Ca^{++}
    d. So^+

145. A patient has night blindness. This may be due to a deficiency in:
    a. vitamin C
    b. vitamin D
    c. vitamin A
    d. vitamin K

146. A patient taking ascorbic acid is taking:
    a. vitamin K
    b. vitamin C
    c. vitamin A
    d. vitamin D

147. An inability of the blood to clot may mean a deficiency of:
    a. vitamin C
    b. vitamin D
    c. vitamin A
    d. vitamin K

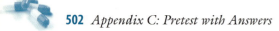

Chapter 32

148. Records of patient demographics, drug history, and therapeutic profile must be kept due to the mandates of the:
    a. Hazardous Substances Act
    b. Controlled Substances Act
    c. Consolidated Omnibus Budget Reconciliation Act
    d. Poison Prevention Packaging Act

149. Patient counseling is mandatory, under the:
    a. Controlled Substances Act
    b. Consolidated Omnibus Budget Reconciliation Act
    c. Food, Drug, and Cosmetic Act
    d. Patient Protection Act

150. A drug causes liver toxicity with therapeutic dose. This would be a violation of the:
    a. Occupational Safety and Health Act
    b. Food, Drug, and Cosmetic Act
    c. Consolidated Omnibus Budget Reconciliation Act
    d. all of the above

Chapter 33

151. When dealing with a spill of a toxic drug on your arm, you should:
    a. immediately rinse your arm under running water
    b. scrub the affected area
    c. gently blot the drug solution from your arm with an absorbent towel before washing
    d. wash the area immediately with soap and water

152. Wearing protective clothing and gloves is sufficient to protect you from the toxic effects of anti-neoplastic drugs, unless:
    a. the gloves are too thin
    b. the sleeves on the coat are too tight
    c. you rub your eyes or nose while working
    d. you are working within 7 inches of the drug material

153. Which of these organizations is a state regulatory agency?
    a. The U.S. Food and Drug Administration
    b. JCAHO
    c. The Consumer Product Safety Commission
    d. The State Board of Pharmacy

154. Childproof caps must be placed on dispensing containers according to legislation produced by the:
    a. Pharmacy and Therapeutics Committee
    b. Joint Commission on Accreditation of Healthcare Organizations
    c. Consumer Product Safety Commission
    d. U.S. Food and Drug Administration

155. Claims of misbranded drugs would be handled by the:
     a. Pharmacy and Therapeutics Committee
     b. Joint Commission on Accreditation of Healthcare Organizations
     c. Consumer Product Safety Commission
     d. U.S. Food and Drug Administration
     e. State Board of Pharmacy

Chapter 34

156. A prescription for Demerol:
     a. must be received on a duplicate or triplicate form (depending on the state)
     b. may be called or faxed in
     c. may be obtained by telephone by the pharmacist in an emergency
     d. both a and c are correct

157. You receive a prescription for meperidine. It contains a corrected date. You should:
     a. alert the pharmacist
     b. call the prescriber
     c. ignore the change in date and fill the prescription
     d. refuse to fill the prescription and give it back to the patient

158. A patient buys a bottle of acetaminophen over the counter. She gives the drug to her child, at an adult dose, as no pediatric dose is specified on the label. The child goes into liver failure. This problem was a result of a violation of the:
     a. Controlled Substances Act
     b. Consolidated Omnibus Budget Reconciliation Act
     c. Federal Hazardous Substances Act
     d. Food, Drug, and Cosmetics Act

159. A patient's confidential information is released to her sister, without the patient's consent. This is a violation of the:
     a. Patient Privacy Act
     b. Board of Pharmacy Ethics Mandates
     c. Health Insurance Portability and Accountability Act
     d. Consolidated Omnibus Budget Reconciliation Act

160. Which of the following personnel, all of whom handle controlled substances, does not require a controlled substance registration?
     a. nurse practitioner
     b. physician
     c. dentist
     d. sales representative for a pharmaceutical company

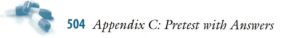

Chapter 35

161. A drug formulary is:
    a. the same thing as a drug inventory
    b. a formula for compounding a drug
    c. a list of all of the drugs carried by a particular pharmacy
    d. a list of brand-name drugs carried by a pharmacy

162. Drug duplication in a pharmacy inventory refers to:
    a. filling two prescriptions for one patient for the same drug
    b. stocking two proprietary-label drugs in identical dosage forms that contain the same drug
    c. taking two drugs that do the same thing
    d. none of the above

163. Ordering Class II drugs:
    a. may be done by the technician
    b. is done by computer
    c. requires a special form
    d. must be done within five days of running out

164. Which of the following does not need to appear on a purchase order for a drug?
    a. the name of the drug
    b. the strength of the drug
    c. the type of packaging and units per package
    d. all of the above must appear on a purchase order

Chapter 36

165. When a drug is recalled due to serious or toxic patient effects, which of the following should occur?
    a. the patients using the drug should be notified
    b. the providers prescribing the drug should be notified
    c. the drug supply with the appropriate lot number should be removed from inventory and returned to the supplier
    d. all of the above

166. A drug is found on the pharmacy shelf that expires in three weeks. This drug:
    a. should be dispensed
    b. should be sent back to the manufacturer
    c. should be marked and reevaluated in three weeks
    d. should be removed from the pharmacy shelf

167. All Schedule II drugs must be:
    a. kept in a marked, locked cabinet
    b. documented carefully, with no mistakes or strikeovers
    c. inventoried at specified, required intervals
    d. All of the above

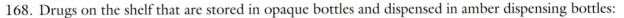

168. Drugs on the shelf that are stored in opaque bottles and dispensed in amber dispensing bottles:
    a. are sensitive to heat
    b. are sensitive to humidity
    c. are sensitive to light
    d. may be unstable

169. A drug label says to store the drug between 15°C and 25°C. The drug should be stored:
    a. on the pharmacy shelf
    b. in the refrigerator
    c. in the freezer
    d. away from bright light

Chapter 37

170. Which of the following is considered computer software?
    a. hard disk
    b. modem
    c. processor
    d. disk operating system

171. Which of the following is a use for computers in the pharmacy?
    a. maintenance of patient information
    b. billing
    c. identification of drug-drug interactions
    d. all of the above

172. An example of an input device would be a:
    a. light pen
    b. printer
    c. modem
    d. monitor

Chapter 38

173. A patient calls the pharmacy and says that her child has taken her medication by mistake. You should:
    a. tell her to call 911
    b. refer her to the nearest poison control center
    c. attempt to counsel her
    d. refer her to the pharmacist

174. The technician is not allowed to:
    a. call the prescriber to clarify a prescription order
    b. offer support to the patient
    c. tell the patient not to take aspirin with her Coumadin prescription
    d. tell the patient that the pharmacy carries a generic drug for her prescription that is considerably cheaper than the proprietary drug

Pretest Answers

1. c	36. d	71. c	106. a	141. b
2. b	37. c	72. b	107. a	142. d
3. d	38. a	73. c	108. b	143. d
4. c	39. a	74. c	109. c	144. b
5. c	40. d	75. b	110. a	145. c
6. d	41. b	76. b	111. c	146. b
7. d	42. b	77. c	112. c	147. d
8. d	43. a	78. d	113. b	148. c
9. a	44. b	79. a	114. c	149. b
10. c	45. c	80. c	115. d	150. b
11. c	46. b	81. a	116. d	151. c
12. d	47. c	82. c	117. a	152. c
13. c	48. c	83. b	118. a	153. d
14. d	49. c	84. c	119. b	154. c
15. a	50. d	85. a	120. c	155. d
16. c	51. c	86. b	121. d	156. d
17. b	52. c	87. c	122. b	157. a
18. c	53. c	88. b	123. b	158. d
19. a	54. b	89. c	124. b	159. c
20. d	55. d	90. c	125. d	160. d
21. d	56. c	91. b	126. b	161. c
22. d	57. d	92. d	127. d	162. b
23. b	58. b	93. c	128. a	163. c
24. d	59. b	94. b	129. b	164. d
25. d	60. c	95. c	130. a	165. d
26. c	61. c	96. c	131. b	166. d
27. d	62. c	97. a	132. b	167. d
28. c	63. a	98. d	133. d	168. c
29. a	64. b	99. c	134. c	169. a
30. d	65. d	100. c	135. b	170. d
31. c	66. c	101. c	136. a	171. d
32. b	67. a	102. c	137. c	172. a
33. d	68. c	103. c	138. b	173. d
34. d	69. c	104. d	139. b	174. c
35. a	70. d	105. d	140. d	

Sample Examination and Answer Sheet

1. An example of a drug that should not be taken with Coumadin would be:
   a. aspirin
   b. alcohol
   c. acetaminophen
   d. penicillin

2. The system of measurement in which liquid is measured in drams is the:
   a. metric system
   b. apothecary system
   c. avoirdupois system
   d. household system

3. A pharmacy receives a shipment of drug product that costs $50 per case of 20 tubes. The price markup is 200%. The selling price per tube is:
   a. $5
   b. $3
   c. $2.50
   d. $7.50

4. Which of the following drugs causes photosensitivity?
   a. ibuprofen
   b. carbamazepine
   c. tetracycline
   d. both b and c

5. You receive an order for Amoxil 200 mg PO qid for 10 days. Your supply is a suspension of 50 mg/2 mL. The quantity dispensed is:
   a. 10 mL
   b. 25 mL
   c. 280 mL
   d. 320 mL

6. The list of drugs that are stocked by the pharmacy and have been decided to be the most efficacious and cost-efficient is called the:
   a. drug list
   b. therapeutic compendium
   c. formulary
   d. inventory

7. The SIG on a prescription reads "i po ac, hs." The drug:
   a. should be taken with food
   b. may cause drowsiness
   c. should be taken on an empty stomach
   d. may cause diarrhea

8. Which of the following drugs should not be stored at 5°C?
   a. Compazine suppositories
   b. amoxicillin suspension
   c. mannitol solution
   d. Phenergan suppositories

9. Which of the following must be on an order for Lasix tablets when it is presented to the pharmacy?
   a. date of birth of the patient
   b. address of the patient
   c. drug strength
   d. allergies

10. An order carries the following SIG: ii gtt au prn. The proper auxiliary label to affix to the labeled container would read:
    a. take with food
    b. for the ear
    c. for the eye
    d. may cause drowsiness

11. Which of the following drugs is a benzodiazepine?
    a. phenobarbital
    b. Phenergan
    c. lorazepam
    d. phenytoin

12. Which of the following is used for congestive heart failure?
    a. Lanoxin
    b. Lomotil
    c. Keflex
    d. Isuprel

13. The appearance of a white, fluffy precipitate in a 500 mL bag of D_5W would indicate that the product:
    a. has been exposed to cold
    b. has been exposed to bright light
    c. is contaminated and should be discarded
    d. should be shaken to disperse the precipitate before dispensing

14. Personnel handling cisplatin should:
    a. wear protective clothing and gloves
    b. work in a well-ventilated area
    c. shake the product well before drawing the dose
    d. keep the product out of bright light

15. Which of the following drugs does not require special handling and/or the wearing of protective clothing?
    a. Methotrexate injection
    b. Adriamycin injection
    c. mannitol injection
    d. vincristine injection

16. An order is for phenobarbital gr iss IV. Available stock is 200 mg/3 mL. The amount dispensed should be:
    a. 2.5 mL
    b. 1.35 mL
    c. 0.67 mL
    d. 1.8 mL

17. An order is for lidocaine 30 mg SC. Available stock is a 1% solution. The amount dispensed is:
    a. 3 mL
    b. 2 mL
    c. 1.5 mL
    d. 0.5 mL

18. 500 mcL of U-100 insulin is equal to:
    a. 5 units
    b. 50 units
    c. 0.5 units
    d. cannot be determined without more information

19. An order is for Synthroid 50 mcg #30, SIG: i qd. The pharmacy has 0.025 mg tablets in stock. The number of tablets dispensed is:
    a. 15
    b. 150
    c. 60
    d. 6

20. The smallest amount that can be accurately measured in a medication dosage cup is:
    a. 5 mL
    b. 2 mL
    c. 4 mL
    d. 10 mL

21. Which of the following is not commercially available?
    a. Tegretol 200 mg tablets
    b. Valium 5 mg tablets
    c. Ritalin 10 mg tablets
    d. Paxil 5 mg tablets

22. Which of the following dosage forms is not commercially available?
    a. amoxicillin tablets
    b. heparin tablets
    c. warfarin tablets
    d. diazepam injection

23. Which of the following is not available by injection?
    a. Zantac
    b. Micronase
    c. Medrol
    d. Lasix

24. Which of the following is available as a sublingual spray?
    a. amyl nitrate
    b. Proventil
    c. Nitrostat
    d. Synthroid

25. Containers used for packaging of parenteral drugs must be:
    a. sterile
    b. made of plastic
    c. pyrogen-free
    d. both a and c

26. Which of the following might be contraindicated in a person with diabetes?
    a. Procardia
    b. Indocin
    c. Isuprel
    d. Micronase

27. Which of the following must be prepared using protective clothing and gloves?
    a. cyclobenzaprine
    b. cyclophosphamide
    c. cyclizine
    d. cycloserine

28. A 1 L IV bag contains 1,000,000 units of penicillin G. The flow rate of the solution is 25 gtt/min, and the infusion set is labeled 15 gtt/mL. The dose that the patient receives per hour is:
    a. 100 units
    b. 1,500 units
    c. 100,000 units
    d. 250,000 units

29. One L of a 10% solution of drug is flowing at a rate of 50 mL/hr. After 2 hours, how much drug has the patient received?
    a. 0.5 g
    b. 1 g
    c. 5 g
    d. 10 g

30. A procedure for compounding cortisone cream specifies that 5 g of cortisone is needed to make 1 kg of cream. What percentage of cortisone will be in the cream?
    a. 5%
    b. 2%
    c. 0.5%
    d. 1%

31. Which of the following would be contraindicated with vitamin K therapy?
    a. Micronase
    b. Coumadin
    c. Heparin
    d. Trental

32. You have a solution of heparin that is 100,000 units/L, with an infusion apparatus labeled 60 gtt/mL. The flow rate required to deliver a dose of 20 units/min would be:
    a. 3 gtt/min
    b. 12 gtt/min
    c. 15 gtt/min
    d. 20 gtt/min

33. With which of the following drugs is it mandatory that a package insert be included with the product?
    a. Vicodin
    b. Roxicet
    c. Premarin
    d. Decadron

34. Which of the following is not a Schedule II drug?
    a. Roxicet
    b. Valium
    c. Demerol
    d. Morphine

35. Which of the following is an oral anticoagulant?
    a. streptokinase
    b. heparin
    c. warfarin
    d. urokinase

36. You prepare a 250 mL bag of NS with 1 g of Kefzol. The patient is to receive a 250 mg dose per hour. The infusion set is calibrated at 10 gtt/mL. The flow rate needed to deliver the dose is:
    a. 1 gtt/min
    b. 10 gtt/min
    c. 20 gtt/min
    d. 15 gtt/min

37. Which of the following would not require potassium supplementation?
    a. Lasix
    b. Diuril
    c. Mevacor
    d. Aquatensen

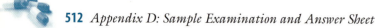
38. An order is for Isuprel 200 mcg IM. Available stock is a 1:5,000 dilution. You dispense:
    a. 0.5 mL
    b. 1.5 mL
    c. 1 mL
    d. 10 mL

39. An order is for 40 mEq of potassium to be administered in 40 mL of orange juice. Your stock of potassium chloride is 20 mEq/5 mL. The amount of solution to be added to the juice would be:
    a. 50 mL
    b. 1 mL
    c. 10 mL
    d. 11.1 mL

40. An order is for Lasix 40 mg bid po for 10 days. You prepare a single unit dose of Lasix solution (10 mg/mL). The amount dispensed would be:
    a. 10 mL
    b. 18 mL
    c. 4 mL
    d. 8 mL

41. An order is for amoxicillin 500 mg po. The drug available is in a suspension of 125 mg/5 mL. The amount of suspension dispensed would be:
    a. 25 mL
    b. 10 mL
    c. 20 mL
    d. 5 mL

42. A patient is prescribed Medrol 0.5 mg po q6h. The pharmacy has 2 mg scored tablets in stock. A unit dose of medication would be:
    a. ¼ tablet
    b. ½ tablet
    c. one tablet
    d. the order cannot be filled

43. The pharmacy receives bottles of amoxicillin labeled 125 mg/5 mL. There is 500 mg of drug in each vial. The amount of water added to each vial should be:
    a. 10 mL
    b. 5 mL
    c. 20 mL
    d. 15 mL

44. Which of the following is an antihistamine?
    a. Adrucil
    b. Allegra
    c. AeroBid
    d. Aldomet

45. A prescription is for Zantac 150 mg #60. The instructions read "i po bid." The total daily dose prescribed is:
   a. 150 mg
   b. 300 mg
   c. 450 mg
   d. cannot be determined

46. Drugs classified as having a high abuse potential and little or no therapeutic benefit are designated as:
   a. Schedule II
   b. Schedule V
   c. Schedule I
   d. Narcotics

47. Which of the following is commercially available?
   a. Zantac 10 mg/mL
   b. Prilosec 25 mg/5 mL
   c. Prozac 50 mg tablet
   d. ibuprofen 800 mg tablet

48. The risk of contamination or infection is greatly reduced by:
   a. wearing a mask and gloves
   b. wearing clean clothing
   c. thorough handwashing and cleaning of equipment before and after use
   d. wearing a lab coat

49. An example of a semisolid dosage form would be a:
   a. cream
   b. pulvule
   c. capsule containing liquid drug
   d. powder for reconstitution

50. A patient is allergic to sulfur. Which of the following drugs in his patient profile should be called to the attention of the pharmacist?
   a. Pen V-K
   b. Bactrim
   c. Toprol
   d. BuSpar

51. A child who weighs 40 kg is prescribed a 10 mg/kg dose of Amoxil. The pharmacy has a 50 mg/mL suspension of Amoxil in stock. The amount dispensed for one dose would be:
   a. 12 mL
   b. 10 mL
   c. 8 mL
   d. 4 mL

52. A child is 10 years old and weighs 80 pounds. The adult dose of phenobarbital is 30 mg. Using Clark's Rule, the child's dose would be:
   a. 3 mg
   b. 16 mg
   c. 25 mg
   d. 20 mg

53. The child in Problem 52 receives cyclizine. The adult dose of cyclizine is 50 mg. According to Young's Rule, the child's dose would be:
   a. 29.4 mg
   b. 26.7 mg
   c. 22.7 mg
   d. 18.8 mg

54. A procedure for making cortisone cream states that the cream contains 200 g of mrystic acid per 1,000 g of cream made. The percentage of mrystic acid is:
   a. 2%
   b. 5%
   c. 20%
   d. 0.5%

55. A patient receives 10 mL of a 20% solution of drug. The drug dose is:
   a. 20 g
   b. 2 g
   c. 20 mg
   d. 200 mg

56. The recommended child's dose of Keflex is 25 mg/kg/day in two divided doses. The correct dose for a 66-lb child would be:
   a. 375 mg
   b. 825 mg
   c. 412 mg
   d. 750 mg

57. A child with a BSA of 0.84 m² is prescribed digoxin 0.75 mg/m². The amount of drug dispensed is:
   a. 630 mcg
   b. 0.89 mg
   c. 1.1 mg
   d. 0.75 mg

58. Which of the following is a local anesthetic?
   a. Lincocin
   b. BuSpar
   c. Xylocaine
   d. Minipress

59. The preparation of a specific dosage form for a patient with specific needs is called:
    a. bulk compounding
    b. bulk manufacturing
    c. extemporaneous compounding
    d. product formulation

60. A SIG that reads "i gtt ad am & hs" instructs the patient to place the medication in:
    a. the right eye
    b. the right ear
    c. both ears
    d. the right arm

61. The encryption of information into a scannable form is called:
    a. programming
    b. bar coding
    c. optic laser coding
    d. data storage

62. An example of a drug that is highly light-sensitive is:
    a. verapamil
    b. nitroglycerin
    c. cefamandole
    d. penicillin

63. Which of the following is a transdermal patch formulation?
    a. MacroBid
    b. Levophed
    c. Nitro-Dur
    d. Micronase

64. Which of the following types of tablets require very careful handling?
    a. tablets for oral use
    b. enteric-coated tablets
    c. sublingual tablets
    d. vaginal tablets

65. A buccal dosage form would be placed:
    a. in the nostril
    b. in the mouth
    c. against the cheek
    d. under the tongue

66. An ophthalmic preparation would be placed in the:
    a. ear
    b. nose
    c. eye
    d. mouth

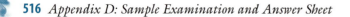

67. Parenteral preparations must be prepared:
    a. quickly
    b. using aseptic technique
    c. under sanitary conditions
    d. in the absence of light

68. One Liter of saline is running through an infusion apparatus delivering 15 gtt/mL. The infusion will go for 5 hours. The flow rate in gtt/min will be:
    a. 100
    b. 150
    c. 50
    d. 95

69. The instructions for storage of a drug product state that the product should be stored at 5–15°C. The product should be stored:
    a. on the pharmacy shelf
    b. in the freezer
    c. in the refrigerator
    d. in a warm room

70. Lanoxin is a proprietary name for:
    a. nitroglycerin
    b. amyl nitrate
    c. digoxin
    d. digitoxin

71. Which of the following is available as an inhaler for use by asthmatics?
    a. Calan
    b. Lopid
    c. Dyazide
    d. Proventil

72. A bottle of Excedrin PM is simply labeled "Aspirin." This would be illegal under the:
    a. Consolidated Omnibus Budget Reconciliation Act
    b. Occupational Safety and Health Act
    c. Food, Drug, and Cosmetic Act
    d. Durham and Humphrey Amendments

73. The patient package insert is:
    a. required to be given directly to the patient or caregiver with every supply of a drug preparation containing estrogen
    b. required to be delivered to the patient at the time of the first dose of a drug containing estrogen
    c. written in scientific terms to best present studies done and facilitate patient comprehension
    d. both a and b are correct

74. Mr. Dan Hill has the following drugs in his patient profile:
    - Diuril
    - Tagamet
    - Xanax
    - Tegretol
    - Lanoxin

He decides to stop taking his medications and "be free." His wife calls 911 two days later, as he is having a grand mal seizure. The deficient drug responsible was most likely:

a. Xanax
b. Tegretol
c. Diuril
d. Lanoxin

75. Which of the following may be used as an antiepileptic agent and an antiarrhythmic agent?
    a. lamotrigine
    b. Paxil
    c. phenytoin
    d. Cardioquin

76. A patient is taking aspirin. He is prescribed the following drugs. Which drug(s) would require that he change his pain reliever to acetaminophen?
    a. Coumadin
    b. Nicardipine
    c. Ticlid
    d. both a and c

77. A diabetic patient is prescribed the following drugs:
    - Theo-Dur
    - Naprosyn
    - Beclomethasone
    - Bumex

    Which of these should be called to the attention of the pharmacist?
    a. Theo-Dur
    b. Bumex
    c. Naprosyn
    d. Beclomethasone

78. Which of the following may cause smooth muscle contraction and possibly premature labor?
    a. Carafate
    b. Misoprostol
    c. Nexium
    d. Citrucel

79. Which of the following would interfere with the effects of an estrogen-based contraceptive?
    a. liotrix
    b. Zithromax
    c. Ogden
    d. Estrovis

80. A patient arrives at the pharmacy window with a prescription for Lomotil. The prescriber is Dr. Tom Nuzecki DDS. You should:
    a. fill the prescription with a smile
    b. call the prescriber
    c. refuse to fill the prescription, as it is not valid
    d. consult the *United States Pharmacopoeia*

81. A patient is to receive atropine for a diagnostic procedure. You look in his patient profile and see the following drugs being administered:
    - Tegretol
    - nifedipine
    - Tofranil
    - Tagamet

    Which drug should you call to the attention of the pharmacist?
    a. Tegretol
    b. nifedipine
    c. Tofranil
    d. the Tagamet/nifedipine combination

82. A patient has a prescription for hydromorphone, written for 10 tablets. The pharmacy has only five in stock. You have the tablets on order for next week. You should:
    a. fill the prescription for five and mark the other five on the form as a refill
    b. fill the prescription for five tablets and tell the patient to come in next week for the rest
    c. refuse to fill the prescription
    d. tell the patient that he can only have five unless he goes to another pharmacy

83. A patient has asthma. Which of the following drugs might be contraindicated?
    a. acetaminophen
    b. Vicodin
    c. Roxicet
    d. Tylenol

84. A patient is prescribed Aldomet. Which of the following drugs in his patient profile should be called to the attention of the pharmacist?
    a. Vicodin
    b. Lasix
    c. Imipramine
    d. Nifedipine

85. A NitroDur patch:
    a. would aid in the treatment of high blood pressure
    b. would show decreased effects with time (tolerance)
    c. contains isosorbide mononitrate
    d. has a duration of action of five days

86. Prandin does not cause hypoglycemia, as it:
    a. does not affect blood sugar
    b. does not work unless sufficient glucose is present in the blood
    c. affects mainly lipids
    d. affects the breakdown and absorption of sugars, not sugar utilization

87. A mildly diabetic patient experiences hypoglycemia. Which of the following drugs is responsible?
    a. glyburide
    b. miglitol
    c. Micronase
    d. both a and c

88. Which of the following is a barbiturate?
    a. alprazolam
    b. phenobarbital
    c. buspirone
    d. carbamazepine

89. A patient who is taking cyanocobalamin is taking:
    a. vitamin A
    b. vitamin B_6
    c. vitamin C
    d. vitamin B_{12}

90. Which of the following is regulated by the FDA?
    a. the purity and efficacy of drug products
    b. the safety of drug products
    c. the standards of manufacture of drug products
    d. all of the above

Examination Answer Sheet

Instructions: Circle the letter corresponding to the correct answer.

1.	a	b	c	d	31.	a	b	c	d	61.	a	b	c	d
2.	a	b	c	d	32.	a	b	c	d	62.	a	b	c	d
3.	a	b	c	d	33.	a	b	c	d	63.	a	b	c	d
4.	a	b	c	d	34.	a	b	c	d	64.	a	b	c	d
5.	a	b	c	d	35.	a	b	c	d	65.	a	b	c	d
6.	a	b	c	d	36.	a	b	c	d	66.	a	b	c	d
7.	a	b	c	d	37.	a	b	c	d	67.	a	b	c	d
8.	a	b	c	d	38.	a	b	c	d	68.	a	b	c	d
9.	a	b	c	d	39.	a	b	c	d	69.	a	b	c	d
10.	a	b	c	d	40.	a	b	c	d	70.	a	b	c	d
11.	a	b	c	d	41.	a	b	c	d	71.	a	b	c	d
12.	a	b	c	d	42.	a	b	c	d	72.	a	b	c	d
13.	a	b	c	d	43.	a	b	c	d	73.	a	b	c	d
14.	a	b	c	d	44.	a	b	c	d	74.	a	b	c	d
15.	a	b	c	d	45.	a	b	c	d	75.	a	b	c	d
16.	a	b	c	d	46.	a	b	c	d	76.	a	b	c	d
17.	a	b	c	d	47.	a	b	c	d	77.	a	b	c	d
18.	a	b	c	d	48.	a	b	c	d	78.	a	b	c	d
19.	a	b	c	d	49.	a	b	c	d	79.	a	b	c	d
20.	a	b	c	d	50.	a	b	c	d	80.	a	b	c	d
21.	a	b	c	d	51.	a	b	c	d	81.	a	b	c	d
22.	a	b	c	d	52.	a	b	c	d	82.	a	b	c	d
23.	a	b	c	d	53.	a	b	c	d	83.	a	b	c	d
24.	a	b	c	d	54.	a	b	c	d	84.	a	b	c	d
25.	a	b	c	d	55.	a	b	c	d	85.	a	b	c	d
26.	a	b	c	d	56.	a	b	c	d	86.	a	b	c	d
27.	a	b	c	d	57.	a	b	c	d	87.	a	b	c	d
28.	a	b	c	d	58.	a	b	c	d	88.	a	b	c	d
29.	a	b	c	d	59.	a	b	c	d	89.	a	b	c	d
30.	a	b	c	d	60.	a	b	c	d	90.	a	b	c	d

Answers for Scoring

1. a	19. c	37. c	55. b	73. d
2. b	20. c	38. c	56. a	74. b
3. d	21. d	39. c	57. a	75. c
4. d	22. b	40. c	58. c	76. d
5. d	23. b	41. c	59. c	77. d
6. c	24. c	42. a	60. b	78. b
7. c	25. d	43. c	61. b	79. b
8. c	26. c	44. b	62. b	80. c
9. c	27. b	45. b	63. c	81. c
10. b	28. c	46. c	64. c	82. d
11. c	29. d	47. d	65. c	83. c
12. a	30. c	48. c	66. c	84. c
13. c	31. b	49. a	67. b	85. b
14. a	32. b	50. b	68. c	86. b
15. c	33. c	51. c	69. c	87. d
16. b	34. b	52. b	70. c	88. b
17. a	35. c	53. c	71. d	89. d
18. b	36. b	54. c	72. c	90. d

Grading: A passing score for this exam is 76.8% or above.

Solutions to the Chapter Review Questions

Chapter 1

1. The paper prescription contains only the information needed to fill the prescription, dosage directions, and information given by the patient. Therefore, the diagnosis and dosage schedule would not be included; however, they would be found on a hospital order. The correct answer is **d**.

2. When the prescription is received, it must contain certain information relating to the patient and prescriber. Information such as the patient's address, age, and allergies may be taken at the time of acceptance. Therefore, the correct answer is **d**.

3. The technician may fill prescriptions that have been properly documented (i.e., a hard-copy prescription). Since refill requests are made on a previously filled (documented) prescription, and prescriptions are normally filled off of hard-copy prescriptions, the technician may do both of these. However, prescriptions submitted by electronic means must be transferred to a hard-copy form by the pharmacist (or intern) before filling, and refill authorizations may only be taken by the pharmacist in most states. The correct answer is **d**.

4. The drug information on a hospital order is essentially the same as the paper prescription; however, a physician practicing in a hospital will have a DEA number on file or may use the DEA number assigned to the hospital. Therefore, the DEA number is not required. The correct answer is **c**.

5. The DEA number always starts with two letters: one represents the status of the prescriber, and the second is the first letter of the last name. Therefore, since the DEA number starts with AU, and the prescriber's name is Smith, the number is invalid. You should alert the pharmacist. The correct answer is **c**.

6. Prescriptions may be received by fax, modem (e-mail), and telephone. The patient may also bring in the prescription, so the correct answer is **d**.

7. All prescriptions dispensed from the pharmacy must be documented. This means that all must have some sort of paper prescription. Thus, prescriptions received over the telephone, by fax, or by e-mail must be transcribed to a hard copy by the pharmacist (or intern) before filling. The correct answer is **c**.

8. Prescriptions for controlled substances (C-II) must be filled within three days of writing depending on the state. Therefore, the prescription is no longer valid. The problem should be referred to the pharmacist. The correct answer is **b**.

9. A prescription that is written for a generic drug may always be filled with a proprietary (brand) name. Thus, you may fill the prescription with the brand name; however, the pharmacist may wish to explain the situation to the patient. The correct answer is **b**.

10. No information is to be added or changed on a prescription for a schedule II drug (e.g., Roxicet). Therefore, the correct answer is **d**.

Chapter 2

1. Emulsions, such as lotions, are delicate mixtures of oil and water. Rapid changes in temperature or prolonged exposure to very hot or cold temperatures will cause them to separate. The correct answer is **d**.

2. Even if you don't remember the notations, your first clue should be the brand name, Tim*optic;* gtt drop, o eye, u both, bid means two times a day. Since the medication is to be placed into the eye, the correct answer is **d**.

3. Solid dosage forms are, in general, those which can be picked up and handled. The only one that cannot be safely handled is a cream. The correct answer is **c**.

4. Most doses to the patient are dispensed using a unit dose cart. Occasionally, individual doses may be ordered, under special circumstances, but normal dosing is done with the use of a unit dose cart. The correct answer is **a**.

5. Procardia and Procardia XL (the extended release form) are not the same. Even though the names look similar, the technician could not dispense this drug for Procardia. The correct answer is **c**.

6. Enteric-coated drugs are designed to dissolve in the intestines. The coating is a protection for the drug against stomach acid in order for it to make it to the intestines safely. The correct answer is **b**.

7. Syrups contain high concentrations of sugar, extracts contain high concentrations of oils or plant portions, and elixirs contain a high concentration of alcohol. The correct answer is **c**.

8. SQ injections are placed just under the skin so a very fine needle is required. The correct answer is **a**.

9. The half-life defines how long a drug is active in the body, so it can be used to determine how often it should be given. The correct answer is **a**.

10. DAW means that no generics may be dispensed. Therefore, the brand name of the drug must be dispensed. The correct answer is **b**.

Chapter 3

1. Concurrent medications are those which the patient is taking at the same time as the prescription drug. These include any medications, whether they are over-the-counter drugs such as aspirin; prescription drugs; or potent herbal medications, such as "herbal Fen-Fen" or goldenseal, both of which mimic the sympathetic nervous system and act as sympathomimetic drugs. The correct answer is **d**.

2. A patient profile must be created for *anyone* receiving prescription drugs from a pharmacy. The correct answer is **d**.

3. A change in demographic information (address, phone number) must be recorded in the profile but is not of sufficient importance to report to the pharmacist. The technician may simply update the profile. The correct answer is **a**.

4. An important change in the reported information on a patient, such as the development of a rash, could be a symptom of a serious drug allergy. The pharmacist should be alerted and the profile should be updated to reflect this information. The correct answer is **d**.

5. The question asks what would be found in the retail setting; those are—**a, c, and d.** But the question asks which of these would **not** be found on a hospital profile. The correct answer is **c**.

6. A therapeutic duplication means two of the same drug, or drugs that do exactly the same thing. Trimethoprim and sulfisoxazole are both antibiotics but may be used together. Antihistamines and aspirin are not related. Tylenol #3 contains acetaminophen, so it would be a duplication to take acetaminophen as well. The correct answer is **b**.

7. Identification information includes name, address, and date of birth. The correct answer is **c**.

8. In order for a prescription to be filled, the co-pay or self-pay information is necessary. The correct answer is **a**.

9. Hospital profiles include labs, diet information, blood work results, diagnosis, and treatment information. The correct answer is **d**.

10. Concurrent medications means that multiple medications are being taken by the patient. The correct answer is **b**.

Chapter 4

1. The instructions are to instill one drop in each eye daily. The correct answer is **d**.

2. Withdrawing and measuring a drug solution while it is cold may cause error, because when the drug is warmed to room temperature, it will expand. Thus, the patient may be given a larger dose than prescribed, because the solution contracted at cold temperature and gave a deceptively low volume, which was actually greater when measured at the proper temperature. *It should be noted,* however, that some suspensions must be kept cold at all times, so some error is expected and factored into the dosage prescribed. The correct answer is **b**.

3. If the tablet is scored so that an accurate measurement of a partial tablet can be made, the prescription may be filled. Since one half of a tablet is needed, the tablets would have to be scored in half. The correct answer is **c**.

4. If the drug only comes in one strength, the strength does not need to be specified on either the prescription or the label. The same applies for combination drugs, which are drugs sold in combination with other drugs (e.g., Tylenol # 3, trimethoprim, with sulfisoxazole, etc.). The correct answer is **d**.

5. Since aseptic means the cleanest possible, all of these practices would be used. The best answer is **d**.

6. While dispensing of any drug should be the cleanest possible, aseptic technique is used only for injectable drugs. Sterility is extremely important for drugs injected into the body, because organisms multiply in the bloodstream, causing sepsis (they are destroyed by the digestive system, if the drugs are taken orally), and these organisms come from the surroundings. The correct answer is **d**.

7. A fine needle could not penetrate muscle tissue. A larger bore needle is required. The correct answer is **a**.

8. A sterile gown, safety glasses and face mask are three required protective items. The correct answer is **b**.

9. Coring is when a small piece of the vial stopper enters the vial along with the needle. Entering at a 45° angle, smoothly and slowly, can prevent coring. The correct answer is **c**.

10. The NDC number identifies the manufacturer, name of the drug, and the package size. The correct answer is **a**.

Chapter 5

1. Each drug has a particular storage requirement (i.e., the conditions under which it will retain the most potency). As a rule, medications will stay potent longer if shielded from light, heat, and humidity. To determine the best conditions for a particular drug and dosage form that it is in, it is best to consult the manufacturer's label. The correct answer is **d**.

2. The stability of a drug refers to how fast it will break down. Once it begins to break down, it loses potency and will not work as well at prescribed doses. The correct answer is **c**.

3. A reconstituted drug in suspension is mixed with water. Hydrating the drug causes the drug to be less stable and lose potency at a faster rate. The storage form that will slow this process is refrigeration. The correct answer is **c**.

4. If the strength of a drug solution or suspension is not given on the label, it can be easily calculated. Simply divide the volume by the total amount of drug. The correct answer is **c**.

5. Contamination of drugs may arise from dust and microorganisms in the air, as well as dirt and other sources. The amount of contamination from room air is not a problem for drugs that are not meant for parenteral use. However, improper cleaning of measuring devices can lead to contamination of a dispensed drug, not with microorganisms but with another drug. The correct answer is **b**.

6. Slow-moving drugs are still prescribed and thus should be kept in inventory. However, to maintain an efficient system of inventory, they should be ordered in smaller quantities and less frequently. The correct answer is **a**.

7. A daily dose is drug sufficient for 24 hours. Since the order is for two capsules taken twice a day, the daily dose is 2 × 2 or four capsules. The correct answer is c.

8. If a drug cannot accurately be measured out and administered as a unit dose, it is packaged as a bulk medication. Since tablets and suppositories can be packaged individually, the correct answer is **c**.

9. 25°C is room temperature, and 5°C is refrigeration. Therefore, 15°C would be a cool room. The correct answer is **d**.

10. All drugs stocked in the hospital are the responsibility of the pharmacy no matter where they are located. The correct answer is **b**.

Chapter 6

1. When a portion of the cost of the medication is paid by the patient, it is called co-pay. When the patient is reimbursed, it is called out-of-pocket, as the patient must pay first before being reimbursed. The correct answer is **b**.

2. The insurance affidavit is a form filled out by the pharmacist. This is then sent to the insurance company by the patient for reimbursement. The patient pays for the prescription when it is dispensed. The correct answer is **c**.

3. A third-party payor is an organization that is in the business of insurance. This would include union plans, employee insurance, health benefits, Medicare, and Medicaid. The correct answer is **c**.

4. To compute the selling price of a medication, we must first take the pharmacy's cost and mark up the price by a percentage of that cost. The correct answer is **c**.

5. A closed formulary is a defined list of drugs. The correct answer is **d**.

Chapter 7

1–4. These all involve multiplication of decimals by a power of 10. All we need to do is move the decimal point. Problems 1 and 2 involve multiplication of a number by a decimal number that is less than one. So, we move the decimal point to the left.

1. (0.01×50.0), 0.01 has two decimal places, so we move the decimal over two places; the correct answer is **0.5**.

2. $0.1 \times 25.0 = 2.50$, as 0.1 only has one decimal place. The correct answer is **2.5**.
   In questions 3 and 4, we are multiplying a decimal by a power of 10. Since a decimal is a fraction of 10 (1/10, 1/100, etc.) and now we are multiplying by tens, we do the opposite of what we did before: we move the decimal to the right.

3. $10 \times 0.25 = 2.50$, as 10 has one zero. The correct answer is **2.5**.

4. 100 has two zeros, so the decimal is moved over two spaces: $100 \times 0.002 = $ **0.2**.

5. Two goes into 4 twice. The common denominator is thus 4. So ½ becomes $1/2 \times 2/2$ or 2/4. Rewrite, and add the top numbers: $1/2 + 2/4 = $ **3/4**.

6. When we divide, the second fraction is flipped over and multiplied. Rewrite: $3/4 \times 2/1 = 6/4 = $ **1 1/2**.

7. x = 10. Translated, these numbers become 21 + 14 (iv is 5 − 1 = 4). Answer: **35 (xxxv)**.

8. L = 50, X = 10, IX = 9; LXXX = 80 + XIX = 19 ➔ 80 + 19 = **99 (XCIX)**.
   9–12. We are rounding to two places, and the numbers in problems 9–12 have four places beyond the decimal. So, we take the last two places and see if they are more than, less than, or equal to 50:

9. 35 < 50, so it rounds to **1.00**.

10. 55 > 50, so this rounds to **0.03**.

11. 50 = 50, so we look at the previous number, which is 5, an odd number. We round up to **0.16**.

12. 50 = 50, and the previous number (4) is even. We round down to **0.14**.

13. $(5 \times 1)/(6 \times 2) = $ **5/12**

14. $(5 − 2)/8 = $ **3/8**

15. $7/8 = 21/24$; $2/3 = 16/24$; $(21 + 16)/24 = 37/24$ or **1 13/24**

16. Invert the second fraction: $2/3 \times 4/1 = (2 \times 4)/(3 \times 1) = 8/3$ or **2 2/3**

17. C = 100, D = 500, L = 50, X = 10; (CD = 400) + 50 + 10 = **460**.

18. M = 1,000, C = 100, V = 5, I = 1; 1,000 + 1,000 + 100 + 5 + 1 + 1 = **2,107**.

19. 2010: 1,000 = M, 10 = X; **MMX**.

20. 678: 600 = DC (500 + 100), 78 = LXXVIII (50 + 10 + 10 + 5 + 1 + 1 + 1) ➔ **DCLXXVIII**.

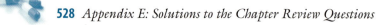

Chapter 8

1. gr i = 60 mg, so gr 1/4 × 60 mg/gr = **15 mg**
2. 5 g × 1,000 mg/g = **5,000 mg**
3. 100 mcg × 1 mg/1,000 mcg = **0.1 mg**
4. $1 g \times \dfrac{1,000 \ mg}{g} \times \dfrac{1,000 \ mcg}{mg} = $ **1,000,000 mcg**
5. gr iss = $1\frac{1}{2}$ grains, so gr iss × 60 mg/gr = **90 mg**
6. gr i = 1 grain, so $gr \ i \times \left(\dfrac{60 \ mg}{gr}\right) \times \dfrac{1 \ g}{1,000 \ mg} = $ **0.06 g**
7. 1 t × 5 mL/t = **5 mL**
8. 5 t × 5 mL/t = **25 mL**
9. $10 \ g \times \dfrac{1 \ kg}{1,000 \ g} = $ **0.01 kg**
10. $0.5 \ L \times \dfrac{1,000 \ mL}{L} = $ **500 mL**
11. gr V = 5 grains, so $gr \ V \times \dfrac{60 \ mg}{gr} = (5 \times 60 \ mg) = $ **300 mg** or

    $$Or \ gr \ V \times \dfrac{65 \ mg}{gr} = (5 \times 65 \ mg) = 325 \ mg$$

12. A dram is 4 mL, but often for calculation purposes it is considered 5 mL, so: 3 dram × 4 mL/dram = **12 mL (or 5 mL/dram × 3 drams = 15 mL)**.
13. This is a two-step problem: 0.5 L × 1,000 mL/L = 500 mL.

    500 mL × 1,000 mcL/mL = **500,000 mcL**

14. 1 t = 5 mL and 1 T = 15 mL. So, 1 T/1 t = 15 mL/5 mL = **3**.
15. 12 fl oz × 30 mL/fl oz = **360 mL**
16. 360 mL are in 12 ounces, from question 15.

    1 dram = 4 mL. 360 mL/4 mL = **90 drams; or**

    1 dram = 5 mL, 360 mL/5 mL = **72 drams**

17. 100 mcg/1,000 = 0.1 mg/1,000 = **0.0001 grams**
18. You are going from smaller to larger numbers, as °F > °C: use °F = °C × (9/5) + 32. Fill in the numbers: °F = 5°C × (9/5) + 32 = 32 + 9 = **41°F**.
19. Use °C = (°F − 32) × (5/9). Fill in the numbers: °C = (86°F − 32) × 5/9 = 6 × 5 = **30°C**. *Hint:* Using this formula is easy, so you can do it in your head. For example, subtracting 32 from 86, we get 54. We have to multiply this by 5/9. That's the same as *dividing* 54 by 9 (9 × 6 = 54) and *multiplying* by **5**! We just multiply **6 × 5** to get **30**.
20. Use °F = °C × (9/5) + 32. Fill in the numbers:

    $$-5°C \times \left(\dfrac{9}{5}\right) + 32 \ \text{and cancel the 5's, which leaves the following:} \ -9 + 32 = 23°C$$

    Hint: Ignore the negative sign until you add the 32, then subtract the 9.

Chapter 9

1. 1:1,000 is 1 gram/1,000 mL. Since 1 g = 1,000 mg, 1:1,000 is also 1,000 mg/1,000 mL = **1 mg/mL**. (It would be wise to memorize this one, as it comes up often.)

2. This is really only a simple conversion problem. 1% is 1 g/100 mL of solution:

$$\frac{0.2\ mL}{eye} \times \frac{1\ g}{100\ mL} = 0.002\ g$$

   It would be easier to express this in mg: 0.002 g × 1,000 mg/g = **2 mg/dose** in each eye.

3. The question here is how many 5 mg doses are in the bottle. First, calculate the amount of drug contained in the bottle.

$$2\% = \frac{2\ g}{100\ mL} = \frac{2,000\ mg}{100\ mL};\ \frac{5\ mL \times 2,000\ mg}{100\ mL} = 100\ mg$$

   Now calculate how many 5 mg doses are in the bottle:

$$\frac{100\ mg/bottle}{5\ mg/dose} = \textbf{20 doses}$$

4. This is a weight per weight (w/w) percent problem. 5% is now 5 g/100 g. The problem is solved in the same way as before:

$$5\ g \times \frac{5\ g}{100\ g} = \frac{25\ g}{100\ g}\ \text{or}\ \textbf{0.25 g (250 mg)}$$

5. We can use alligation for this problem. First we make the chart:

More concentrated stock

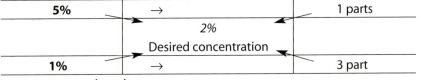

Less concentrated stock

   The solutions in stock are **1%** and **5%**, so these are put on the left. You want a *2%* solution, so 2% goes in the middle.
   Subtract 5 − 2 = 3 on the bottom right and 2 − 1 = 1 on the top right. These numbers refer to the relative amounts of the two solutions used.
   According to the chart, you need one part of the 5% solution to three parts of the 1% solution. Since you need 80 mL total, you determine how much a part is by dividing 80 mL by 4 (1 part + 3 parts, from the chart). One part = 80/4 or 20 mL.
   Answer: Mix **20 mL of the 5%** solution (1 part × 20 mL) + **60 mL** (3 parts × 20 mL) of the **1%** solution.

6. Percentage is in g/100 mL, so you need to get the ratio given into g/100 mL.

$$200\ mg \times \frac{1\ g}{1,000\ mg} = 0.2\ g\ \text{cortisone}$$

If there are 200 mg cortisone (0.2 g) per 1 mL of cream, there must be:

$$\frac{0.2 \ g}{1 \ mL} \times 100 \ mL = 20 \text{ g per 100 mL of cream}$$

$$20 \text{ g}/100 \text{ mL} = \textbf{20\%}$$

7. 20 g of lactic acid/1,000 mL (or 1 L) is given in the problem. Simply cancel zeros:

$$\frac{20 \ g}{1,000 \ mL} = \frac{2 \ g}{100 \ mL}$$

The answer is **2%**.

8. 5 g/500 mL 1 g/100 mL. Answer: **1%**

9. A 2% solution is 2 g/100 mL. You need 1,500 mL, so you must multiply:

$$\frac{2 \ g}{100 \ mL} \times 1,500 \ mL = \textbf{30 g}$$

10. $5\% = \dfrac{5 \ g}{100 \ mL}$

Do the problem:

$$15 \ mL \times \frac{5 \ g}{100 \ mL} = \textbf{0.750 g} \text{ or } \textbf{750 mg}$$

11. You have 2 g/25 mL. To have percent, you need g/100 mL. So, you multiply by $\dfrac{4}{4}$.

$$\frac{2 \ g}{25 \ mL} \times \frac{4}{4} = \frac{8 \ g}{100 \ mL} = \textbf{8\%} \text{ or } \frac{2 \ g}{25 \ mL} = \frac{x}{100 \ mL} = 8 \ g \text{ or } \textbf{8\%}$$

12. The easiest way to do this one is by ratio/proportion (Chapter 9). However, you can also do the problem using simple division and multiplication.
    Saline is 0.9 g of sodium chloride per 100 mL (0.9%). Dividing the 5 g by 0.9 g/100 mL gives the volume that you can make: (5 g/0.9 g) × 100 mL= **555.6 mL** (see Division by Fractions in Chapter 7).

13. 7% is 7 g/100 mL. Convert the 7 g to mg:

$$7 \ g \times \frac{1,000 \ mg}{g} = 7,000 \ mg$$

Rewrite and cancel:

$$\frac{7,000 \ mg}{100 \ mL} = \textbf{70 mg/mL}$$

14. 2% = 2 g/100 mL
    Expressed as a ratio, this would be **2:100** or reduce to 1:50.

15. This problem would require alligation. Fill in the chart:

10%	→	3 parts
	5%	
2%	→	5 parts

According to the chart, you would need 3 parts of the 10% solution and 5 parts of the 2% solution. That makes 8 parts. These eight parts must equal 100 mL as stated by the problem. 100 mL/8 parts 12.5 mL/part. You would then need 3 parts × 12.5 mL = 37.5 mL of the 10%, and 5 parts 12.5 mL = 62.5 mL of the 2% solution. You have 60 mL of the 10% and need only 37.5 mL, but you need 62.5 mL of the 2% and have only 50 mL.

Answer: **No**, you cannot make the solution.

16. 5 g cream × 1 g of cortisone/100 g cream 0.05 g cortisone

$$0.05 \text{ g cortisone} \times 1{,}000 \text{ mg/g} = \textbf{50 mg}$$

(You could also do this problem by the ratio/proportion method (see Chapter 9)):

17. A percentage is an amount per *100*. Therefore, you must multiply:

$$\frac{50 \; mg}{mL} \times \frac{100}{100} = \frac{5{,}000 \; mg}{100 \; mL} = \frac{5 \; g}{100 \; mL}$$

The solution is a **5%** solution.

18. 1:100 = 1 g/100 mL = 1,000 mg/100 mL = 10 mg/mL
    5 mL × 10 mg/mL = **50 mg** of drug

19. The order is for 0.5 g, so to compute the volume needed, we multiply:

$$0.5 \; g \times \frac{100 \; mL}{50 \; g} = 1 \; mL$$

A 3 mL syringe could be used.

20. 0.25% of a 10 g suppository is 10 g × 0.25g/100 g = 0.025 g per suppository = **25 mg per dose**

Chapter 10

1. You want to measure the liquid in a device that is of the closest possible size. The best answer would be a 20 mL graduated cylinder, as it is closest to 15 mL. The correct answer is **c**.

2. A solution taken from the refrigerator will be condensed, due to the cold. When the solution is measured cold and then allowed to warm to room temperature, it will expand. The patient may receive too much drug and may be overdosed. The correct answer is **a**.

3. A household eyedropper is not calibrated; the drop size varies from dropper to dropper. To receive an accurate dose of medication, the patient would need to receive a dropper that is calibrated for the medication. A syringe is calibrated but would be awkward to use. The correct answer is **c**.

4. A glass cylinder refracts light and makes the top of the solution appear curved (the meniscus). Thus, you would want to look at the markings on the cylinder where the bottom of the meniscus falls. The correct answer is **c**.

5. The weight of water at 25°C is important for calibration of measuring equipment. Water weighs 1 g/mL at 25°C. The correct answer is **d**.

6. All of the statements are true. The correct answer is **d**.

7. If the calculations were performed correctly and the scale was used correctly, it is possible that there was a temperature difference between the cortisone and the scale. The drug scale may have been in a cold room. The correct answer is **b**.

8. The household teaspoon varies between 4 mL and 8 mL. The correct answer is **b**.
9. To measure insulin accurately, an insulin syringe should be used. The correct answer is **a**.
10. Class A scales are required by all state boards of pharmacy. The correct answer is **d**.

Chapter 11

1. First, convert the order to match the stock:

$$1.5 \text{ mg} \times 1{,}000 \text{ mcg/mg} = 1{,}500 \text{ mcg}$$

   Do the problem:

$$\text{order} \div \text{stock} = 1{,}500 \text{ mcg} \div 750 \text{ mcg/tablet} = \textbf{2 tablets dispensed}$$

2. First, convert:

$$0.005 \; g \times \frac{1{,}000 \; mg}{g} = 5 \; mg/dose$$

   Do the problem:

$$\frac{5 \; mg/dose}{5 \; mg/tablet} = \textbf{1 tablet per dose dispensed}$$

3. First, convert:

$$125 \; mcg \times \frac{1 \; mg}{1{,}000 \; mcg} = 0.125 \; mg/dose$$

   Do the problem:

$$\frac{0.125 \; mg}{0.25 \; mg/tablet} = \textbf{1/2 tablet per dose dispensed}$$

4. First, convert:

$$\text{gr ss} = \text{½ grain}$$

$$1/2 \; gr \times \frac{60 \; mg}{gr} = 30 \; mg$$

   Do the problem:

$$\frac{30 \; mg}{30 \; mg/tablet} = \textbf{1 tablet dispensed per dose}$$

5. No conversion necessary:

$$\frac{80 \; mg}{40 \; mg/tablet} = \textbf{2 tablets per dose}$$

   A daily dose is the dose × number of doses per day = 2 tablets/dose × 2 doses/day = **4 tablets**

6. No conversion necessary. 60 mg ÷ 30 mg/capsule = **2 capsules per unit dose**

   A daily dose would be 2 capsules/dose × three doses/day = **6 capsules**

7. First, convert:

$$250 \ mg \times \frac{1 \ g}{1,000 \ mg} = 0.25 \ g$$

   Do the problem

$$\frac{0.25 \ g}{0.5 \ g/dose} = \textbf{1/2 tablet per dose}$$

8. Conversion here is done using information from the label: 400,000 U = 250 mg

$$\frac{600,000 \ units/dose}{400,000 \ units/tablet} = \textbf{1.5 tablets per dose}$$

9. First, convert:

$$0.1 \ mg \times \frac{1,000 \ mcg}{50 \ mcg/tablet} = 100 \ mcg/dose$$

   Do the problem:

$$\frac{100 \ mcg}{50 \ mcg/tablet} = \textbf{2 tablets}$$

10. First, convert:

$$gr \ v = 5 \ grains, \ so \ gr \ v \times 60 \ mg/gr = 300 \ mg$$

    Do the problem:

$$\frac{300 \ mg}{300 \ mg/tablet} = \textbf{1 tablet per dose}$$

11. First, convert:

$$gr \ i \ ss = 1.5 \ grains, \ so \ 1.5 \ grains \times 60 \ mg/grain = 90 \ mg$$

    Do the problem:

$$\frac{90 \ mg}{30 \ mg/tablet} = \textbf{3 tablets per dose}$$

12. No conversion necessary:

$$\frac{20 \ mEq}{10 \ mEq/tablet} = \textbf{2 tablets per dose}$$

13. 1 gr = 60 mg; so 60 mg/30 mg per tablet = **2 tablets per dose**

14. gr iss = 1 $\frac{1}{2}$ grains. Convert grains to mg:

$$1 \ \tfrac{1}{2} \ grains \times 60 \ mg/grain = \textbf{90 mg/dose}$$

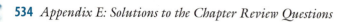

The question asks how many doses are in a vial containing 500 mg.

$$\frac{500 \ mg}{90 \ mg/dose} = \textbf{5.5 or 5 doses per vial}$$

15. You need 40 mg per dose and have 20 mg tablets. You would dispense **2 tablets per dose**.

Chapter 12

Many of the problems are calculated in the same way, so only some of them will be calculated out. These problems may be done in two ways: dividing the order by the stock available, or using ratio-proportion. Both will be demonstrated.

1. The calculation is asking you to determine the amount dispensed for *one* dose. We can calculate this by using either of two ways:

   "*Order over stock*" *method*: Both order and stock are expressed in the same units (mg), so no conversion is necessary.

   $$\frac{12.5 \ mg}{6.25 \ mg/5 \ mL} = \frac{12.5 \ mg \times 5 \ mL}{6.25 \ mg} = 10 \ mL$$

   Ratio/proportion method:

   Step 1. Set up the problem:

   $$\frac{6.25 \ mg}{5 \ mL} = \frac{12.5 \ mg}{x}$$

   Step 2. Cross-multiply:

   $$12.5 \ mg \times 5 \ mL = 6.25 \ x$$
   $$62.5 = 6.25x$$

   Step 3. Divide both sides of the equation by 6.25 mg to get x:

   $$\textbf{10 mL} = \textbf{x}$$

2. First, *convert* the order into milligrams, to match the stock.

   $$0.75 \ g \times 1,000 \ mg/g = 750 \ mg \ ordered$$

   Next, *simplify* the stock. This will make the calculation easier:

   $$\frac{200 \ mg}{5 \ mL} = 40 \ mg/mL$$

   Now *calculate*.

   $$\frac{750 \ mg}{40 \ mg/mL} = \textbf{18.75 mL dispensed}$$

Ratio/proportion method:

$$\frac{750\ mg}{x} = \frac{200\ mg}{5\ mL}$$

Cross-multiply:

$$750\ mg \times 5\ mL = 200\ mg \times x$$

$$3{,}750 = 200x$$

Divide both sides by 200 mg:

$$\textbf{18.75 mL} = x$$

3. **6 mL**

$$\frac{300\ mg\,(order)}{250\ mg/5\ mL\,(stock)} = 6\ mL$$

4. **1.5 mL**

$$\frac{150\ mg}{100\ mg/mL} = 1.5\ mL$$

5. **15 mL**

$$\frac{30\ mg}{10\ mg/5\ mL} = 15\ mL$$

6. **7.5 mL**

$$\frac{40\ mg}{80\ mg/15\ mL} = 7.5\ mL$$

7. First, convert. The order is in grams; the stock is in milligrams.

$$0.5\ g \times 1{,}000\ mg/g = 500\ mg\ \text{of ampicillin ordered}$$

Then, simplify the stock concentration:

$$250\ mg/5\ mL = 50\ mg/mL$$

Finally, calculate:

$$\frac{500\ mg}{50\ mg/mL} = \textbf{10 mL}$$

8. **2.5 mL**

$$\frac{10\ mg}{20\ mg/5\ mL} = 2.5\ mL$$

9. **7.5 mL**

$$\frac{120\ mg}{80\ mg/5\ mL} = 7.5\ mL$$

10. **4 mL**

$$\frac{40 \; mg}{10 \; mg/mL} = 4 \; mL$$

Chapter 13

1. The BSA is 0.6 m². Multiply the dose by the BSA to get the dose for the child:

$$40 \text{ mg/m}^2 \times 0.6 \text{ m}^2 = \textbf{24 mg}$$

2. First, convert pounds to kilograms:

$$66 \text{ lbs}/2.2 \text{ kg} = 30 \text{ kg body weight}$$

Then, divide dose by the body weight:

$$250 \text{ mg}/30 \text{ kg} = 8.34 \text{ mg/kg}$$

Multiply this by 4 (q6h is four times per day): 8.34 mg/kg × 4 = 33.3 mg/kg. This number falls below the safe dosage guideline on the label (50 mg/kg), so **the dose is safe**.

3. Note that only the child's weight and the adult dose are given. Use Clark's Rule:

$$\frac{22 \; lb}{150 \; lb} \times 100 \; mg = \textbf{14.6 mg}$$

4. $\dfrac{15 \; mg}{kg} \times 22 \; kg = \textbf{330 mg}$

5. Use Clark's Rule:

$$\frac{25 \; lb}{150 \; lb} \times 1{,}000 \; mg = \textbf{166.7 mg or 167 mg rounded}$$

6. 5,500 g = 5.5 kg; $5.5 \; kg \times \dfrac{0.5 \; mg}{kg} = \textbf{2.75 mg}$

7. Convert pound to kg: $\dfrac{88 \; lb}{2.2 \; lb/kg} = 40 \; kg$

$$\frac{20 \; mg}{kg} \times 40 \; kg = 800 \; mg \;\; \text{drug ordered}$$

$$\frac{800 \; mg}{300 \; mg/mL} = \textbf{2.67 mL}$$

8. 22 lb = 10 kg body weight. $\dfrac{0.25 \; mg}{kg} \times 10 \; kg = 2.5 \; mg/dose$

Calculate the stock concentration:

$$\frac{5 \; mg}{2 \; mL} = \frac{2.5 \; mg}{mL}; \quad \frac{2.5 \; mg}{2.5 \; mg/mL} = \textbf{1 mL dispensed}$$

9. Use BSA formula for pounds/inches:

$$\sqrt{\frac{36\ in \times 50\ lb}{3131}} = \sqrt{0.5749} = \textbf{0.76 m}^2$$

10. Young's Rule:

$$\frac{8\ yrs}{8\ yrs + 12} \times 250\ mg = \textbf{100 mg}$$

Clark's Rule:

$$\frac{50\ lb}{150\ lb} \times 250\ mg = \textbf{83.3 mg}$$

Chapter 14

1. There are several ways to do this. First, reduce the stock concentration to make the problem simpler:

$$\frac{50\ mg}{5\ mL} = 10\ mg/mL$$

Then, do the problem using the "order over stock" method.

$$\frac{20\ mg}{10\ mg/mL} = \textbf{2 mL}$$

Using the ratio/proportion method,

Cross-multiply: $\dfrac{20\ mg}{X} \bowtie \dfrac{50\ mg}{5\ mL}$ and divide:

$$20\ mg \times 50\ mg = 50x$$

$$100\ mg/50\ mg = \textbf{2 mL}$$

2. gr ss = $\frac{1}{2}$ grain; $\frac{1}{2}$ gr $\times$ 60 mg/gr = 30 *mg*.

$$\frac{30\ mg}{6\ mg/mL} = \textbf{5 mL}$$

3. Simplify the stock:

$$\frac{10,000\ units}{5\ mL} = \frac{2,000\ units}{mL}$$

Divide:

$$\frac{4,000\ units}{2,000\ units/mL} = \textbf{2 mL}$$

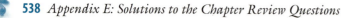

4. A 1 cc syringe holds 100 U of regular (U100) insulin:

$$1 \text{ mL} = 100 \text{ units, so, by ratio/proportion: } \frac{100 \text{ } units}{mL} = \frac{50 \text{ } units}{x} = \textbf{0.5 mL insulin}$$

5. $1 : 1{,}000 = \dfrac{1 \text{ } g(1{,}000 \text{ } mg)}{1{,}000 \text{ } mL} = 1 \text{ } mg/mL$, so a 1 mg dose = **1 mL**

6. Ratio proportion:

$$\frac{500 \text{ } mg}{20 \text{ } mL} = \frac{50 \text{ } mg}{x} = (50 \text{ } mg \times 20 \text{ } mL)/500 \text{ } mg = \textbf{2 mL}$$

7. Ratio proportion:

$$\frac{100 \text{ } mg}{mL} = \frac{150 \text{ } mg}{x} = \textbf{1.5 mL}$$

8. First convert 0.2 g × 1,000 mg = 200 mg
   Ratio proportion:

$$\frac{500 \text{ } mg}{5 \text{ } mL} = \frac{200 \text{ } mg}{x} = \textbf{2 mL dispensed}$$

9. Convert 0.2 mg × 1,000 mcg = 200 mcg

$$\frac{400 \text{ } mcg}{mL} = \frac{200 \text{ } mcg}{x} = \textbf{0.5 mL}$$

10. For an IM injection, you want a volume of around 2 mL to inject. Do the "order over stock" calculation for each concentration given on the label. The concentration that gives an injection volume that is closest to 2 mL is the concentration that you want. In this case, the injection volume closest to the volume calculated (2 mL) is from the 250,000 units/mL concentration, which we would get by adding 18.2 mL to the bottle. Now, you must calculate the exact volume to draw up for the dose:

$$\frac{350{,}000 \text{ } units}{250{,}000 \text{ } units} = 1.4 \text{ } mL$$

Add 18.2 mL of diluent to the vial and then draw up 1.4 mL to fill the order.

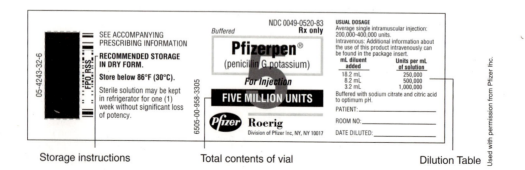

Storage instructions   Total contents of vial   Dilution Table

Chapter 15

1. (a) 1 L = 1,000 mL; $\dfrac{1,000\ mL}{10\ hr}$ = **100 mL/hr**

   (b) $\dfrac{100\ mL}{hr} \times \dfrac{1\ hr}{60\ min}$ = **1.67 mL/min**

2. The flow rate in mL/min is 1.67 (problem 1)

$$\dfrac{1.67\ mL}{min} \times \dfrac{15\ gtt}{mL} = \textbf{25 gtts/min}$$

3. $\dfrac{500\ mL}{4\ hr}$ = 125 mL/hr; $\dfrac{125\ mL}{hr} \times \dfrac{1\ hr}{60\ min}$ = 2.08 mL/min

4. 40 min × 1 hr/60 min = 0.67 hr, so the running time 16.67 hr 1 L 1,000 mL
   Dividing:

$$\dfrac{1,000\ mL}{16.67\ hr} = \textbf{60 mL/hr}$$

   and $\qquad\qquad\qquad\qquad \dfrac{60\ mL}{hr} \times \dfrac{1\ hr}{60\ min} = \textbf{1 mL/min}$

5. Ignore the drug, as it is not pertinent to the problem; the question merely asks for the flow rate of the saline. $\dfrac{250\ mL}{8\ hr}$ = 31.25 mL/hr

$$\dfrac{31.25\ mL}{hr} \times \dfrac{1\ hr}{60\ min} = \dfrac{0.52\ mL}{min} \times \dfrac{60\ gtts}{mL} = \textbf{31 gtts/min}$$

6. $\dfrac{150\ mL}{3\ hr} = \dfrac{50\ mL}{hr} \times \dfrac{1\ hr}{60\ min} = \dfrac{0.83\ mL}{min} \times \dfrac{60\ gtts}{mL} = \textbf{50 gtts/min}$

7. 1 L = 1,000 mL

$$\dfrac{1,000\ mL}{100\ mL/hr} = \textbf{10 hours}$$

8. $\dfrac{300\ mL}{5\ hr} = \dfrac{60\ mL}{hr} \times \dfrac{1\ hr}{60\ min} = 1\ mL/min$

   Since we want gtt/mL, arrange the numbers so that the minutes cancel:

$$\dfrac{15\ gtts/min}{1\ mL/min} = \textbf{15 gtts/mL}$$

9. Simply figure the flow rate in mL/hr, then divide by the flow rate in gtt/hr:

$$\dfrac{1,000\ mL}{10\ hr} = 100\ mL/hr$$

   To get gtt/mL, we want the hours to cancel:

$$\dfrac{1,000\ gtts/hr}{100\ mL/hr} = \textbf{10 gtts/mL}$$

10. This is done the same way as question 9. Flow rate = 600 mL/10 hr = 60 mL/hr

$$\frac{60 \; mL}{hr} \times \frac{1 \; hr}{60 \; min} = 1 \; mL/min$$

$$\frac{60 \; gtts/min}{1 \; mL/min} = \textbf{60 gtts/mL}$$

11. Flow rate (gtt/time)/drop factor = flow rate (mL/time):

$$\frac{60 \; gtts/min}{15 \; gtts/mL} = 4 \; mL/min$$

The hourly rate of infusion is the amount infused per hour, so:

$$\frac{4 \; mL}{min} \times \frac{60 \; min}{hr} = \textbf{240 mL/hr}$$

12. 1 L = 1,000 mL, and 6 hr = 360 min

$$\text{Flow rate} = \frac{1,000 \; mL}{360 \; min} = 2.78 \; mL/min$$

(a) $\dfrac{10 \; gtt}{mL} \times \dfrac{2.78 \; mL}{min} = \textbf{28 gtts/min}$

(b) $\dfrac{15 \; gtt}{mL} \times \dfrac{2.78 \; mL}{min} = \textbf{42 gtts/min}$

13. $\dfrac{100 \; mL}{hr} \times \dfrac{1 \; hr}{60 \; min} \times 40 \; min = \textbf{66.67 mL}$

14. First, calculate the flow rate in mL/min. Volume/time = 120 mL/30 min = 4 mL/min. Next, calculate flow rate in gtt/min:

$$\frac{4 \; mL}{min} \times \frac{15 \; gtt}{mL} = \textbf{60 gtts/min}$$

15. Similar to Problem 14:

$$\frac{300 \; mL}{90 \; min} \times \frac{10 \; gtt}{mL} = \textbf{33 gtts/min}$$

Chapter 16

1. The problem states how much to put in the bag: 250 mg. No further calculation is necessary. To do order/stock, first reduce the stock:

$$\frac{500 \; mg}{5 \; mL} = 100 \; mg/mL$$

Then, do order over stock:

$$\frac{250 \; mg}{100 \; mg/mL} = \textbf{2.5 mL added}$$

2. Concentration is always expressed in amount per volume (amount = 250 mg, volume = 500 mL).

$$\frac{250\ mg}{500\ mL} = \textbf{0.5 mg/mL}$$

3. First, figure how much drug is added:

$$10\ mL \times \frac{10\ g}{100\ mL} = \textbf{1 g drug added}$$

Next, figure the concentration:

1 g = 1,000 mg and 1 L = 1,000 mL, so $\dfrac{1{,}000\ mg}{1{,}000\ mL} = \textbf{1 mg/mL}$

4. For this, you must know that D_5 is 5% dextrose.

$$\frac{5\ g}{100\ mL} \times 300\ mL = \textbf{15 g}$$

5. 1:1,000 is

$$\frac{1\ g}{1{,}000\ mL} = \frac{1{,}000\ mg}{1{,}000\ mL} = \textbf{1 mg/mL}$$

You should memorize this! Amount × concentration: 10 mL × 1 mg/mL = **10 mg** of drug in a 1:1,000 solution.

6. Because the drug in the vial was diluted with a greater amount of saline than the instructions called for, the final concentration will be less than 250 mg/mL. Set up the problem:

$$\frac{correct(8\ mL)}{actual(13\ mL)} \times 250\ mg/mL = \textbf{153.8 mg/mL}$$

Or:

$$\frac{drug(2{,}000\ mg)}{volume(13\ mL)} = \textbf{153.8 mg/mL}$$

7. $\dfrac{2{,}500{,}000\ units}{2.5\ mL} = \textbf{100,000 units/mL}$

8. The problem states that there are 20 mEq in 5 mL of solution, so 20 mEq was added to the 1 L bag.

The final concentration is therefore

$$\frac{20\ mEq}{1{,}000\ mL} = \textbf{0.02 mEq/mL}$$

9. $\dfrac{1{,}000{,}000\ units}{20\ mL} = \textbf{50,000 units/mL}$

10. 5 mL × 250 mg/mL = 1,250 mg of drug added to 250 mL saline.
    The concentration is then 1,250 mg/250 mL = **5 mg/mL**

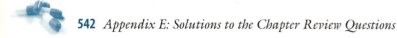

Chapter 17

1. The 250 mL infusion is to run for 5 hours, so the flow rate is:

$$\frac{250 \; mL}{5 \; hr} = \frac{50 \; mL}{hr(60 \; min)} = 0.833 \; mL/min$$

   a.   Flow rate × drop factor = gtt/time, so

$$\frac{0.833 \; mL}{min} \times \frac{60 \; gtt}{mL} = \textbf{50 gtts/min}$$

   b.   Dose per minute = $0.833 \; mL/min \times \left(\dfrac{500 \; mg}{250 \; mL}\right) = \textbf{1.67 mg/min}$

2. The long way to approach this problem:

$$C = \frac{5,000 \; units}{500 \; mL} = 10 \; units/mL$$

$$F = \frac{500 \; mL}{2 \; hr} = 250 \; mL/hr$$

$$D/t = \frac{10 \; units}{mL} \times \frac{250 \; mL}{hr} = 2,500 \; units/hr \; \text{ or } \textbf{1,250 units in 30 minutes}$$

Shortcut: 5,000 U infuse in 2 hours, so ½ of that, or 2,500 U infuse per hour. Therefore, 1,250 U would infuse in a half-hour (30 minutes).

3. $C = \dfrac{10 \; units}{mL}$ and D/t = 1,000 units/hr, so using C × F = D/t:

$$F = \frac{1,000 \; units/hr}{10 \; units/mL} = \textbf{100 mL/hr}$$

4. The amount of drug added to the bag is:

$$10 \; mL \times \frac{10 \; g}{100 \; mL} = 1 \; g \; \text{ added to 500 mL}$$

The concentration (C) is $\dfrac{1,000 \; mg}{500 \; mL} = 2 \; mg/mL$

The flow rate (F) is $\dfrac{30 \; gtt/min}{15 \; gtt/mL} = 2 \; mL/min$; $\dfrac{2 \; mL}{min} \times \dfrac{60 \; min}{hr} = 120 \; mL/hr$

Therefore, the dose per hour is: $\dfrac{2 \; mg}{mL} \times \dfrac{120 \; mL}{hr} = \textbf{240 mg/hr}$

5. $\dfrac{40 \; mEq}{1,000 \; mL} = 0.04 \; mEq/mL \times 50 \; mL = 2 \; mEq/hr$; 2mEq/hr × 2 hours = **4 mEq**

6. $\dfrac{10,000 \; units}{8 \; hr} = \textbf{1,250 units/hr}$

7. 5 g = 5,000 mg, so C = 5,000 mg/1,000 mL or 5 mg/mL. D/t = 250 mg/hr, so

$$F = \frac{250 \; mg}{5 \; mg/mL} = \textbf{50 mL/hr}$$

Or

$$\frac{5,000 \; mg}{1,000 \; mL} = \frac{250 \; mg}{x} = \textbf{50 mL/hr}$$

At 50 mL/hr, the 1,000 mL IV will run:

$$\frac{1,000 \; mL}{50 \; mL/hr} = \textbf{20 hours}$$

8. 1 g = 1,000 mg and 1 L = 1,000 mL, so

$$C = \frac{1,000 \; mg}{1,000 \; mL} = 1 \; mg/mL$$

The hourly dose (*D/t*) = 50 mg/hr, so using **C × F = D/t:**

$$F = \frac{50 \; mg/hr}{1 \; mg/mL} = \textbf{50 mL/hr}$$

9. $C = 0.5\% = \dfrac{(0.5 \; \cancel{g})500 \; mg}{100 \; mL} = 5 \; mg/mL$

$$F = 100 \; mL/hr$$

$$5 \; mg/mL = 100 \; mL/hr = \textbf{500 mg/hr}$$

10. 80 mL × 20 gtts = 1,600 gtts/hr; 1,600 gtts/60 minutes = **26.67 gtts/minute**

Chapter 18

1. The procedure calls for 500 g of psyllium and makes 1,000 g of laxative. 500 g/1,000 g = **50%**
2. The procedure makes 1,000 g using 500 g of psyllium. Using ratio-proportion:

$$\frac{500 \; \cancel{g}}{1,000 \; \cancel{g}} = \frac{x}{500 \; \cancel{g}}$$

Cross-multiply and divide: X = **250 g**

3. The procedure calls for 5 g of bicarbonate to make 1,000 g of laxative:

$$100\% \times \frac{5 \; \cancel{g}}{1,000 \; \cancel{g}} = \textbf{0.5\%}$$

4. Do the problem by ratio-proportion, as in question 3. Calculate the amount of each ingredient as follows:

   To make 250 g, the reduced amounts correctly calculated will look like this:

   250 g is 4 times smaller than 1,000, so divide all ingredients by 4.

psyllium	500 g/4 = 125 g
dextrose	487 g/4 = 121.75 g
citric acid	5 g/4 = 1.25 g
sodium bicarbonate	5 g/4 = 1.25 g
lemon flavoring	3 g/4 = 0.75 g
Psyllium	**125 g**
Dextrose	**121.75 g**
Citric acid	**1.25 g**
Sodium bicarbonate	**1.25 g**
Lemon flavoring	**0.75 g**

5. Percentage is g/100 mL.

$$\frac{5\ g}{1,000\ mL} = \frac{0.5\ g}{1,000\ mL} = \textbf{0.5\%}$$

6. The procedure makes 1 L, so we must multiply by (5 L/1 L) 5. We need 5 g × 5 = **25 g**

7. The procedure calls for 80 g, so (60 g/80 g) × 1 L = **0.75 L or 750 mL**

8. $\dfrac{240\ mL}{1,000\ mL} \times 20\ g = \textbf{4.8}$

9. We q.s. to 1,000 mL, so if the ingredients take up 50 mL of volume, we are actually adding 1,000 mL − 50 mL = **950 mL** of calcium hydroxide solution. The correct answer is **c**.

10. Use ratio/proportion:

$$\frac{2\ g}{100\ mL} = \frac{x}{200\ mL}$$

Cross-multiply and divide: X = 4 g. The correct answer is **c**.

Chapter 19

1. Use the formula: Cost + Markup = Selling Price

   cost = unknown

   markup = 200% (two times the cost)

   selling price = **$6.90**

Fill in the equation with the available information:

Cost + markup (2 cost) = selling price (3 × cost) = $6.90

Divide $6.90 by 3 to get the cost:

Cost is then $6.90 ÷ 3 or **$2.30 per tube**

2. Remember: *Gross profit* and *markup* are the same thing. If the original selling price is $6.90, half off of that (50% off) would be the new price, or $3.45. The cost price never changes—it is still $2.30. Therefore, the gross profit per tube is:

$$\$3.45 - \$2.30, \text{ or } \$1.15$$

There are 50 tubes total profit is 50 × $1.15 = **$57.50**.

3. a. Remember: A 200% markup means the same as 2 times the cost.

$$\text{Cost of the vial} + \text{Markup} = \text{Selling Price for the vial}$$

$$\$15 + (2 \times \$15) = \textbf{\$45 per vial}$$

$$\text{Cost} \quad \text{Markup} \qquad\qquad \text{Selling Price}$$

b. The gross profit made on one vial the markup 2 × $15 = $30.

4. The vial contains 5 g of drug. The order is for 1 g, so: $\dfrac{1\ g}{5\ g/vial} = 1/5\ vial$ to be dispensed for the patient (the vial sells for $45), so: 1/5 = 0.2 × $45 = **$9 per dose**.

Since the patient receives the dose twice per day, the daily-dose charge would be $9 × 2, or **$18**.

5. To figure the selling price (charged to the patient):
   Remember that a 10% solution is 10 g per 100 mL.
   A 1 g dose would be 1/10 of that 100 mL, or 10 mL.
   The solution is priced at $2 per 10 mL, and since 10 mL = the 1 g dose, the patient would be charged $2.

To figure the profit made, we use the formula:

$$\text{Cost} + \text{Markup} = \text{Selling Price}$$

Fill in the numbers: Cost = x

$$\text{Cost} + (2 \times \text{cost}) = \$2, \text{ so } x + 2x = \text{selling price } (\$2)$$

$$3x = \$2; x = \$2/3$$

The cost to the pharmacy is $2 ÷ 3, or 67 cents. Since we are charging $2 per dose, the profit is $2 − $0.67, or **$1.33**.

Chapter 20

1. 50 mL × 1 L/1,000 mL = 0.05 L = 50,000 mcL. **d.**
2. 50 g = 50,000 mg, so 10% (0.1) × 50 g either 5 g or 5,000 mg. **d.**
3. **d.**

4. gtt = drop, A = ear, U = each, qod = every other day. **c.**
5. The largest amount is 5 g. **a.**
6. The smallest is one dram, which is 4 mL. **a.**
7. The best answer is **b**.
8. Order: 2.5 mg twice a day. Stock: 5 mg/mL.

$$\frac{2.5\ mg}{5\ mg/mL} = 0.5\ mL/dose$$

    A daily dose = 1 mL. **a.**

9. gr i = 60 mg, or two tablets per dose. **c.**
10. 15 mL = 1 T. **a.**
11. ss = 1/2, so gr ss = 60 mg/2 = 30 mg. **c.**
12. ℥ is one ounce, which is 30 mL. **d.**
13. **d.**
14. **c.**
15. Reconstitution refers to the addition of an appropriate solution to the drug. **c.**
16. **c.**
17. 2.5 mL two times a day = 5 mL. **b.**
18. Both A and B. A: 10 g/100 mL = 10%. B: 100 g/L = 100 g/1,000 mL = 10 g/100 mL = 10%. **d.**
19. **c.**
20. 60 mg × 20 mg/mL = 3 mL. **b.**
21. **a.**
22. **c.**
23. **b.**
24. **d.**
25. **d.**
26. $20\ mL \times \dfrac{10\ g}{100\ mL} = 2\ g$ **c.**
27. **d.**

    For Problems 29–34, *dose* is in mg, g, etc. The *form* is the tablet, syrup, etc. *Supply dose* is mg/tablet, mg/mL, etc.

28. **b.**
29. **b.**
30. **a.**
31. **c.**
32. **b.**
33. **c.**
34. **c.**
35. **a.**
36. **b.**
37. **b.**
38. First, calculate flow rate in mL/min:

    2,000 mL is infused in 12 hr (720 min). $\dfrac{2,000\ mL}{720\ min} = 2.78$ mL/min.

Next, multiply by the drop factor: $\dfrac{2.78\ mL}{min} \times \dfrac{10\ gtt}{mL} = 27.8$ **round to 28**.

Since you cannot have part of a drop, the answer is 28 gtt/min. **c.**

39. The correct answer is **b**.

$$\frac{500\ mL}{5\ hr} = 100\ mL/hr$$

$$\frac{100\ mL/hr \times 60\ gtts/mL}{60\ min} = \textbf{100 gtts/min};\ \frac{100\ gtt/min}{60\ gtts/mL} = \textbf{1.67 mL/min}$$

40. $C \times F = D/t$, so:

$$F = \frac{D/t}{C}$$

Because $= D/t = 75,000$ units/4 hr $= 18,750$ units/hr, and $C = \dfrac{150,000\ units}{1,000\ mL} = 150\ units$

$$F = \frac{18,750\ units/hr}{150\ units/mL} = \textbf{125 mL/hr. c.}$$

41. 66 lb/2.2 = 30 kg body weight. Dose = 25 mg/kg $\times$ 30 kg= 750 mg/day. In two doses, each is 375 mg. **a.**

42. 10 mg/m² $\times$ 0.8 m² = 8 mg. **c.**

43. $2\% = \dfrac{2\ g}{100\ mL}$, at 100 mL/hr, 2 g is the hourly dose. **c.**

44. D/t = 100,000 units, C = 1,000,000 units/1,000 mL or 1,000 units/mL, so F = 100 mL/hr. **c.**

45. $\dfrac{66\ lb}{150\ lb} \times 500\ mg = \textbf{220 mg. c.}$

46. $\dfrac{8\ yrs}{8\ yrs + 12} \times 500\ mg = \textbf{200 mg. c.}$

47. 62 lb/2.2 = 28.18 kg.

$$40\ mg/kg \times 28.18\ kg = 1,127.20\ mg\ (adult\ dose).$$

$$1,127.20\ mg/1.7 = 663\ mg.\ \textbf{b.}$$

48. Use Clark's Rule: $\dfrac{50\ lb}{150\ lb} \times 100\ mg = \textbf{33 mg. d.}$

49. Use Young's Rule: $\dfrac{10\ yrs}{10\ yrs + 12} \times 100\ mg = \textbf{45.45 mg. c.}$

50. 12 hr = 720 min. $\dfrac{2,000\ mL}{720\ min} = 2.78\ mL/min$ **round to 2.8 mL/min. d.**

51. Answer **c**.

$$\frac{500\ mL}{4\ hr} = 125\ mL/hr;\ \frac{125\ mL/hr \times 10\ gtts/mL}{60\ min} = 20.8\ gtt/min\ \textbf{round to 21 gtts/min.}$$

52. $C = \dfrac{100{,}000 \ units}{1{,}000 \ mL} = 100 \ units/mL$; $\dfrac{75{,}000 \ units}{100 \ units/mL} = 750 \ mL$ used in 8 hr, so 750 mL/8hr = 94 mL/hr. **c**.

53. 100,000 units/5 hr = 20,000 units/hr. **b**.

54. D_5W is 5% dextrose. concentration. **5% = 5 g/100 mL, at 100 mL/hr the patient receives a 5 g dose of dextrose. d**.

55. $1\% = \dfrac{1 \ g(1{,}000 \ mg)}{100 \ mL} = 10 \ mg/mL$

   10 mg/mL × 500 mL= 5,000 mg infused in 2 hr = 2,500 mg/hr.

   2,500 mg/hr/60 min = 41.67 mg/min. **d**.

56. 73 lb/2.2 = 33.2 kg = 25 mg = 830 mg/day = two doses of 415 mg/dose. **b**.

57. 50 mL; 1:100 = 1 g/100 mL, so 0.5 g = 50 mL.

58. The whole 500 mL is infused: 500 mL/4 hours = 125 mL/hr.

59. 30 mEq/6 hours = 5 mEq/hr.

60. 4 oz bottle = 120 mL. **b**.

Chapter 21

1. The mechanism of action of a drug refers to how it acts at a cellular or biochemical level. The first two answers reference cellular or biochemical mechanisms, the third does not—inflammation is a physiological manifestation of cellular and biochemical processes. The correct answer is **d**.

2. An adverse effect is an undesirable effect produced by a drug. These effects may be toxic to the body (e.g., hearing loss or liver damage). These effects can occur at therapeutic doses. The correct answer is **d**.

3. A toxic effect is one in which damage occurs to an organ or system. All three of the answers describe a condition in which an organ has been damaged. The correct answer is **d**.

4. Drugs of a class produce similar effects, including adverse effects, and have similar mechanisms of action. The correct answer is **a**.

5. Drugs of choice are the most effective drugs for a condition. They are the first drugs to be prescribed, but *only* if the patient does not have a sensitivity to the drug. The correct answer is **b**.

6. In an elderly patient, renal clearance and hepatic function are decreased. The correct answer would be The correct answer is **c**.

7. With each successive dose of drug, plasma levels rise, as the drug enters the bloodstream, and then fall, as the drug is distributed within the tissues (e.g., bound to proteins, stored in fat, etc.). The correct answer is **c**.

8. A fat-soluble drug would likely be metabolized in the liver. A patient with cirrhosis would not be able to adequately metabolize the drug and it could build up to toxic levels in the plasma. Many drugs are also enzymatically activated in the liver. The correct answer is **d**.

9. The term *absorption* only applies to a drug which is applied *outside* of the body (which includes the digestive tract). By definition, drugs injected directly into the blood are not absorbed. The correct answer is **d**.

10. A weak base will most likely be absorbed in a basic environment, such as the duodenum. The correct answer is **c**.

11. A lipid-soluble drug will not be compatible with water. Thus, it will head for the fatty tissues. The correct answer is **b**.

12. A vasoconstrictor is added to slow absorption, by constricting blood vessels in the area. The correct answer is **b**.

13. To be active in the body, a drug must be free in the plasma. The correct answer is **c**.

14. The large dose is a loading dose. The correct answer is **b**.

15. The prefix *cefa* designates a cephalosporin and *bid* means twice a day. The correct answer is **d**.

Chapter 22

1. These drugs are both antidepressants. They should not be used together. The correct answer is **a**.

2. Valium (diazepam) and alcohol are CNS depressants. They will, therefore, cause excessive sedation that can progress through the usual stages of hypnosis, coma, and death. The correct answer is **d**.

3. Phenobarbital is a barbiturate with a long half-life. The correct answer is **c**.

4. For this condition, we are looking for a long half-life. Lorazepam and diazepam both fit the bill, but only lorazepam is used as a hypnotic. The correct answer is **c**.

5. The only one listed that is prescribed as an anxiolytic is Xanax, or alprazolam. The correct answer is **d**.

6. Paxil is a proprietary name for paroxetine. Therefore, we are looking for the generic of Lamictal, which is lamotrigine. The correct answer is **d**.

7. Nardil is phenylzine, an MAO inhibitor. Wine and cheese contain tyramine, and excessive blood pressure would be produced. The correct answer is **c**.

8. Mr. Hill gets an anxiolytic, an analgesic, an antidepressant, and an anticonvulsant—BUT (there is always a "but") carbamazepine (Tegretol) is also used in the therapy of trigeminal neuralgia. We don't know which of these conditions he has. We do know that he is prescribed alprazolam, which is used for anxiety. Note that the answer is **chronic** anxiety—if the word *chronic* were not included, the answer would not have been correct. The correct answer is **b**.

9. Tegetrol and alprazolam both may cause sedation. The correct answer is **c**.

10. MAO inhibitors are contraindicated with increased levels of thyroid. The correct answer is **c**.

11. The correct answer is **d**.

12. Haldol (haloperidol) blocks dopamine receptors. The correct answer is **c**.

13. Bromocriptine should be stored below room temperature. The correct answer is **b**.

14. Tolcapone can cause severe liver failure. The correct answer is **a**.

15. Aripiprazole is the generic name for Abilify. The correct answer is **b**.

16. Paxil is paroxetine, an SSRI. Zoloft is also an antidepressant of the same class. The correct answer is **c**.

17. The geriatric dose of Pamelor is limited to 35 to 50 mg/day. The correct answer is **b**.

18. Lorazepam solution for injection must be stored refrigerated. The correct answer is **c**.

19. Depakene is a brand name for valproic acid. The correct answer is **a**.

20. SSRI include citalopram and sertraline. The correct answer is **c**.

Chapter 23

1. These can be symptoms of opiate intoxication. To determine this, one may use a short-acting opiate antagonist, such as naloxone (Narcan), to see if the patient improves. The correct answer is **b**.
2. The key word here is "interaction," not "duplication." The oxycodone would potentiate the respiratory depressant actions of the phenobarbital. The correct answer is **b**.
3. The daily dose of Tylenol (APAP) is 1,000 mg × 4 = 4 grams of acetaminophen per day, which is the maximum dose. Vicodin also contains APAP, so this combination causes an overdose to be given. This amount may cause hepatotoxicity. The correct answer is **a**.
4. Most of these drugs would be inappropriate for a patient with liver damage—the acetaminophen may rise to toxic levels, and the phenobarbital is also metabolized by the liver. The correct answer is **c**.
5. Tylenol is acetaminophen, and Vicodin is a combination drug containing acetaminophen. The correct answer is **d**.
6. This question requires an understanding of the mechanisms involved. In order to promote stomach ulcers, the drug must inhibit prostaglandin synthesis *and* be absorbed through the gastric mucosa *in an active form*. Acetaminophen does not affect prostaglandin synthesis, and ibuprofen is absorbed in the duodenum. Sulindac is a "pro-drug" and is activated *after* absorption. The correct answer is **d**.
7. Acetaminophen is not anti-inflammatory. The correct answer is **c**.
8. The antithrombotic effect of aspirin and other COX-1 inhibitors would interact with other antithrombotic agents, and with anticoagulants. The correct answer is **c**.
9. The total effects of ibuprofen and ketoprofen are delayed, and that of naproxen is delayed by several weeks. Aspirin has immediate effects. The correct answer is **b**.
10. The pro-drug here is sulindac. The correct answer is **b**.

Chapter 24

1. Drugs that affect the beta receptor will affect blood sugar. The correct answer is **b**.
2. Digoxin is a cardiac glycoside. The correct answer is **d**.
3. Nifedipine is a dihydropyridine-class calcium channel blocker. These have little or no effect on the heart, but a major effect on vessels. The correct answer is **c**.
4. Direct vasodilators effect arteries and arterioles. The correct answer is **c**.
5. Severe bradycardia is the hallmark of early glycoside toxicity. The correct answer is **b**.
6. Drugs that affect veins cause postural hypotension. Alpha receptor blockers prevent compensation when blood pools in veins, and venodilators have the same effect. 1 and 2 are alpha receptor blockers and 3 is a venodilator. The correct answer is **d**.
7. Clonidine and captopril both affect arteriolar diameter, and furosemide affects fluid volume. The patient appears to be hypertensive. The correct answer is **b**.
8. Atropine inhibits parasympathetic effects, so sympathetic effects are seen. It also blocks reflex parasympathetic action, as the receptors for acetylcholine are blocked. Isoproterenol is a sympathetic agonist. These two drugs could have fatal consequences if given together. The correct answer is **a**.
9. This drug is nifedipine, which has mainly vascular actions. Primary action is on arteries and arterioles. The correct answer is **c**.

10. Coumadin is warfarin, which has a delayed onset. Enalapril is a pro-drug, so it also must be converted before it has pharmacological action. The correct answer is **d**.

11. Capoten is captopril, which decreases the formation of angiotensin II. Candesartan is an antagonist at the angiotensin II receptor. Thus, the effects of the drugs will be similar (but not entirely the same!). The correct answer is **b**.

12. Warfarin may be given orally. The correct answer is **d**.

13. TPA is an effective lysis agent, and the smaller clots produced may occlude small vessels. The correct answer is **b**.

14. This sounds like postural hypotension, caused by a nitrate. The correct answer is **b**.

15. The correct answer is **c**.

Chapter 25

1. Medrol is methylprednisone, which is given orally. The correct answer is **a**.

2. All of these have a delayed onset, except for albuterol, which is immediate-acting. The correct answer is **a**.

3. Serevent is salmeterol, which is a beta$_2$ agonist. The correct answer is **b**.

4. Caffeine is a methylxanthine, as is theophylline. The correct answer is **b**.

5. Both beclomethasone and fluticasone are inhaled. The correct answer is **d**.

6. Singulair is montelukast, a leukotriene receptor antagonist. The correct answer is **d**.

7. One action of corticosteroids is the inhibition of the immune system. The correct answer is **c**.

8. The correct answer is **c**.

9. Albuterol is classified as a beta adrenergic agonist. The correct answer is **a**.

10. Mast cells are affected by steroids and anti-inflammatories. The correct answer is **d**.

Chapter 26

1. This would be a broad-spectrum antibiotic. The correct answer is **c**.

2. A bacterio**cidal** drug kills directly. The correct answer is **b**.

3. Antibiotics will cause an increased rate of growth of yeast and viruses, due to the death of bacteria, which results in increased availability of nutrients. The correct answer is **b**.

4. Antibiotics have no effect on a virus and taken when not needed can cause a superinfection. The correct answer is **c**.

5. Cephalosporins can cause reactions in penicillin-allergic patients. The correct answer is **b**.

6. Antibiotics interfere with estrogen-based contraceptives. The correct answer is **c**.

7. Tazobactam is an inhibitor of penicillinase, which is a form of penicillin resistance. The correct answer is **d**.

8. Polymox is amoxicillin. It is acid-stable and is thus orally active. The correct answer is **c**.

9. Procaine decreases vessel size so that the penicillin is absorbed slowly. It is a way to administer a higher dose that is absorbed over a longer period of time. The correct answer is **c**.

10. The correct answer is **b**.

11. The correct answer is **d**.

12. Gentamicin is an aminoglycoside; erythromycin is a macrolide. Increased plasma concentrations of either drug due to dehydration could cause ototoxicity. The correct answer is **b**.

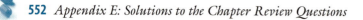

13. Sulfa drugs will precipitate out and damage kidney tubules if the urine is concentrated, which is possible in dehydrated patients. The correct answer is **a**.
14. **Ocu**flox. The correct answer is **c**.
15. Isoniazid can cause severe hepatotoxicity. The correct answer is **a**.
16. The correct answer is **b**.
17. The correct answer is **d**.
18. The correct answer is **d**.
19. The correct answer is **c**.
20. Cephalosporins are similar in structure and action to penicillin. The correct answer is **a**.

Chapter 27

1. Anthracycline antibiotics are cardiotoxic. The correct answer is **b**.
2. Cytoxan and Reglan are available in oral form. The correct answer is **d**.
3. Both Reglan and Compazine are used for nausea. The correct answer is **d**.
4. The only agent listed that is given subcutaneously is Bleomycin. The correct answer is **c**.
5. Methotrexate inhibits the conversion of folic acid to folinic acid. Administration of folinic acid would counteract this effect. The correct answer is **b**.
6. Central-line administration of 5-FU dramatically reduces adverse effects. The correct answer is **b**.
7. Procrit is a parenteral product, available in multidose vials. The correct answer is **b**.
8. Methotrexate is useful in the therapy of rheumatoid arthritis because it depresses the immune system. The correct answer is **c**.
9. Leucovorin is used to "rescue" normal cells while still allowing treatment to affect the tumor cells. The correct answer is **a**.
10. Cyclophosamide is one of the agents derived from nitrogen mustard. The correct answer is **d**.

Chapter 28

1. Imodium is an opiate, and both Prilosec and Nexium are proton pump inhibitors. Axid is nizatidine, an H_2 blocker. The correct answer is **b**.
2. Cimetidine interferes with cytochrome P_{450} metabolism. The correct answer is **a**.
3. The patient has a transient increase in stomach acid, so a simple antacid would be best. The correct answer is **a**.
4. Only Zantac is available for injection. The correct answer is **c**.
5. Prevacid is delayed release. The correct answer is **c**.
6. Uterine contraction may be caused by misoprostol, which is a prostanoid and may contract uterine smooth muscle. The correct answer is **b**.
7. These drugs are stool softeners, or demulcents. The correct answer is **a**.
8. Imodium is loperamide, which is a non-narcotic opiate. The correct answer is **b**.
9. Lomotil contains atropine, which could cause tachycardia. The correct answer is **c**.
10. Mintezol is mebendazole, an anthelmintic. The correct answer is **b**.
11. Lomotil and OxyContin both contain opiates, and the potential for additive respiratory depression is increased. The correct answer is **a**.
12. Since the phenobarbital is a weak acid, it will ionize in the basic environment created by the Alka-Seltzer. This means that the absorption of the drug from the stomach will be decreased,

and the elimination increased. Thus, his serum levels of phenobarbital might decrease, and the seizures increase. The correct answer is **c**.

13. The sucralfate may bind drugs in the stomach, preventing absorption. The correct answer is **d**.

14. Tagamet is an H_2 antagonist. Dulcolax is a laxative. Imodium is an anti-diarrheal. The correct answer is Protonix. The correct answer is **a**.

15. Lomotil has an opiate (diphenoxylate) which is in schedule 5. The correct answer is **b**.

Chapter 29

1. The largest complex has the longest duration, as it takes time to extract the insulin from the protamine and zinc. The correct answer is **d**.

2. We want the fastest action possible. A and C are agents for type II diabetes. Humalog is human insulin and would be acceptable, but Novolog is a rapid-acting form of insulin and would be the best choice. The correct answer is **d**.

3. Lantus insulin is a zinc complex insulin. The correct answer is **d**.

4. Micronase is an oral sulfonylurea for the treatment of type II diabetes. The correct answer is **d**.

5. Prandin blocks carbohydrate absorption and should be taken immediately before a meal. The correct answer is **b**.

6. Methimazole can cause mental abnormalities in the fetus. The correct answer is **a**.

7. The insulin aspart is rapid-reacting and the NPH insulin is long-acting. The correct answer is **c**.

8. The most common way of administering insulin is with the use of an insulin syringe. We now have the refillable cartridge "pen," as well. The correct answer is **c**.

9. The patient may be allergic to pork and should be switched to human insulin. The correct answer is **b**.

10. The correct answer is **b**.

11. Oral sulfonylureas can cause severe hypoglycemia. The correct answer is **d**.

12. The correct answer is **c**.

13. Levemir is indicated for both Type I and Type II diabetes. The correct answer is **b**.

14. This drug is triggered by the presence of glucose. The correct answer is **b**.

15. Thyroid hormone will increase the sensitivity of the heart to catecholamines. This may cause tachycardia and cardiac arrhythmias. The correct answer is **b**.

16. The correct answer is **c**.

17. The correct answer is **b**.

18. Estrogens have no effect on lipids. The correct answer is **d**.

19. The correct answer is **c**.

20. Tamoxifen is an estrogen antagonist. The correct answer is **b**.

Chapter 30

1. Folic acid is required for the construction of red blood cells. The correct answer is **a**.

2. Vitamin B_{12} is involved in myelination. The correct answer is **c**.

3. Cyanocobalamin is vitamin B_{12}, a water-soluble vitamin. The correct answer is **d**.

4. Tocopherols form vitamin E. The correct answer is **d**.

5. The retinoids (beta carotene derivatives) form vitamin A. The correct answer is **b**.

6. Vitamins A, D, and K are fat soluble. The correct answer is **c**.

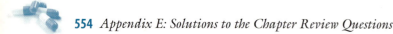

7. Vitamin D, or specifically D$_3$ (the activated form), is required for bone mineralization. The correct answer is **b**.

8. Vitamins B and C are water soluble. Vitamin D does not have any anti-oxidant properties. The correct answer is **b**.

9. Vitamin A is required for proper night vision. The correct answer is **d**.

10. Riboflavin is required for the conversion of glucose to energy, in the mitochondrial citric acid cycle. The correct answer is **b**.

11. Iron is abbreviated Fe. The correct answer is **b**.

12. Potassium is an absolute requirement for the heart, and is also required for proper nerve function. The correct answer is **d**.

13. Pantothenic acid is a B-vitamin, B-5. The correct answer is **d**.

14. Calcium is a key player in muscle control and properly functioning nerves. The correct answer is **c**.

15. Vitamin K plays a major role in blood clotting so lack of it can lead to bruising and bleeding. The correct answer is **a**.

Chapter 31

1. Norvasc is a calcium channel blocker (amlodipine). The correct answer is **a**.

2. Keflex and Ceclor are cephalosporin antibiotics, and Polymox is amoxicillin. The correct answer is **d**.

3. Lasix is the only diuretic. The correct answer is **b**.

4. Choices B and C are SSRIs. Elavil is a tricyclic, which has both antimuscarinic and antihistamine actions. The correct answer is **a**.

5. Drugs that affect the cardiovascular system often have some form of "cardio" in the name, much like the ones that affect the vessels have "vaso." *Cardi*zem, a calcium channel blocker, would affect both the heart and the vessels, while *Card*ura, an alpha receptor blocker, would affect the vessels and speed up the heart by reflex action. The question asks which drug has a *direct* effect on the heart. The effects of Cardura are *indirect*. The correct answer is **a**.

6. Antifungal drugs (generic names) often end in "ole." The only possible answers are A and B. (However, cefamandole [B] begins with "cef," so it is a good bet that it's a cephalosporin antibiotic.) The correct answer is **a**.

7. This is a good example of look-alike and sound-alike drugs. Three of these names contain "pen," and one contains "cillin." Of the "pen" drugs, the only one with "pen" in the beginning is pentoxifylline. This drug actually lowers the blood viscosity. The correct answer is **c**.

8. Here we are looking for something that is long-lasting. All of them start with "Nitro," but the only one that ends in "dur" (as in "durable") is Nitro-Dur. The correct answer is **c**.

9. Nitropress is nitroprusside. The correct answer is **d**.

10. Antibiotics can destroy vitamin K–producing bacteria in the gut. The correct answer is **b**.

11. Percodan contains aspirin, which would synergize with the Coumadin. The correct answer is **c**.

12. Of the drugs listed, nitroglycerine dilates veins, which would be synergistic with the vasodilation produced by nifedipine. The correct answer is **b**.

13. Atropine increases heart rate and conduction; verapamil decreases it. The correct answer is **b**.

14. Antibiotics decrease vitamin K and would potentiate the actions of warfarin. The correct answer is **a**.

15. These are oral sulfonylureas used for type II diabetes. The correct answer is **b**.

16. The correct answer is **d**.
17. Lasix and gentamicin have synergistic effects and can produce ototoxicity and deafness. The correct answer is **b**.
18. The calcium and magnesium in Rolaids would chelate the tetracycline and inactivate it. The correct answer is **c**.
19. The correct answer is **c**.
20. The correct answer is **c**.
21. The correct answer is **b**.
22. Verapamil would decrease both cardiac conduction and cardiac output, which would decrease the potential for arrhythmia and would lower blood pressure. The correct answer is **c**.
23. The SSRI and MAO inhibitor will both produce large amounts of free catecholamines and serotonin. Cardiac stimulation could result. The correct answer is **c**.
24. Cephalosporins have cross-sensitivity with penicillins. The correct answer is **d**.
25. The correct answer is **b**.
26. It does contain atropine, but the classification is due to the opiate diphenoxylate. The correct answer is **a**.
27. Atropine increases sympathetic activity, and the thyroid hormone sensitizes the heart to norepinephrine. Severe arrythmias could result. The correct answer is **a**.
28. Aspirin allergy is a problem with cyclooxygenase inhibitors, particularly naproxen. Combinations should be with drugs that do not inhibit cyclooxygenase (e.g., acetaminophen). The correct answer is **c**.
29. Nitroglycerin dilates veins and will cause orthostatic hypotension. Prazosin blocks alpha receptors and inhibits the compensatory response. The correct answer is **c**.
30. While Reglan is used as a gastrointestinal agent (GERD), it also has anti-emetic effects for chemotherapy patients. The correct answer is **d**.
31. The correct answer is **t**.
32. The correct answer is **g**.
33. The correct answer is **q**.
34. The correct answer is **d**.
35. The correct answer is **h**.
36. The correct answer is **c**.
37. The correct answer is **l**.
38. The correct answer is **j**.
39. The correct answer is **r**.
40. The correct answer is **i**.
41. The correct answer is **m**.
42. The correct answer is **o**.
43. The correct answer is **b**.
44. The correct answer is **n**.
45. The correct answer is **a**.
46. The correct answer is **f**.
47. The correct answer is **s**.
48. The correct answer is **e**.
49. The correct answer is **p**.
50. The correct answer is **k**.

Chapter 32

1. The only act that specifically addresses contaminants is the Federal Food, Drug, and Cosmetic Act. The correct answer is **d**.

2. Childproof packaging is required on all drugs and hazardous substances, unless the package is specifically intended for use by adult handicapped persons. Aspirin may be packaged in non-childproof containers intended for arthritic adults, etc., if the label bears a warning. This is not true of children's aspirin. All prescription drugs would automatically be packaged in child-resistant packaging. The exception would be the drug intended for the arthritic patient, to whom it would be permissible to dispense a drug in non-child-resistant packaging with a signed waiver. All of the drugs except those for the arthritic person are required to have child-resistant packaging. The correct answer is **d**.

3. Safety and efficacy are determined by clinical studies in humans. Additional studies, using animals, are also required. The correct answer is **b**.

4. Over-the-counter drugs must, by definition, have no abuse potential and be of low strength. *Low abuse potential* (#1) is not acceptable. The correct answer is **d**.

5. Drugs classified as Schedule I have no proven therapeutic benefit and are highly addictive. **c**.

6. Schedule II drugs include strong opiates with proven therapeutic benefits. These would include morphine and meperidine. Heroin has no proven therapeutic benefit and is highly addictive. It is classified as Schedule I. The correct answer is **d**.

7. Xanax is a C-IV(C-III in some states). It can thus be written on a regular prescription form and filed with prescriptions for non-Schedule drugs. It must, however, be marked as a prescription for a controlled substance, commonly by marking it with a red "C" or noting the "C" class. The correct answer is **d**.

8. Mandatory patient counseling may be done only by the pharmacist and must be given to whoever is responsible for having the prescription filled, whether patient or caregiver. It is required with all prescriptions, whether new or refilled. The correct answer is **d**.

9. This statement is legally called a *transfer warning* and is found on prescription drug labels. The correct answer is **c**.

10. This warning appears on the label of an over-the-counter product that does not have child-resistant packaging (e.g., intended for adult handicapped or arthritic patients). The correct answer is **a**.

11. The label on a drug product must carry *all* of this information. The correct answer is **d**.

12. Patient counseling **must** be done by the pharmacist or licensed intern. It may include instructions for taking the drug, importance of dosage intervals, self-monitoring techniques, and any adverse effects to be expected. The correct answer is **c**.

13. Therapeutic duplication is when two or more prescriptions have the same therapeutic use. The correct answer is **a**.

14. The record described refers to the patient profile, which is necessary for therapeutic monitoring and mandated by the Consolidated Omnibus Budget Reconciliation Act. The correct answer is **c**.

15. Therapeutic monitoring applies to the specific therapy of a single patient. It does not include prevention of improperly administered drugs or drug "mix-ups." Ultimate responsibility for the monitoring lies with the pharmacist, but the technician also assists. The correct answer is **a**.

16. The best way to dispose of a syringe and needle is to place both the syringe and needle in an autoclavable sharps container. The correct answer is **b**.

17. Care should be taken to keep noxious drugs away from skin or mucous membranes. Thus, adequate clothing should be worn. A paper coat is preferable to a cloth coat as it can be thrown away, causing less risk of contamination of the surrounding area. The correct answer is **d**.

18. With a flammable substance spill, you should always be sure to keep it away from electrical outlets and ensure that nothing is present to cause ignition (e.g., a flame or electrical appliance that might spark). The correct answer is **d**.

19. Under the new HIPAA laws, a patient may request communication by a particular means that ensures confidentiality. The correct answer is **c**.

20. According to the new HIPAA privacy regulations, a privacy policy must be available to both patients and staff, must be enforced by a particular individual on the staff who is responsible for the protection of patient confidentiality, and must contain a list of staff who have access to such confidential information. The correct answer is **d**.

Chapter 33

1. The Joint Commission is an independent agency, the Pharmacy and Therapeutics Committee is institutional, and the FDA and CPSC are federal agencies. The only state agency is the State Board of Pharmacy. The correct answer is **d**.

2. All of these things fall under FDA jurisdiction. The correct answer is **d**.

3. Investigations into claims of misbranded drugs are handled by the FDA. The correct answer is **d**.

4. A package insert contains information necessary for the pharmacist to counsel the patient. This includes results of studies showing the drug's efficacy and toxicity. The correct answer is **d**.

5. A **PPI** is written in layperson's terms and must be given to the patient with the first dose of a drug containing estrogen and every refill thereafter (as long as therapy continues). The correct answer is **d**.

6. Investigations into consumer product-related deaths are done by the Consumer Product Safety Commission. The correct answer is **b**.

7. The Poison Prevention Packaging Act is a statute produced from the Consumer Product Safety Commission. The correct answer is **c**.

8. The correct answer is **b**.

9. While herbal products are used as medications, they are still considered food supplements. The correct answer is **b**.

10. The P&T committee operates in a hospital setting and consists of physicians and pharmacists who determine the formulary for their pharmacy. The correct answer is **a**.

Chapter 34

1. Dr. Dee does not prescribe benzodiazepines in the course of his practice. The prescription is not legally valid. You should decline to fill the prescription and alert the pharmacist. The correct answer is **d**.

2. Patient counseling involves a discussion of the drug action, adverse effects, food and drug contraindications, and dosing. All of the answers are appropriate. The correct answer is **d**.

3. A medical student may prescribe drugs only under the DEA number of the hospital and under supervision. The correct answer is **d**.
4. Keflex is not a controlled substance. The prescription is therefore good for a year. It does, however, have to be presented for filling within six months depending on the state. The correct answer is **d**.
5. Demerol (meperidine) is a C-II. It must therefore be submitted on a triplicate form. It can, however, be obtained by a telephone order in an emergency, provided the telephone order is followed by a hard copy within three days. The correct answer is **d**.
6. Prescriptions for C-II drugs are not allowed to have extra writing or corrections on the form. Do not return the form, as the person will simply attempt to have the prescription filled at another pharmacy. Alert the pharmacist. The correct answer is **a**.
7. Valium is a C-IV (or C-III, depending on the state). It therefore does not have to be on the triplicate form. Prescriptions for controlled substances other than C-II are valid for six months, and five refills are allowed. The correct answer is **d**.
8. The entire prescription of a C-II has to be filled at one time, as no refills are allowed. The remainder could be supplied within 72 hours, but the pharmacy will not get the drug in until the following week. Therefore, the patient should be told to go to another pharmacy, unless he or she wants to settle for only five tablets. The correct answer is **d**.
9. All of the above professionals work under a DEA number that is assigned to them or their institution. The only person who does not require registration is the pharmaceutical representative. The correct answer is **d**.
10. The prescription is still valid for one year, so no changes would be made in the filling or expiration date. The correct answer is **b**.

Chapter 35

1. The pharmacy chain or the institutional therapeutics committee or institution chooses which drugs to stock and includes them in the *formulary*. The correct answer is **b**.
2. The vendor who supplies the pharmacy with most of its formulary is called the **prime vendor**. Thus, the contract is called the **prime vendor agreement**. The correct answer is **c**.
3. When an investigational study concludes, the remaining drug is to be removed from the pharmacy shelves and returned to the sponsor of the study. The correct answer is **c**.
4. When the supply of medication drops below the PAR level, the medication is automatically reordered. The correct answer is **c**.
5. Controlled substances, particularly Schedule II drugs, must be ordered by the pharmacist using a triplicate DEA 222 form. The correct answer is **c**.

Chapter 36

1. In case of a drug recall, affected drugs are identified by lot number and removed from the shelves to be returned to the supplier. The patient and prescriber of the drug must be notified. The correct answer is **d**.
2. Unit dose medications, if unopened (and thus not contaminated), may be returned to inventory. The correct answer is **c**.

3. Regular prescription drugs must be inventoried one – two times a year. The correct answer is **c**.
4. Controlled substances must be inventoried every two years. They must also be kept separate, in a locked cabinet, and carefully documented. The correct answer is **d**.
5. Opaque bottles are used to protect the drug from light. The correct answer is **c**.

Chapter 37

1. Storage in random-access memory is temporary. The correct answer is **a**.
2. Output goes from the computer to the user. This would include the monitor, printer, and graphics device (plotter), but an optical scanner sends information to the computer. The correct answer is **c**.
3. The disk operating system is a set of instructions for the computer that tells it what to do. The correct answer is **d**.
4. This is a trick question. Computers do not generate prescriptions, prescribers do. The correct answer is **c**.
5. All of these devices send information *out*, except for the light pen. The correct answer is **a**.

Chapter 38

1. Emergency calls are always referred to the pharmacist. The correct answer is **d**.
2. The technician may not offer advice regarding drug-drug interactions. The correct answer is **c**.
3. It would be acceptable for the technician to provide source information (reading material) for the patient. The correct answer is to refer the patient to the pharmacist. The correct answer is **b**.
4. Communication from computer to computer is accomplished by the use of a *modem*. The correct answer is **c**.
5. Good communication is based on confidence and trust. Knowledge on the part of the technician will increase confidence of the patient in the technician's abilities. A neat appearance always inspires a professional attitude and facilitates communication as it facilitates trust and confidence. The correct answer is **d**.
6. A lack of cooperation and anger could be a result of any of these things. The correct answer is **d**.
7. Under federal law, all counseling and professional explanation must be done by the pharmacist. State laws differ in the latitude of responsibilities and duties. You should not tell a patient that you do not know something, as this inspires a lack of confidence. You should refer the patient to the pharmacist. The correct answer is **a**.
8. The technician is openly discussing the use and care of the medication that the patient is to take. This is confidential information. HIPAA amendments implemented in 2003 state that confidential information cannot be audibly discussed in a public place. The correct answer is **c**.
9. It is important to consider all these when talking to customers, so you do not anger or offend them. The correct answer is **d**.
10. A technician may not counsel patients, take authorizations from physicians, or offer medical advice on procedures or supplements. These are all items that require clinical judgment. A technician may share information with insurance companies. The correct answer is **a**.

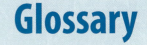

Glossary

absorption: how the drug gets into the bloodstream

abusable drug: a drug that is psychologically addictive

accreditation: the process by which an agency or organization evaluates and recognizes a program of study or an institution as meeting predetermined qualifications

ACE: angiotensin converting enzyme. This enzyme converts a blood protein, angiotensin, to a potent vasoconstrictor, angiotensin II.

acid-labile: easily destroyed by stomach acid

addiction: a need to continually use a drug. Addiction has two forms—physical addiction and psychological addiction.

additive effect: when two drugs have the same effect. The effect of one will be added to the effect of the other.

adjunct therapy (also called adjuvant therapy): an additional drug that is added to the therapeutic regimen for a specific disease or condition. This drug may increase the effect of the primary drug therapy, or may provide an additional effect.

administration (or route of administration): refers to how a drug or therapy is introduced into the body. The effects of most therapies depend upon the ability of the drug to reach the target area, thus the route of administration and consequent distribution of a drug in the body is an important determinant of its effectiveness.

admixture: a drug or other therapeutic substance added to a large-volume IV

ADT: computer program for admission/discharge and transfer that provides significant demographic and clinical information for each patient

adulteration: consisting in whole or in part of any filthy, putrid, or decomposed substance, ones prepared, packed, or held under unsanitary conditions; purporting to be or represented as drugs recognized in an official compendium, but differing in strength, quality or purity from said drugs

adverse effect: a negative effect produced by the drug (e.g., fluid retention)

aerosol: finely nebulized medication for inhalation therapy

agonist: mimics the actions of the endogenous substance

AIDS: acquired immune deficiency syndrome

alligation: the mathematical process by which the correct amounts of two different drug concentration may be mixed to form a solution or solid of a desired percentage (e.g., mixing a 2% solution and a 10% solution to obtain a 7% solution)

ambulatory care: care provided on an outpatient basis

American Council on Pharmaceutical Education: the accrediting body for colleges of pharmacy by which high educational standards are established and monitored

American Druggist Blue Book: provides prices and other miscellaneous information about prescription drugs, over-the-counter products, cosmetics, toiletries, and other items sold in pharmacy stores

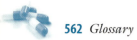

American Society of Hospital Pharmacists (ASHP): a national organization established in 1942 that presently includes pharmacists in various institutional health care settings. It currently contains a section for pharmacy technicians.

analgesic: a drug that relieves pain

anaphylaxis: a life-threatening condition characterized by wheezing and severe hypotension (shock)

anhydrous: containing no water

anionic: carrying a negative charge

antagonistic: which will either destroy or stop the growth of bacteria

anticoagulant: a substance that interferes with the formation of clotting factors in the blood

anticonvulsants: drugs used to decrease seizures

antidote: a remedy for counteracting a poison

antineoplastic agent: agent used in cancer chemotherapy

antineoplastic drug: an anticancer drug (cancer chemotherapeutic)

antiretroviral drug: an agent used to combat the activity of a retrovirus (e.g., HIV)

antiseptic: a substance used to destroy pathogenic organisms on living organisms

antithrombotic: a substance that interferes with platelet function

antithrombolytic agents: drugs that aid in preventing or interfering with the formation of thrombus or blood clots

antitussive: cough suppressant

anxiolytic: a drug that decreases anxiety

apothecary system of measurement: an antiquated system that is rarely used. Units of volume include the dram, minim, and (fluid) scruple. Units of weight include the grain and scruple.

application software: referred to as programs that accept data from the user. It calculates, stores user-specific data, and presents information according to the prescribed instructions.

arachidonic acid: a fatty acid found in cell membranes. This molecule is acted upon to form prostaglandins, prostacyclines, and thromboxanes.

arrhythmia: abnormal heart function (abnormal beat), arising from an abnormal conduction rate in the heart

aseptic: a condition in which there are no living microorganisms; free from infective agents

aseptic technique: practice of cleanliness and disinfection designed to prevent bacterial contamination of drug products, particularly IV drugs

aspirin allergy: a condition in which a patient is hypersensitive to aspirin. This hypersensitivity causes a decreased synthesis of a protective prostanoid in the lungs that normally functions to keep airways open. A patient "allergic" to aspirin may thus experience shortness of breath and severe wheezing.

automated pharmacy systems: mechanical systems that perform operations and activities relative to storage, packaging, dispensing, and distribution of medications. These systems may also collect, control, and maintain transaction information (e.g., payment and billing).

autonomic nervous system (ANS): the part of the nervous system that regulates unconscious body functions (e.g., heart rate, blood pressure). The ANS originates at the level of the spinal cord and radiates throughout the body.

auxiliary label: pictorial label placed on the dispensing bottle to alert the patient to important information (e.g., proper usage of the drug, side effects, food interactions, special instructions)

avoirdupois system of measurement: one that is used by the patient at home. Units include the teaspoon, tablespoon, fluid ounce, cup, pint, quart, gallon, pound, and ounce. This system is used to buy medication by weight.

backup systems: alternate procedures in the event the computer system should fail

bacteriocidal drug: an agent that kills the bacteria directly

bacteriostatic drug: one that halts the metabolism and/or reproduction of bacteria. These do not kill the bacteria directly, but prevents cell function and replication. The bacteria will thus die out within one generation, as long as the drug is present.

bar coding: a series of vertical bars and spaces of varying thicknesses and heights that represent coded information

beta receptor antagonist (beta blocker): a drug that selectively blocks beta receptors in the autonomic nervous system

bile: a fluid secreted by the liver

bioavailability: term used to indicate the rate and relative amount of administered drug that reaches the circulatory system intact

biodegradable: can be broken down by living organisms

bioengineered therapies: the process used in the manufacture of therapeutic agents through recombinant DNA (deoxyribonucleic acid) technology

biological equivalents: those chemical equivalents that, when administered in the same amounts, will provide the same biological or physiological availability

biological fluids: body fluids, such as blood, serum and plasma, etc.

biologicals: medicinal preparations made from living organisms or their products; include serums, vaccines, antigens, and antitoxins

biopharmaceutics: the branch of pharmaceutics that concerns itself with the relationship between physiochemical properties of a drug in a dosage form, and the pharmacologic, toxicologic, or clinical responses observed after drug administration

biotechnology (biotech) drugs: genetically engineered therapeutic agents

biotechnology: the application of biological systems and organisms to technical and industrial processes

blister packages: plastic material with a cardboard support that is heat-sealed to individually package medication

body surface area (BSA): the total area of the body (i.e., the area covered by skin)

bolus: a dose of drug administered at one time (e.g., as a single injection)

bradycardia: slow heart rate

broad-spectrum antibiotic: one that has activity against both g$^+$ and g$^-$ organisms

bronchoconstriction: narrowing of the airways (bronchioles)

buccal: administered at the inside of the cheek

bulk compounding: preparation of a medication from a standardized written procedure

bulk laxative: something that adds fiber to the stool, making it easier to pass

bulk manufacturing: preparation of a large volume of medication from a standardized written procedure

calibrate: to standardize the accuracy of a measuring device

calibrated: accurately marked for precise measurement

candida: a type of yeast found in moist areas of the body at times of immune suppression (e.g. body cavities, external genitalia)

caplet: tablet shaped like a capsule

capsule: a gelatin container enclosing medicine

cardiac glycosides: drugs that are used in cardiac failure, to increase the amount of calcium available to the heart muscle, thus increasing the force of contraction

cardiac output: the amount of blood delivered into the circulation by the heart in one beat

cardiotonic: an agent that has the effect of producing or restoring normal heart activity

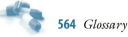

cardiotoxic: causes damage to the heart

cathartic: an agent that causes bowel evacuation

catheter: a tubular device used for the drainage or injection of fluids through a body passage; made of silicone, rubber, plastic, or other materials

cationic: carrying a positive charge

cell cycle: a representation of the process by which cells divide. The cell cycle begins with a preparatory phase, in which components are gathered for the synthesis of cellular proteins and DNA. It then moves into a synthesis phase, in which the components are used to make DNA and proteins. It is followed by a third phase, in which chromosomes divide, and a fourth phase, in which cell division occurs. By interfering with any stage of the cell cycle, cellular division can be disrupted.

cell cycle–specific drug: a drug that works only in one phase of the cell cycle

central-line infusion: when drug is infused directly into large veins or arteries in the chest, rather than into a peripheral vein in the arm or hand

central processing unit (CPU): the unit of the computer that accomplishes the processing or execution of given calculations or instructions

chelating: forming an insoluble complex with something

chemotherapeutic agent: any drug or chemical that is used to treat a disease or condition by destroying the cell

chemotherapy: the treatment of an illness with medication

cholinergic agonist: a drug that mimics the effects of acetylcholine

chronic illness: a disturbance in health that persists for a long time

chronotropic agent: a substance that changes heart rate. A *positive* inotropic agent would increase heart rate, whereas a *negative* inotropic agent would decrease it.

Class A prescription balance: a sensitive balance scale with a range of 6 mg to 120 g

clearance: removal of a drug from the plasma

clinical: involving direct observation of the patient

clinical pharmacokinetics: that branch of pharmacology that deals with the movement of drugs through the body

clinical pharmacy: patient-oriented pharmacy practice that is concerned with health care through rational drug use

clinical pharmacy practice: the application of knowledge about drugs and drug therapy to the care and treatment of patients

combination therapy: when two or more drugs that have different mechanisms of action and/or adverse effects are used in the therapeutic regimen

common denominator: a number that is common to two or more fractions, allowing addition and subtraction of the fractions

compliance: act of adhering to prescribed directions when taking medications

compounding: the preparation of a drug product from a *written procedure*

computer application: a series of computer programs written for a particular function (e.g., inventory management)

computer network: the technology that supports the connection of multiple computers, including applications, processors, printers, and computers

computer server: a central computer that collects and stores information for use by other computers

concentration: the amount of drug contained in a set volume of liquid or mass

concurrent: occurring at the same time

concurrent medication: any drug or herbal medication that is taken by the patient, in addition to a prescribed medication

contaminated: unclean; when drugs, pollutants, or microorganisms have been introduced into a drug, drug product, or area where they can cause harm

continuous infusion: when drug is administered to the patient over a period of time (e.g., over a period of days)

contraindicate: to advise against a form of treatment or a drug for a specific condition

control documents: forms, such as records, sheets, logs, or checklists, that track conformance with standards that have been established to reduce the likelihood of an error or negative outcome

controlled substances: drugs, regulated by the federal and/or state Drug Enforcement Agency, which have a potential for abuse (e.g., narcotics, select psychotropics, steroids)

Controlled Substances Act: federal law regulating the manufacture, distribution, and sale of drugs that have the potential for abuse

co-payment (co-pay): the amount a patient pays for a prescription in a third-party plan

coring: when the insertion of a needle through the rubber septum of a drug vial results in some of the rubber from the septum becoming lodged in the needle. The rubber fragment may then be ejected into the vial or drawn up with the drug, causing contamination.

corticosteroid: a substance similar in structure to cortisol, a steroid released from the adrenal gland

cost price: the wholesale cost of the medication to the pharmacy

counterbalance: a double-pan balance capable of weighing relatively large quantities

counterirritant: an agent (e.g., capsaicin) that is applied locally to produce an inflammatory reaction for the purpose of bringing blood to the area

CPU: central processing unit of the computer hardware; the brain of the computer

cream: emulsified, semisolid dosage form

cross-contamination: when residue left behind from the preparation of one prescription contaminates another prescription (e.g., if improper cleansing techniques have been followed)

cross-linking agent: a drug that binds together the two strands of DNA in a "criss-cross" manner, preventing DNA replication

cross-multiplication: multiplying the numerators and denominators of two fractions and setting them equal to determine an unknown quantity (e.g., $2/3 = 4/X$ becomes $2 \times X = 3 \times 4$ so $X = 6$)

cross-sensitivity: when a patient is allergic to one class of drugs (e.g., penicillins) and experiences an allergic reaction to a drug with a similar chemical structure (e.g., cephalosporins)

cyclooxygenase (COX): an enzyme that acts on arachidonic acid to begin the synthesis of prostanoids (e.g., prostaglandins, prostacyclines). This enzyme has two isomers (COX-1 and COX-2), which result in different physiological effects.

cytochrome P_{450}: a group of enzymes that aid in drug metabolism

cytoprotective agent: something that protects cells from damage

cytotoxic: a substance that causes cell death

data entry: the input of information into a computer

DAW (dispense as written): this designation entered on the prescription form mandates that the prescription should be filled exactly as stated on the medication order (e.g., brand name, dosage, and form specified). No substitutions of any kind may be made.

DEA number: an alphanumeric nine-digit number issued to the prescriber or the institution by the Drug Enforcement Agency (DEA). Possession of this number indicates that the prescriber or institution has registered with the DEA and is authorized to prescribe or dispense drugs by prescription.

degrade: decompose, break down

demulcent: a substance that absorbs moisture

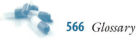

diabetes mellitus: a metabolic disorder in which a lack of insulin or insulin receptors inhibits the proper utilization of carbohydrates

diagnosis: the determination of the nature of a disease or symptom through physical examination and clinical tests

diluent: liquid mixed with drug to create a solution or suspension

disinfectant: a substance used to destroy surface pathogens on inanimate objects

dispensing: the process of selecting, preparing, checking, and delivering prescribed medication and associated information (must be under the supervision of a pharmacist)

dispensing fee: an amount added to the price of the prescription to cover the cost of dispensing. This may be a percentage or a flat fee.

dissolution: the act of dissolving

distribution: the process by which a drug gets into the bloodstream

diuresis: increased urination

diuretic: an agent that causes an increase in the production of urine

dosage: the amount of a drug given

dosage conversion: the determination of the correct amount of drug to dispense per the physician's order relative to the drug strength and dosage form on hand

dosage form: the way in which a drug is dispensed (e.g., tablet, capsule, cream, liquid)

dosage schedule: the specific times that a medicine is to be administered

dosage strength: the quantity of a drug present in a given dosage form

dose: a quantity of drug to be given at one time

double-pan balance: two pans that hang opposite each other and works on gravity

dromotropic agent: a substance that changes the rate of electrical conduction in the heart

drop factor: the number of drops per milliliter dispensed by an IV tubing

drug: any substance approved by the FDA to be used in the treatment or prevention of pathological conditions

drug administration: process by which a drug is given to the patient (e.g., orally, by injection, topical application, etc.)

drug-drug interaction: when two or more drugs interfere with each other. This may occur when more than one drug binds to the same proteins as another, uses the same enzymes for metabolism, changes the elimination of another drug, is antagonistic or synergistic with another drug, etc.

drug duplication: when the same drug appears under two different labels (e.g., Clavamox and Polymox)

drug formulary: a list of medicinal agents stocked by the pharmacy that are considered to be the most useful in patient care

drug information: information about drugs and the effects of drugs on people. The provision of this is a part of each pharmacist's practice.

drug label: information placed on a drug container that includes data required by drug regulations

drug of choice (DOC): the drug that is most effective in the therapy of a particular condition

drug order: a course of medication therapy ordered by a medical practitioner in an organized health care setting

drug recall: removal of a drug from sale, due to a health-hazard potential or false information

drug regimen review: process to provide appropriate drug therapy for patients

Drug Topics Red Book: reference guide listing all pharmaceuticals, medicinals, and sundries sold in drugstores, with currently available prices

drug-use control: the system of knowledge, understanding, judgments, procedures, skills, controls, and ethics that ensures optimal safety in the distribution and use of medication

duodenum: the first section of the small intestine after the stomach; responsible for significant drug absorption

edema: fluid retention

efficacy: the maximum effect that can be achieved by a drug, regardless of dose

electrolytes: naturally occurring ions in the body that play an essential role in cellular function by maintaining fluid balance and establishing acid-base balance; an ionizable substance in solution (e.g., sodium, potassium chloride)

elimination: removal of the drug from the blood. This may be by removal from the body, sequestering of the drug into fat, or chemical inactivation of the drug.

elixir: a sweetened liquid containing the drug and flavoring that contains a high percentage of alcohol

embolism: obstruction or occlusion of a blood vessel by a transported blood clot

emesis: vomiting

emetic: an agent that causes vomiting

endogenously: originating within the body

enteral dosing: route of medication that passes through the digestive tract

enteric-coated tablet: a special tablet coating that prevents the release of a drug until it enters the intestine

enterohepatic recycling: when drug or drug metabolites are secreted into the bile, enter the small intestine, and are reabsorbed back into the body

epidural: administration of a drug into the space surrounding the spinal cord

epinephrine: a substance released from the adrenal gland that increases heart rate, cardiac output, blood pressure (a *biphasic* effect), and blood sugar

etiology: the causes involved in the development of a disease or condition

euphoria: an exaggerated feeling of well-being

excretion: the process whereby drugs leave the body

expectorant: a substance that promotes the ejection of mucus or an exudate from the lungs, bronchi, and trachea

expiration date: the last date of sale as determined by the manufacturer. Any sale after this date is illegal and may result in a levy of fines by pharmacy and/or health inspectors.

extemporaneous compounding: the preparation of a customized drug product or dosage form for a specific patient where no written procedure exists. This may only be done by the *pharmacist.*

extended-release capsules: capsules that are formulated in such a way as to gradually release the drug over a predetermined time period

extract: the oil or active portion of a plant or herb

Federal Food, Drug, and Cosmetic Act: the federal statute through which the FDA enforces its rules and regulations

first-line drug: a drug that is chosen as the first choice in primary therapy if the drug of choice is not suitable for administration

first-pass effect: the extent to which a drug is immediately metabolized following oral administration. A high first-pass effect means that a large portion of the drug dose is immediately metabolized on the first passage through the liver, before it can be presented to the body. A drug with a high first-pass effect is not suitable for oral administration, and must be administered intravenously.

fixed disk: the installed data storage within a computer ("hard" disk)

floor staff: the health care providers and practitioners who work in a particular area of the hospital (e.g., nurses, physicians, patient care technicians)

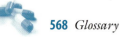
floor stock: drugs stocked within a particular unit or patient floor for administration to the patient by the nurse, who is responsible for preparation and administration

floppy disk: removable data storage medium

flow rate: the rate in mL/hr or drops/min that an IV fluid is administered to the patient

fluid extract: a liquid preparation of an herb containing alcohol as a solvent or preservative

Food and Drug Administration (FDA): a federal organization that creates rules, regulations, and standards with regard to drug or food products; and inspects drug and food facilities to ensure the purity of such products

food supplement: a nutritional aid. Herbal drugs are also classified as food supplements.

formulary: a list of drugs currently stocked in the pharmacy

generic drugs: drugs that are not sold under a proprietary label

generic name: the generally accepted name of the drug (e.g., penicillin). This name is not owned by any particular company, and is separate from the chemical name of the drug.

geriatric pharmacy practice: pharmacy practice that focuses on the medical and pharmaceutical care of the elderly

gingival hyperplasia: swelling of the gums

glaucoma: eye condition where the fluid pressure in the eye increases

graduated cylinder: a glass or plastic cylinder used for the measurement of liquids

gram-negative bacterium (g⁻): a bacterium that does not absorb a special stain ("gram" stain). This type of organism has a very dense cell wall and is thus more difficult to treat with antibiotics.

gram-positive bacterium (g⁺): a bacterium that has a less-developed cell wall and thus absorbs the gram stain

habituation: acquired tolerance for a drug

hardware: the physical working parts of the computer

health care clearinghouse: an organization that processes or facilitates the processing of health care information, for transmission to another aspect of the health care system (e.g., an insurance company)

health care delivery: organized programs developed to provide physical, mental, and emotional health care in institutions for homebound and ambulatory patients

health care provider: a physician, nurse, pharmacy, or any other person or organization who furnishes, bills for, or is paid for rendering health care in the normal course of business

health information: any information, whether oral or recorded in any form or medium, that: (1) is created or received by a health care professional or organization; and (2) relates to the past, present, or future physical or mental health or condition of an individual; the provision of health care to an individual, or the payment for these services

health maintenance organization (HMO): a prepaid health insurance plan that provides comprehensive health care for subscribers, with emphasis on the prevention and early detection of disease and continuity of care. HMOs are either not-for-profit or for-profit, are designated as either an independent practice association (IPA) or a staff model, and are often owned and operated by insurance carriers. HMOs were developed as a means to control health care delivery, access, and cost.

hemodialysis: procedure by which impurities or wastes are removed from the blood

hemophilia: hereditary blood-coagulation disorder

hemostatic: an agent that stops blood flow

herb: a plant used as a healing remedy

high-efficiency particulate air (HEPA) filter: an air-filtering device used in laminar flow hoods

HIPAA (Health Insurance Portability and Accountability Act): regulations that provide for privacy and confidentiality of personal health information

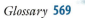

HIV: human immunodeficiency virus

homeostasis: maintaining stability in the internal body environment; a state of equilibrium

home pharmaceutical service: dispensing and delivery of medications to patients who have their clinical status monitored at home

homogeneous: of uniform composition throughout

hormone: a chemical substance, produced by a particular type of cell, that has a specific regulatory effect in the body

hospice: an institution that provides a program of palliative and supportive services to terminally ill patients and their families in the form of physical, psychological, social, and spiritual care

hospital information systems (HIS): systems that integrate information from many parts of the hospital

hydrolysis: any reaction in which water is one of the reactants and breaks up a substance

hydrophilic: water-loving

hydrophobic: lipid-loving (or water-hating)

hygroscopic: moisture-absorbing

hypercalcemia: a condition in which calcium levels in the blood are too high

hyperglycemia: high serum blood glucose level

hyperkalemia: a condition in which potassium levels in the blood are too high

hypernatremia: a condition in which sodium levels in the blood are too high

hypersensitivity: excessive response to a sensitizing agent

hypersensitivity reaction: a severe allergic reaction to a small amount of drug

hypertension: high blood pressure

hyperthyroid: relating to the overproduction of thyroid hormone

hypnotic agent: a drug that induces sleep

hypocalcemia: a condition in which calcium levels in the blood are too low

hypoglycemia: low blood sugar

hypoglycemic agent: a drug that lowers the level of glucose in the blood; used primarily by diabetics

hypokalemia: a condition in which potassium levels in the blood are too low

hyponatremia: a condition in which sodium levels in the blood are too low

hypotension: low blood pressure

hypotensive crisis: when blood pressure goes so low that the blood does not circulate properly and tissues become ischemic

hypothyroid: relating to the underproduction or no production of thyroid hormone

hypovolemia: a condition of decreased fluid volume in the body (i.e., a state of severe dehydration)

immunity: resistance to a particular disease

immunomodulators: agents that modulate the activity of the immune system to a desired level

immunosuppression: a decrease in function of the immune system

improper fraction: a fraction in which the top number is larger than the bottom number (e.g., a number that is greater than one that is written improperly as a fraction)

incompatibility: producing an undesirable effect when mixed or used together

independent pharmacy: privately owned pharmacy

infection: the state or condition in which the body (or part of it) is invaded by a microorganism that multiplies and produces an immune response and certain physiological effects

infiltration: occurs when an intravenous solution leaks into the surrounding tissues instead of directly into the vein as intended

infusion: the slow, constant introduction of a drug or solution into the bloodstream

infusion pump (controller): regulates the flow of an intravenous solution

injection: the introduction of a fluid substance into the body by means of a needle and syringe

inotropic agent: a substance that increases the force of contraction of heart muscle

inpatient: a patient confined to an institution for care (e.g., a patient admitted to a hospital)

input device: something that feeds information to a computer's CPU, such as keyboards, light pens, optical scanners, bar-code readers

institutional pharmacy: pharmacy services provided in hospitals, nursing homes, health maintenance organizations, prisons, mental retardation facilities, or other settings wherein groups of patients are provided formal, structured pharmacy programs

institutional setting: a pharmacy practice within a patient care setting or health care organization (e.g., hospital pharmacy, nursing home)

insulin syringe: a device calibrated in international units specific for the measurement of insulin. Insulin syringes come in two sizes—the low-dose syringe (capacity of 30 units) and the high-dose syringe (capacity of 100 units, or 1 mL of regular U-100 insulin). These syringes have a permanently attached 30-gauge needle.

insurance affidavit: a form used to transfer information regarding a claim for payment of a dispensed prescription from the pharmacy to the insurance provider

intermittent injection: repeated intravenous administration of a drug at specified time intervals

international unit (IU or U): an arbitrary measurement of drug concentration. The amount of drug per unit varies by drug.

intoxication: state of being poisoned by a drug or toxin

intraarterial injection: administration of drug or fluid directly into an artery

intracardiac injection: administration of a drug directly into the heart

intradermal: administered into the dermal layer of the skin

intraocular: within the eye

intrasynovial (IS): injection directly into joint fluid

intrathecal (IT): injections into the fluid in the space between the spinal cord and the spinal meninges

intravenous (IV): within a vein; administering drugs or fluids directly into the vein

inventory: a complete listing of the exact amounts of all the drugs in stock at a particular time

investigational drugs: drugs that are undergoing clinical trials but have not received approval for marketing by the Food and Drug Administration

iontophoresis: use of an electric current to cause an ionized drug to pass through the skin into the systemic circulation

irritant laxative: something that increases secretions from the intestinal lining, making the stool softer and more watery

ischemia: a condition in which there is a lack of oxygen to the tissues

isotonic: having the same osmotic pressure as plasma

IV drip: a bag or bottle of sterile liquid infused over a long period

JCAHO: *See* Joint Commission on Accreditation of Healthcare Organizations

Joint Commission on Accreditation of Healthcare Organizations (JCAHO): not-for- profit organization whose standards are set to ensure effective, quality services (e.g., optimal standards for the operation of hospitals)

lacrimal fluids: tears

laminar flow hood: a forced-air device that allows a sterile workspace. The forced-air currents form a barrier between the user and the workspace by pushing sterile filtered air across the opening of the hood to maintain a particulate-free working environment.

leaching: the slow movement of a substance from one area into a surrounding area

liability: that responsibility imposed upon a party who breaches a duty owed to another person

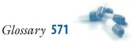

lipid-soluble: able to mix with fats

lipophilic: fat-loving

liposome: a fatty substance that encapsulates and slowly releases a drug

loading dose: larger than normal dose at the beginning of a drug regimen

local administration: when the drug is applied or introduced into a specific area

local area network (LAN): electronic connections that permit different systems (mainframe, minicomputers, and microcomputers), as well as computers made by different manufacturers, to communicate and share data

long-term care: health care provided in an organized medical facility for patients requiring chronic or extended treatment

long-term care facility: a resident facility for individuals who need constant care

lotions: emulsified preparations intended for external application

lymphocytic: dealing with the lymph system

mainframe: the largest, most powerful type of computer system; is able to service many users at once and process several programs simultaneously; has large primary and secondary storage capacities

malpractice: a deviation from the standard of care that arises out of a professional relationship; also called professional negligence

managed care: provision of health care services in the most cost-effective way

manufacturer's label: the labeling on a container of medication as it comes from the manufacturer (i.e., the label on a stock bottle or vial of drug)

markup: the difference between the cost and selling price of a drug. This is normally an increase in price expressed as a percentage of the cost of the drug to the pharmacy.

materials management: the division of a hospital pharmacy responsible for the purchasing, control, storage, and distribution of drugs and pharmaceutical products

mechanism of action: how the drug works, on a cellular and biochemical level

Medicaid: a state health care coverage program with some federal funding assistance for those with low income, minimal assets, and no health care coverage, as mandated by Title XIX of the Social Security Act. Medicaid may go by different names in different states; often known as medical assistance programs.

medical records department: the hospital department responsible for the maintenance and review of patients' medical charts

Medicare: a federal health care coverage program for those 65 years of age and over, certain disabled persons, and persons with end-stage renal disease, as mandated by Title XVIII of the Social Security Act of 1965. Medicare includes Part A and Part B, which cover both hospital care and outpatient services.

medication administration record (MAR): the document used by the nursing department to document the administration of medication to the patient

medication cart: a free-standing, computerized cart containing the daily medications for patients on a particular floor in an institutional setting

medication order: the list of drugs and drug doses to be prepared for a particular patient in an institutional setting

medium: solvent used to dissolve a substance

meniscus: the curved surface of a liquid seen when measuring liquid in a glass graduated cylinder

metabolism: the chemical alteration of a drug by the body

methylxanthines: a class of drugs that inhibits the actions of phosphodiesterase and increases levels of cAMP

metric system of measurement: one that is used internationally, or in a medical or scientific setting within the United States. Units of weight include the microgram, milligram, gram, kilogram, and

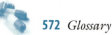

more rarely, the picogram and fentogram. Units of volume include the microliter, milliliter, liter, and deciliter.

micronized drug particles: very small drug particles that have a diameter in the micrometer size range

milliequivalent (mEq): a numerical quantity based on molar concentrations of charged ions in solution

miosis: pinpoint pupils of the eye

misbranding: when the label of a drug container does not accurately reflect what is in the container

mixed fraction: whole number and fraction written together (e.g., 1½)

mnemonic codes: abbreviations of longer instructions that are easy to remember

monoamine oxidase: an enzyme that breaks down epinephrine and norepinephrine (*monoamine oxidase "A"*) or dopamine (*monoamine oxidase "B"*)

monotherapy: treatment with a single drug

morbidity: a disease state; the ratio of the sick to the well in a given area

mortality: occurrence of death; the ratio of deaths to the living in a given area

muscarinic antagonist: a drug that inhibits the actions of acetylcholine at the muscarinic receptor

myelosuppression: a decrease in the formation of bone marrow cells, particularly white blood cells and red blood cells

myocardial infarction: a blockage within a blood vessel that supplies blood to the heart, resulting in decreased flow of oxygen to the heart muscle

narcotic: a physically and psychologically addictive drug that relieves pain

narcotic antagonists: agents that oppose the effects of a narcotic

national drug formulary: a list of all drugs manufactured that meet federal criteria for therapeutic effectiveness

NDC number: a number found on the drug label that contains codes that denote the generic name of the drug, manufacturer, proprietary label, dosage form, and strength

neonatal: refers to an infant

neuroleptic malignant syndrome: a life-threatening condition produced with certain antipsychotics, characterized by an increase in fever, muscle rigidity, and cardiovascular instability

new drug application (NDA): papers that a pharmaceutical company must file with the FDA, with data from supporting studies, before the company is allowed to manufacture and test the drugs

nitrogen mustard: a type of drug that is made from toxic nitrogen and sulfur compounds

nomogram: a chart that relates the height and weight of a person to the person's body surface area

norepinephrine: a substance released from nerve terminals in the sympathetic autonomic nervous system that increases heart rate, blood pressure, and blood sugar

nosocomial: a disease or infection originating in the hospital

NSAID: nonsteroidal anti-inflammatory drug. These drugs are unrelated to corticosteroids, and act to decrease pain and inflammation.

objective: the purpose or goal toward which effort is directed

OBRA90 (Omnibus Budget Reconciliation Act): regulations that required pharmacists to counsel patients on their medications, also requires drug suppliers to provide fair pricing to all facilities

Occupational Safety and Health Act: federal law that assures every worker in the nation safe and healthful working conditions; established the Occupational Safety and Health Administration (OSHA)

ointment: semisolid, external dosage form

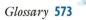

oncology: the study or knowledge of tumors; commonly referred to as the study of cancer and related diseases

operational manual: lists only those policies and procedures that affect the internal working of the pharmacy department

oral syringe: a calibrated device for measuring liquids to be taken orally. It may appear similar to the parenteral syringe or may be a calibrated plastic barrel attached to a rubber bulb for suction.

osteomalacia: a softening of the bone due to decreased calcium storage

osteoporosis: disorder characterized by the degeneration of bone matrix, prevalent in older people particularly women

ostomy: an artificial opening into the body (e.g., opening in the trachea or intestine)

OTC: over the counter (i.e., prescription is not required)

ototoxicity: damage to the ear

out-of-pocket: the patient pays for the medication directly, and the pharmacy submits claims to the insurance company for patient reimbursement

output device: something that displays information received from a computer's CPU, such as video display terminal (VDT), cathode ray tube (CRT), printer, or plotter

package insert: information included with the stock of drug that describes the effects of the drug and adverse effects that have been reported. This document, which is written in technical terms, also presents the studies done on the drug, with results of those studies.

parasympathetic nervous system: the portion of the ANS that releases acetylcholine as a neurotransmitter. This portion of the ANS regulates day-to-day activities of the body.

parenteral dosing: route of medication that bypasses the digestive tract (e.g., rectal suppository, injection, transdermal patch)

PAR level: the minimum amount of a particular medication remaining in stock in the pharmacy. Once this level is reached, the drug is automatically reordered.

passive diffusion: movement of drug molecules from an area of high concentration to one of lower concentration

pathology: study of the characteristics, causes, and effects of disease

patient counseling: the teaching of the patient, by the pharmacist, regarding the drugs that the patient will be taking. This includes mechanism, adverse effects, and self-monitoring techniques.

patient package insert: an informational document written for the lay public describing the benefits and risks of medications; it describes why the drug is given, and the effects and adverse effects that can be expected. Long-term effects (e.g., promotion of breast, ovarian, or cervical cancer, in the case of an estrogen) are also laid out in a way that the patient can understand.

patient profile: a document that is used to incorporate patient information, allergies, sensitivities, and all medications the patient is receiving, both active and discontinued

PCA: patient-controlled analgesia

pediatric: normally considered to be a person under 12 years of age

peptide: small chain of amino acids

percentage: a drug concentration expressed as amount per 100 (e.g., 5 g per 100 mL expressed as 5%). Percentage may be expressed in weight per volume (*w/v*), weight per weight (*w/w*), or volume per volume (*v/v*).

percutaneous: through the skin

peripheral unit: a device that attaches to a computer's CPU and sends or receives information

personally identifiable patient: a person who may be identified by the information communicated between parties. This information may be a name, address, birth date, or other information that could link the patient with the transmitted confidential information.

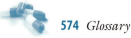

Pharm.D. degree: the doctor of pharmacy degree

pharmaceutical care: the responsible provision of drug therapy to achieve definite outcomes that improve a patient's quality of life

pharmaceutical services: focus on rational drug therapy and include the essential administrative, clinical, and technical functions to meet this goal

pharmaceutics: that area of the pharmaceutical sciences that deals with the chemical, physical, and physiological properties of drugs and dosage forms and drug-delivery systems

pharmacist: a person who (1) has completed a formal course of education in a pharmacy school and (2) is licensed to prepare and distribute drugs and counsel on the use of medication in the state in which he or she practices

pharmacognosy: the study of the biologic and biochemical features of natural drugs

pharmacokinetics: that branch of pharmacology that deals with a mathematical description of drug absorption, distribution, metabolism, and excretion and their relationship to the dosage form

pharmacology: the science that deals with the origin, nature, chemistry, physiological effects, mechanism of action, administration therapy, and uses of drugs

pharmacopoeia: a listing of drugs containing information on drugs and their purity, preparation, and standards

pharmacotherapy: the treatment of disease with medications

pharmacy: the professional practice of a pharmacist; preparing, dispensing, monitoring, and public education

Pharmacy and Therapeutics Committee: a group of health care professionals that regulate the standards for the operation of the pharmacy, in an institutional setting; the liaison between the department of pharmacy and the medical staff. It consists of physicians, nurses, and pharmacists who represent the various clinical aspects, and select the drugs to be used in the hospital.

Pharmacy Code of Ethics: rules established for the profession by pharmacists that guide proper conduct for pharmacists

pharmacy technician: a person skilled in various pharmacy service activities not requiring the professional judgment of the pharmacist; who has received training to competently perform numerous pharmacy activities under the supervision of a registered pharmacist

phlebitis: inflammation of a vein

phosphodiesterase: an enzyme that breaks down a physiologically active chemical called cyclic AMP (cAMP) and decreases its actions. In the cardiovascular system, cAMP increases the heart's force of contraction and causes vasoconstriction.

photosensitivity: a severe sensitivity to sunlight. Patients (particularly light-skinned patients) who are photosensitive may experience severe sunburn with very little exposure to the sun.

physician: an authorized practitioner of medicine

physician assistant: an authorized practitioner of medicine who works under the responsible supervision of a licensed physician

phytochemist: person who studies plant chemistry and applies these chemicals to science

piggyback IV: a small-volume intravenous solution (25–250 mL) that is run into an existing infusion line over a brief period of time (e.g., 50 mL over 15 minutes)

placebo: a dose that has no drug in it at all

pneumonia: inflammation of lungs, usually due to infection

podiatrist: a practitioner specializing in foot care

Poison Prevention Packaging Act: federal law mandating special packaging requirements that make it difficult for children under the age of five to open the package or container

policy: a defined course to guide and determine present and future decisions; established by an organization or employer who guides the employee to act in a manner consistent with management philosophy

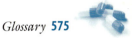

polymer: a high-molecular-weight substance made up of repeating base units

polymorphic state: a condition in which a substance occurs in more than one crystalline form

postural hypotension: a rapid drop in blood pressure upon standing

potency: the degree of therapeutic effect that can be achieved with a drug, relative to dose

PPN: peripheral parenteral nutrition

preferred provider organization (PPO): an insurance plan that provides comprehensive health care through contracted providers

prescriber: a person in health care who is permitted by law to order drugs that legally require a prescription; includes physicians, physician assistants, podiatrists, dentists, optometrists, and nurse practitioners

prescription: permission granted orally or in writing from a physician for a patient to receive a certain medication on an outpatient basis that will help relieve or eliminate the patient's problem

prescription balance: a device used to measure very small quantities of drug

prescription order: an order for an individual drug that is to be dispensed in proper dosage amount and form to a patient from a retail (outpatient) pharmacy

preservatives: substances used to slow the growth of microorganisms

prime vendor: drug wholesaler who contracts directly with hospital pharmacies as the primary source of pharmaceuticals

procedures: guidelines on the preferred way to perform a certain function; particular actions to be taken to carry out a policy

prodrug: a drug that must is converted to its active form after absorption

propellant: substance used to help expel the contents of a pressurized container

prophylaxis: prevention of or protection against disease

proprietary drug name: the commercial designation for a drug or drug product that is owned by a particular company (e.g., Celebrex). This is also called a *brand name* or *trade name*.

protein binding: when a drug molecule is chemically attracted to tissue or plasma proteins and binds to them, effectively creating a storage site for the drug

proteins: macromolecules consisting of amino acids

protocol: a written description of how an activity, procedure, or function is to be accomplished

proton pump: the cellular transport system that is used to make gastric acid

pyrogen-free: free of fever causing agents

psychiatric: relating to the medical treatment of mental disorders

psychosis: a psychiatric condition in which a patient is dissociated from reality and is often difficult to control

psychotropic: a drug used to treat mental and emotional disorders

purchase order: a form that is used to order drugs and supplies from a wholesaler

purified protein derivative (PPD): the antigen used in the skin test for tuberculosis

quality assurance: a method of monitoring drug integrity to ensure a certain level of quality that meets predetermined criteria

quality standards: the minimum results needed to achieve a desired level of quality

random-access memory (RAM): the temporary memory of the computer (buffer)

ratio: a relationship between two numbers; an expression of the amount of drug as a fraction of the total (e.g., 5 g in 100 mL). Ratios may be expressed in weight of drug per total volume (w/v), weight of drug per total weight (w/w), or volume of solution per total volume (v/v).

ratio-proportion: a calculation method involving cross-multiplication

read-only memory (ROM): the portion of the computer or peripheral device where information is permanently saved, and cannot be altered (written to)

reconstitute: add a sterile solvent to a sterile active ingredient for injectable purposes

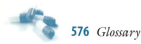

refill authorization: the extending of a prescription, in time or amount, by the prescriber directly. This can only be done by the pharmacist or licensed pharmacy intern.

regulation: an authoritative rule dealing with details of procedure

regulatory law: the area of law that deals with governmental agencies and how they enforce the intent of the statutes under which they operate

renal: pertaining to the kidney

drug resistance: when an antibiotic is used too frequently, an organism may mutate to develop a defense against the drug, becoming resistant

respiratory depression: a decrease in the rate of respiration, usually mediated at the level of the brainstem

retrovirus: a virus that is able to use viral RNA to make viral DNA, which then gets inserted into the DNA of the host (patient)

robotics: technology based on a mechanical device, programmed by remote control to accomplish manual activities such as picking medications according to a patient's computerized profile

route of administration: how a drug enters the body (oral, injection, etc.)

sanitation: cleaning and disinfection of drug apparatus to protect against bacterial contamination or cross-contamination with other drugs

satellite pharmacy: where distribution occurs from a decentralized pharmacy staffed by at least a pharmacist and a technician. The satellite usually handles all the needs of the units for which it is responsible.

schedule drug: a controlled substance that is classified as Schedule II–V by the DEA under the Controlled Substance Act of 1974

scored: a tablet with a groove down the center that allows the tablet to be easily broken

secondary storage: data and programs maintained on tapes or disks

second-line drug: that which is used if the first-line drug is not available or cannot be used

sedative: a drug that has a calming effect

self-monitoring: the attention paid by the patient to changes in body function, which may indicate that the drug dosage is too high or too low

self-pay: the patient pays for the medication directly to the pharmacy

selling price: the amount charged to the consumer for the drug or device

sepsis: blood toxicity due to the presence of pathogenic organisms and toxins in the blood. It is also known colloquially (and inaccurately) as blood poisoning.

septum: the rubber top of the drug vial where the syringe needle is inserted

serotonin: a neurotransmitter in the brain that has been shown to elevate mood

shelf life: how long the drug remains potent and in its proper form

site survey: the visit by representatives of ASHP to review the training program to ascertain compliance with the standards

software: the actual programs for the computer system

solution: water containing dissolved drug particles; a homogeneous mixture of one or more substances dissolved in water

solution balance: hanging pan balance used for weighing large amounts

solvation: process by which a solute is incorporated into the solvent

SSRI: a selective serotonin reuptake inhibitor

stability: a condition that resists change; for example, a drug maintains potency

standard: a reference to be used in evaluating institutional programs and services

standard of care: the acceptable level of professional practice by which the actions of a professional are judged

standards of practice: rules that pharmacists establish for the profession that represent the preferred way to practice

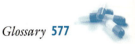

staphylococcus (plural: staphylococci): a virulent microorganism that is the most common cause of many localized infections (e.g., skin infections)

stat (statim): perform immediately

state board of pharmacy: an agency that regulates the conduct and educational level of the pharmacist and pharmacy staff, and ensures proper pharmacy practice. This may include spot checks to evaluate proper temperature control and sanitation, as well as documentation that proper procedures are being followed.

status asthmaticus: a life-threatening condition in which the bronchioles constrict and airways are blocked

status epilepticus: a life-threatening seizure condition that may be caused by abrupt withdrawal of anticonvulsant therapy

sterile: free from microorganisms

steroid: a substance with a particular chemical structure (a steroid nucleus). Steroids are lipid-based and many are anti-inflammatory agents.

stop order: the date and time when therapy is to end. An automatic stop order requires a physician's renewal order for the medication to be reinstated.

subcutaneously: under the skin; introduced beneath the skin (e.g., subcutaneous injections)

sublingual tablet: a soft tablet that is meant to be dissolved under the tongue

superinfection: where an antibiotic selectively destroys only certain populations of bacteria in the intestine, leaving other, more virulent organisms to proliferate into potentially lethal numbers, causing a secondary infection

suppositories: semisolid dosage forms for insertion into body cavities (e.g., rectum, vagina, urethra), where they melt at body temperature, releasing drug

surfactants: surface active agents, commonly known as wetting agents

suspending agents: chemical additives used in suspensions to thicken the liquid and retard settling of particles

suspension: liquid containing finely divided drug particles that are not dissolved but are uniformly distributed

sympathetic agonist: a drug that mimics the effects of epinephrine

sympathetic nervous system (SNS): the portion of the ANS that releases norepinephrine. Epinephrine and the adrenal gland, where it comes from, may also be considered part of the sympathetic nervous system. This SNS regulates the response of the body to stress (e.g., increased heart rate, pupillary dilation, etc.).

sympatholytic: a substance that blocks the activity of the sympathetic nervous system

sympathoplegic: a substance that impedes the activity of the sympathetic nervous system

synergistic effect: when two drugs have the same physiological effect but different mechanisms, and one potentiates the effects of the other such that the combined effect is greater than the sum of both drugs' effects

synthesize: to produce by bringing elements together to form a chemical compound

syringe: a calibrated device for measuring liquids. It consists of a barrel, plunger, and tip with needle attachment.

syrup: a sweetened solution containing drug

system software: contains the operating system that includes master programs for coordinating the activities of the hardware and software in a computer system

systemic: relating to the body as a whole, rather than locally applied

systemic action: affects the body as a whole

systemic administration: when the drug goes throughout the body (usually carried in the bloodstream)

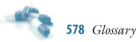

systemic side effect: an effect on the whole body, but secondary to the intended effect

tablet: a pressed powder dosage form of varying weight, size, and shape that contains a medicinal substance

tablet-splitter: a device that cuts tablets in half

tachycardia: rapid heart rate

tardive dyskinesia: motor skills disorder that is characterized by lip-smacking

tare: a weight used to counterbalance the container holding the substance being weighed

tax-free alcohol: ethyl alcohol obtained at cost under applicable federal regulations, to be used only for diagnostic and therapeutic purposes

teratogenic: causes birth defects

therapeutic: effective in treatment of a disease, infirmity, or symptom by various methods

therapeutic alternates: drug products that contain different drugs but that are of the same pharmacologic and/or therapeutic class

therapeutic duplication: when a patient has been prescribed two drugs that do the same thing, or are the same drug under different names (e.g., Ceclor and Pen-V K)

therapeutic effect: a healing, curative, or palliative effect

therapeutic equivalent: a drug product that, when administered in the same amount, will provide the same therapeutic effect and pharmacokinetic characteristics as another drug to which it is compared

therapeutic monitoring: the supervision of a patient with regard to the drugs that he or she has been prescribed. This includes analysis for therapeutic duplication, allergies, and other contraindications.

therapy: treatment of a disease or condition

third-party payor: medication is paid for in full or in part by an insurance company or institution

thrombi: blood clot

thrombocytopenia: a deficiency in platelets

thrombolytic agent: agents that break up blood clots

thrombolytic drug: one that acts to dissolve a clot that has already formed

thrombosis: development or presence of a blood clot

thymidine kinase: an enzyme involved in the synthesis of DNA

tincture: an alcohol-based solution containing a medicinal substance

tocolytic: substance that delays or prolongs the birth process

tolerance: a gradual decrease in the effect of a drug, due to biological adaptation of tissues

topical: pertaining to the surface of a part of the body

torsion balance: one weigh pan that hangs of the end of the scale; it is not very accurate, so not used to measure small quantities

total parenteral nutrition (TPN): a balanced nutritional mixture of sugars, proteins, electrolytes, and fats to be administered intravenously

toxic effect: an adverse effect where the drug damages an organ or system (e.g., ototoxicity)

toxicity: degree to which something produces organ damage

toxicology: the scientific study of poisons and their actions and detection, as well as the treatment of conditions caused by them

toxin: a poisonous substance

TPN: total parenteral nutrition

transdermal: entering through the dermis or skin, as in administration of a drug applied to the skin in ointment or patch form

triplicate form: also called a DEA222 form; used to order Schedule II narcotics

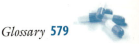

unit dose: a single use package of a drug. In a unit dose distribution system, a single dose of each medication is dispensed prior to the time of administration.

unit dose cart: concise way to organize and distrubute individual doses for patients. The pharmacy prepares a unit's medication orders and labels with individual patient identification; the medication is then distributued by the nurses atprescribed times

universal claim form (UCF): a pharmacy prescription claim form that is utilized to serve as the basis for reimbursement of prescriptions dispensed

urticaria: hives

USP: *United States Pharmacopeia*

utilization review: work of committee that determines how the use of resources meets criteria and standards

vaccination: introduction of a vaccine into the body to produce immunity to a particular disease (e.g., smallpox inoculation)

vaccine: a suspension of attenuated or killed organisims (e.g., bacteria, viruses, or rickettsia) administered for the prevention of infectious diseases (e.g., tetanus)

vascular: related to or containing blood vessels

vasoconstrictor: a substance that causes smooth muscle in arterial walls to contract and constricts arteries

vasodilator: a substance that relaxes smooth muscle in arterial walls, thus dilating arteries

venodilators: a substance that relaxes the veins and increases myocardial perfusion

volatile: evaporates at low temperature

volume of distribution: volume of space that a drug occupies within the body

Suggested Reading

Physiology

Introduction to the Human Body: The Essentials of Anatomy and Physiology,
5th Edition
Authors: Gerald Tortora and Sandra Grabowski
ISBN 047136777X

Fundamentals of Anatomy & Physiology, 6th Edition
Author: Frederic Martini
ISBN 0130615684

Pharmacology

Beginning

Basic Pharmacology for Health Occupations, 3rd Edition
Authors: Henry Hitner and Barbara Nagle
ISBN 0028006798

Intermediate

Essentials of Pharmacology
Editors: Cedric Smith and Alan Reynard
ISBN 0721655319

Advanced

Pharmacology Secrets
Author: Patricia K. Anthony
ISBN 1560534702

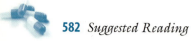

Pharmacy Mathematics

Dosage Calculations, 7th Edition
Author: Gloria Pickar
ISBN 076680542

Medical Terminology

Taber's Cyclopedic Medical Dictionary, 19th Edition
ISBN 0803606540

Index

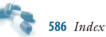

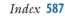

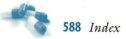

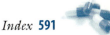

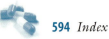

Practice Exam Software to Accompany Pharmacy Technician Certification Exam Review, Third Edition

IMPORTANT! READ CAREFULLY: This End User License Agreement ("Agreement") sets forth the conditions by which Cengage Learning will make electronic access to the Cengage Learning-owned licensed content and associated media, software, documentation, printed materials, and electronic documentation contained in this package and/or made available to you via this product (the "Licensed Content"), available to you (the "End User"). BY CLICKING THE "I ACCEPT" BUTTON AND/OR OPENING THIS PACKAGE, YOU ACKNOWLEDGE THAT YOU HAVE READ ALL OF THE TERMS AND CONDITIONS, AND THAT YOU AGREE TO BE BOUND BY ITS TERMS, CONDITIONS, AND ALL APPLICABLE LAWS AND REGULATIONS GOVERNING THE USE OF THE LICENSED CONTENT.

1.0 Scope of License

1.1   *Licensed Content.* The Licensed Content may contain portions of modifiable content ("Modifiable Content") and content which may not be modified or otherwise altered by the End User ("Non-Modifiable Content"). For purposes of this Agreement, Modifiable Content and Non-Modifiable Content may be collectively referred to herein as the "Licensed Content." All Licensed Content shall be considered Non-Modifiable Content, unless such Licensed Content is presented to the End User in a modifiable format and it is clearly indicated that modification of the Licensed Content is permitted.

1.2   Subject to the End User's compliance with the terms and conditions of this Agreement, Cengage Learning hereby grants the End User, a nontransferable, nonexclusive, limited right to access and view a single copy of the Licensed Content on a single personal computer system for noncommercial, internal, personal use only. The End User shall not (i) reproduce, copy, modify (except in the case of Modifiable Content), distribute, display, transfer, sublicense, prepare derivative work(s) based on, sell, exchange, barter or transfer, rent, lease, loan, resell, or in any other manner exploit the Licensed Content; (ii) remove, obscure, or alter any notice of Cengage Learning's intellectual property rights present on or in the Licensed Content, including, but not limited to, copyright, trademark, and/or patent notices; or (iii) disassemble, decompile, translate, reverse engineer, or otherwise reduce the Licensed Content.

2.0 Termination

2.1   Cengage Learning may at any time (without prejudice to its other rights or remedies) immediately terminate this Agreement and/or suspend access to some or all of the Licensed Content, in the event that the End User does not comply with any of the terms and conditions of this Agreement. In the event of such termination by Cengage Learning, the End User shall immediately return any and all copies of the Licensed Content to Cengage Learning.

3.0 Proprietary Rights

3.1   The End User acknowledges that Cengage Learning owns all rights, title and interest, including, but not limited to all copyright rights therein, in and to the Licensed Content, and that the End User shall not take any action inconsistent with such ownership. The Licensed Content is protected by U.S., Canadian and other applicable copyright laws and by international treaties, including the Berne Convention and the Universal Copyright Convention. Nothing contained in this Agreement shall be construed as granting the End User any ownership rights in or to the Licensed Content.

3.2   Cengage Learning reserves the right at any time to withdraw from the Licensed Content any item or part of an item for which it no longer retains the right to publish, or which it has reasonable grounds to believe infringes copyright or is defamatory, unlawful, or otherwise objectionable.

4.0 Protection and Security

4.1   The End User shall use its best efforts and take all reasonable steps to safeguard its copy of the Licensed Content to ensure that no unauthorized reproduction, publication, disclosure, modification, or distribution of the Licensed Content, in whole or in part, is made. To the extent that the End User becomes aware of any such unauthorized use of the Licensed Content, the End User shall immediately notify Cengage Learning. Notification of such violations may be made by sending an e-mail to infringement@cengage.com.

5.0 Misuse of the Licensed Product

5.1   In the event that the End User uses the Licensed Content in violation of this Agreement, Cengage Learning shall have the option of electing liquidated damages, which shall include all profits generated by the End User's use of the Licensed Content plus interest computed at the maximum rate permitted by law and all legal fees and other expenses incurred by Cengage Learning in enforcing its rights, plus penalties.

6.0 Federal Government Clients

6.1   Except as expressly authorized by Cengage Learning, Federal Government clients obtain only the rights specified in this Agreement and no other rights. The Government acknowledges that (i) all software and related documentation incorporated in the Licensed Content is existing commercial computer software within the meaning of FAR 27.405(b)(2); and (2) all other data delivered in whatever form, is limited rights data within the meaning of FAR 27.401. The restrictions in this section are acceptable as consistent with the Government's need for software and other data under this Agreement.

7.0 Disclaimer of Warranties and Liabilities

7.1   Although Cengage Learning believes the Licensed Content to be reliable, Cengage Learning does not guarantee or warrant (i) any information or materials contained in or produced by the Licensed Content, (ii) the accuracy, completeness or reliability of the Licensed Content, or (iii) that the Licensed Content is free from errors or other material defects. THE LICENSED PRODUCT IS PROVIDED "AS IS," WITHOUT ANY WARRANTY OF ANY KIND AND CENGAGE LEARNING DISCLAIMS ANY AND ALL WARRANTIES, EXPRESSED OR IMPLIED, INCLUDING, WITHOUT LIMITATION, WARRANTIES OF MERCHANTABILITY OR FITNESS FOR A PARTICULAR PURPOSE. IN NO EVENT SHALL CENGAGE LEARNING BE LIABLE FOR: INDIRECT, SPECIAL, PUNITIVE OR CONSEQUENTIAL DAMAGES INCLUDING FOR LOST PROFITS, LOST DATA, OR OTHERWISE. IN NO EVENT SHALL CENGAGE LEARNING'S AGGREGATE LIABILITY HEREUNDER, WHETHER ARISING IN CONTRACT, TORT, STRICT LIABILITY OR OTHERWISE, EXCEED THE AMOUNT OF FEES PAID BY THE END USER HEREUNDER FOR THE LICENSE OF THE LICENSED CONTENT.

8.0 General

8.1   *Entire Agreement.* This Agreement shall constitute the entire Agreement between the Parties and supercedes all prior Agreements and understandings oral or written relating to the subject matter hereof.

8.2   *Enhancements/Modifications of Licensed Content.* From time to time, and in Cengage Learning's sole discretion, Cengage Learning may advise the End User of updates, upgrades, enhancements and/or improvements to the Licensed Content, and may permit the End User to access and use, subject to the terms and conditions of this Agreement, such modifications, upon payment of prices as may be established by Cengage Learning.

8.3   *No Export.* The End User shall use the Licensed Content solely in the United States and shall not transfer or export, directly or indirectly, the Licensed Content outside the United States.

8.4   *Severability.* If any provision of this Agreement is invalid, illegal, or unenforceable under any applicable statute or rule of law, the provision shall be deemed omitted to the extent that it is invalid, illegal, or unenforceable. In such a case, the remainder of the Agreement shall be construed in a manner as to give greatest effect to the original intention of the parties hereto.

8.5   *Waiver.* The waiver of any right or failure of either party to exercise in any respect any right provided in this Agreement in any instance shall not be deemed to be a waiver of such right in the future or a waiver of any other right under this Agreement.

8.6   *Choice of Law/Venue.* This Agreement shall be interpreted, construed, and governed by and in accordance with the laws of the State of New York, applicable to contracts executed and to be wholly preformed therein, without regard to its principles governing conflicts of law. Each party agrees that any proceeding arising out of or relating to this Agreement or the breach or threatened breach of this Agreement may be commenced and prosecuted in a court in the State and County of New York. Each party consents and submits to the nonexclusive personal jurisdiction of any court in the State and County of New York in respect of any such proceeding.

8.7 *Acknowledgment.* By opening this package and/or by accessing the Licensed Content on this Web site, THE END USER ACKNOWLEDGES THAT IT HAS READ THIS AGREEMENT, UNDERSTANDS IT, AND AGREES TO BE BOUND BY ITS TERMS AND CONDITIONS. IF YOU DO N   ONS, YOU MUST NOT ACCESS THE   LICENSED PRODUCT TO CENGAGE   OF THE END USER'S PURCHASE) W   CENGAGE LEARNING, FOR A CREDIT   estions/comments regarding this Agreem   @cengage.com.

Minimum System

Operating systems: Mi   , Windows 7
Processor: Minimum r
Memory: Minimum re
Hard Drive Space: 500
Screen resolution: 102
CD-ROM drive
Sound card & listening
Flash Player 10. The A   m
    http://www.adobe.

Setup Instruction

1. Insert disc into   rt automatically. If it does not, go to step
2. From My Comp
3. Double-click th

Technical Suppo

Telephone: 1-800-64
8:30 A.M.–6:30 P.M. E
E-mail: delmar.help@cengage.com
Microsoft© and Windows© are registered trademarks of the Microsoft Corporation.
Pentium© is a registered trademark of the Intel Corporation.